Body Trainer for Men

Ray Klerck

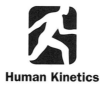

Human Kinetics

Library of Congress Cataloging-in-Publication Data

Klerck, Ray, 1979-
  Body trainer for men / Ray Klerck.
      pages. cm
  Includes bibliographical references.
  1. Personal trainers. 2. Physical fitness for men. 3. Exercise for men. I. Title.
  GV428.7.K54 2013
  613.7'1--dc23
                              2013014338
  ISBN-10: 1-4504-1970-4 (print)
  ISBN-13: 978-1-4504-1970-3 (print)

Acquisitions Editor: Tom Heine; **Developmental Editor:** Cynthia McEntire; **Assistant Editor:** Elizabeth Evans; **Copyeditor:** Mandy Eastin-Allen; **Permissions Manager:** Martha Gullo; **Graphic Designer:** Nancy Rasmus; **Graphic Artist:** Kim McFarland; **Cover Designer:** Jonathan Kay; **Photograph (cover):** Fotosearch/age fotostock; **Photographs (interior):** Greg Smith/© Human Kinetics; **Visual Production Assistant:** Joyce Brumfield; **Photo Production Manager:** Jason Allen; **Art Manager:** Kelly Hendren; **Associate Art Manager:** Alan L. Wilborn; **Illustrations:** © Human Kinetics; **Printer:** United Graphics

We thank Coyne Conditioning in Burleigh Heads, Queensland, Australia, for assistance in providing the location for the photo shoot for this book.

Human Kinetics books are available at special discounts for bulk purchase. Special editions or book excerpts can also be created to specification. For details, contact the Special Sales Manager at Human Kinetics.

Printed in the United States of America   10 9 8 7 6 5 4 3 2 1

The paper in this book is certified under a sustainable forestry program.

Human Kinetics
Website: www.HumanKinetics.com

United States: Human Kinetics
P.O. Box 5076
Champaign, IL 61825-5076
800-747-4457
e-mail: humank@hkusa.com

Canada: Human Kinetics
475 Devonshire Road Unit 100
Windsor, ON N8Y 2L5
800-465-7301 (in Canada only)
e-mail: info@hkcanada.com

Europe: Human Kinetics
107 Bradford Road
Stanningley
Leeds LS28 6AT, United Kingdom
+44 (0) 113 255 5665
e-mail: hk@hkeurope.com

Australia: Human Kinetics
57A Price Avenue
Lower Mitcham, South Australia 5062
08 8372 0999
e-mail: info@hkaustralia.com

New Zealand: Human Kinetics
P.O. Box 80
Torrens Park, South Australia 5062
0800 222 062
e-mail: info@hknewzealand.com

E5583

Thank you to my wonderful wife Natalie
for putting up with my late nights, and thank you
to my beautiful children Carter, Tyla and Asher
for providing the motivation and inspiration.

Contents

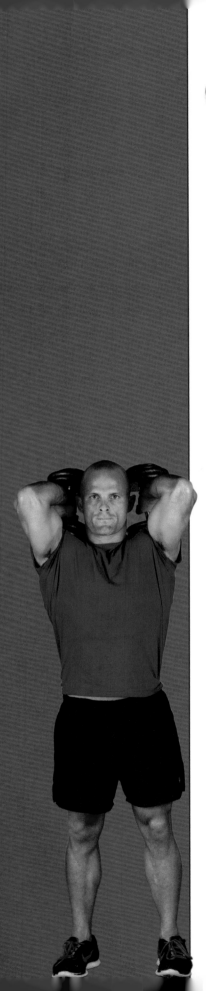

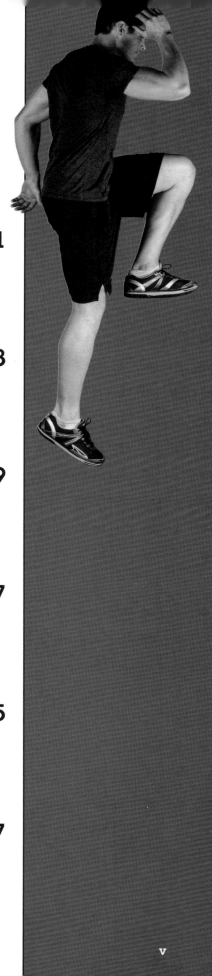

Preface

Today, life happens in an instant. Chores that used to take days or years can now be ticked off in seconds. People expect immediate results in every part of their lives. Push a pedal, go faster. Pop a pill, get healthy. Click *accept*, gain a friend. Immediate results.

But some of life's more significant quests, such as looking awesome, aren't accomplished so simply or swiftly. Changing your metabolism, muscle size and physique takes time. So please resist the urge to shake this book: It contains no magic pills or instant solutions that'll change your body by tomorrow. Sure, plenty of fitness-in-a-bottle potions out there promise to turn wimps into hulks in a snap, but the negative consequences of these get-stacked or get-ripped-quick schemes outweigh any real and lasting benefits.

Fortunately, a far better solution exists, and you're holding it. The following chapters offer a depth and breadth of expertise that will help you achieve specific and desired body changes in the shortest time possible without any risk to your health. The well-researched programmes are built on the latest scientifically proven methods that will markedly improve your physique. The principles behind the programmes are easy to understand yet offer powerful long- and short-term results.

If you're a guy who's taken a sabbatical from regular exercise and proper nutrition (or perhaps you never started), this book is for you. These words understand that you're rushed off your feet with work, play and family commitments. They know that several time-thieving elements in your life have prevented you from dedicating more of your day to your health and well-being. These words know that you probably don't like the idea of boot camp-style group exercise or the idea of having a personal trainer bark instructions down your throat. They're cool with that because, despite what the advertising execs would have you believe, those aren't the only ways to earn a body you can be proud of.

Just by reading this you've declared that you're the type of guy who likes to take charge of all areas in his life. You don't like the idea of becoming mass produced by a glossy gym chain. And you certainly don't like wasting your time because there's probably preciously little of it to go around. This book is aimed directly at you: the guy trying to achieve unlimited things with limited time. This is where you'll get reliable, long-term fitness strategies that the latest issue of a fitness magazine or a free Internet column simply can't deliver. Trust me; I've been there and written that. You've decided to take action and this is your first step.

You've obviously started to ask questions about your health and physique—questions you've probably found difficult to answer. The first question should not be about you; it should be about me. What do I know that you and other experts don't? As an internationally recognised fitness and nutrition expert, writer, consultant and personal trainer, I've figured out through my practise and studies what approaches best conquer the most common body challenges men face. As a devoted fitness enthusiast and former *Men's Health* cover model, I've gained considerable firsthand knowledge in developing programmes for everything from sculpted abs to becoming team MVP. This rare blend of experience and science has been so positively received by the men who read my work in the top-flight men's magazines that I wanted to offer a comprehensive fitness guide that addresses every single aspect of crafting the best-looking and best-functioning body possible.

During my nine years as the chief fitness advisor for *Men's Health*, I've fielded hundreds of questions from every type of man and written about nearly every fitness issue. This allowed me to understand the goals everyday guys face, and I discovered how to combine science and practicality to help them achieve their ambitions in the easiest ways possible. Using my specialised techniques, I have advised and trained numerous *Men's Health* cover models, readers and celebrities and helped them achieve world-class physiques. Thanks to these well-received successes, I now contribute monthly to major magazines such as *GQ*, *Fighters Only*, *Runner's World* and *Men's Fitness*. My easy-to-understand features and routines will help the man on the street use cutting-edge scientific research for his personal benefit. And at all times I push the motto 'small steps, big results.'

But that's the last you'll hear about anyone other than yourself because this book has set a journey specifically for you. Like all expeditions, the road ahead can seem unfathomably long and full of unknowns. To ease any travel sickness you might feel as you venture from your comfort zone, the book is divvied into a clear beginning, middle and end.

The beginning (chapter 1) teaches you why you should exercise. The remunerations are far greater than a decent set of guns that will impress your nephew. The benefits will quickly convince you that sweating regularly is as important as breathing. You'll also learn how to take a long, hard look at yourself. Yes, you've probably already looked at yourself and longed for improvement. That's probably part of the reason you're reading this. This is where you'll find out what these improvements should look like. You'll do a few self-tests that'll tell you what your ideal weight is and how strong and fit you are. This will deliver a clear picture of where you are and what you're capable of so that you can set goals and determine how quickly you'd like to progress.

Chapter 1 also includes a step-by-step planning process that will give you the confidence to know where you're headed and how to reward yourself once you've achieved certain milestones. But just because you know where

you are and where you're going doesn't mean you'll hit the ground running. The conviction to get started can actually be the hardest part, and you may need a little encouragement to get out of the blocks. To assist you, this chapter includes some of the best motivational tips for changing your life and well as case studies of guys just like you who overcame their trouble self-starting.

Chapter 2 teaches you about your muscles' pit crew: the kitchen. This chapter outlines the rules for eating to gain muscle and burn fat and provides solid dietary plans that'll dramatically accelerate your results. Up to 70 per cent of all your improvements can be attributed to what you do in the kitchen. Good nutrition comes before training, both in this book and in the real world.

Taking the first steps towards a better you involves working your eyes. Chapter 3 is a meet-and-greet session with your most vital muscles. You'll learn how and why your muscles grow, what their intricacies are and how you can make them work for you. You may think you already know all this but you'll probably find a few surprises that will help you reach your goals faster, even if your goal is to lose as much weight as possible and not build any muscle. Learning about your inner workings will help you tackle the fat-burning section of this book with greater understanding and thereby make losing weight easier. Finally, before you graduate to the workouts, you need a little lesson about stretching. Chapter 4 explains how to rest properly to recover from any tightness experienced in the past few months of training.

Chapter 5 presents total-body training plans for beginners. These programmes, which include both muscle-building and fat-burning elements, are mapped out week for week and progress you towards becoming an intermediate lifter—the middle point of your journey.

Once you complete the intermediate-level workouts in chapter 6 you'll have progressed into a man who is probably pretty happy with what he sees in the mirror. But you now likely have a taste for improvement. At this point you'll have to make a decision: Either move onto chapter 7 for the more advanced workouts or move onto chapters 8 or 9 for fat-burning workouts. This is a fork in the road. One way leads to further fat burning whereas the other leads to further brawn building. Unfortunately, no self-test can tell you which road to choose. That decision lies solely with you and your preference about how you want to look. Fortunately, your decision is not locked in stone and you can change course at any time.

If you've chosen to burn fat, chapters 8 and 9 answer the most common question about fat burning: How do I lose body fat the fastest? These chapters rank and explain all of the most common fat-burning techniques and approaches so that you know what you're up against. They also explain how to put it all together into a cohesive plan. If you want to shed only a few kilos of fat, there's a plan for you as well as a maintenance plan to back it up when you're finished. If you have a bit more to lose, the six-month plan will help you progress from fat to fit.

Once you've traversed your muscle-building or fat-burning journeys, you'll learn how to adapt your programmes to fit your ever-changing lifestyle. Those who adapt to the changes in life achieve the most successful results. Chapters 10 and 11 provide workouts that will help you train during your lunch hour and fix some of life's quirky little problems such as beating a hangover or improving your sex life. This final stretch of road affords you this luxury because you will have developed a baseline of fitness over the previous 6 to 12 months. You'll be in great shape and can at that point afford to tweak things.

There's also a very good chance that during this final stretch you'll want to put your new body to the test. What better place than the sport field? To help you along with this endeavour, chapter 12 offers workouts for the most popular sports. Here you'll get the baseline of fitness to tackle any challenge and test your mettle against your fellow man. At this final step you'll have progressed from a spectator to a participant. Your journey will be complete because you will have traversed the roadmap to the new you. It's much easier than you think, and at the end you'll come away with a new body and a newly confident mindset.

With these practises in mind, *Body Trainer for Men* offers solutions to the most common issues faced in the gym and out. The methods and training plans are interlinked and long term so that rather than forcing you into one particular goal, several improvements can be made concurrently. Now you can prepare to meet all the demands of an energy-sapping work schedule while sculpting the muscle you need to look stellar on the beach. Whatever your present needs or forthcoming goals may be, you'll find the advice in this manual 100 per cent user friendly, result driven and effective. Consider it the perfect exercise partner: one who is never late and has the answers to your questions. Embrace your impatience because you're about to get the physique and health you've always wanted. Not just for an instant but for a lifetime. Keep reading to find out what you've been missing out on.

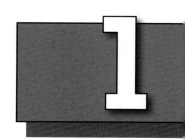

Getting Started

Dogs. If you've ever thought about getting one, or perhaps already have one, you undoubtedly have a rough idea how to look after it. The rules for keeping a pup's tail wagging are all but common sense. Feed it plenty of protein-rich foods—no breads or cakes. Give it plenty of water, not fizzy drinks or beer. And, most important, take it for plenty of long walks and runs. If you didn't have time to walk your pooch, you'd feel pretty damn guilty and probably wouldn't consider befriending man's best friend in the first place. As you've probably heard, fat dogs beget fat owners.

Taking care of your body is no different from owning a dog: Feed it, water it and make sure it gets plenty of exercise. But you don't need to work, well, like a dog to live a healthy, long life. All you need to do is clue in to the benefits of exercise. Exercise is better than the latest prescription drug, offers more pronounced results than the most expensive therapies and is the closest thing we have to a cure-all health elixir. Here are the top 10 benefits of exercise.

1. Longevity

If one thing matters more than anything, it's staying alive. We fortunately have evolved to link our longevity with the amount of sweat that passes our brows. Just how many years can exercise buy you? In a well-known study that examined mortality rates over 26 years in more than 17,000 men who had attended Harvard University, life expectancy was about 2 years longer in those who expended 2,000 calories per week during exercise compared with those who couch surfed (Paffenbarger et al., 1986). A fairly modest investment brings a large return when you consider that the extra years were full of a high-quality, active lifestyle, not just bingo halls.

2. Disease Prevention

Exercise fends off disease better than anything pharmaceutical companies could ever hope to sell. People have tried to bottle and sell it, but there's simply no substitute for the real thing. The healing properties of exercise are so powerful that they strike fear into the heart of more ailments than anything else. They tackle diabetes, heart disease, cancer, kidney disease, liver disease, lung disease, lymphoma, migraines . . . well, you get the picture. Exercise is a powerful immunization against almost every disease.

3. Brain Health

When you exercise to keep your body in rude health, your control centre also gets an upgrade. Not only will regular exercise help you coast into your golden years, it'll help you maintain your faculties and fend off dementia. What's more, exercise keeps your brain and cognitive abilities razor sharp throughout your life. Research has found that regular exercise improves memory, multitasking and planning abilities. As you can see, dumbbells might not be so dumb after all.

4. Improved Sense of Well-Being

You've seen them: the sickeningly smiling people advertising gyms and fitness equipment on the home-shopping channel. Love them or hate them, they're not faking it. Exercise really does lift mood, mostly because you're doing something to take your body a step closer to improvement. Exercise is better than a jumbo box of antidepressants. And your body is kind enough to throw in a bonus: the exercise high. During and after exercise, you manufacture feel-good chemicals and hormones like a built-in motivational aquifer. Your body actually rewards you for looking after it. Talk about taking care of your own.

5. Better Joint Health

It's true that sportsmen often injure themselves doing the things they love. Exercise can be risky business, but it's less risky than not exercising because getting your body moving lubes up your joints. Research in *Journal of Anatomy* found that exercise does no harm to your joints, whereas being overweight and sedentary is more likely to make your knees and hips go rusty (Hunter and Eckstein, 2009). Every joint in your body follows one principle: Use it or lose it. Get moving if you want to keep moving. Keep in mind that exercise has some risk if you perform it improperly, don't follow the principle of progressive overload or just have some bad luck.

6. Improved Self-Confidence

Looking in the mirror and seeing something you—and other people—like is a powerful ego booster. Just don't take it too far or you'll end up like one of the Jersey Shore crew. Whether you're trying to impress the redhead in accounts, interviewing for a new job or convincing the hotel front desk to give you a room upgrade, more confidence comes in handy. Those with low confidence can gain confidence by simply doing a bit of light exercise, such as walking, jogging or even working in the yard. The simple act of doing something healthy and productive for yourself can ramp up your self-esteem. But that doesn't mean that it's a good strategy to run around your office just before you ask out the redhead.

7. Higher Bone Density

Exercise will help you develop a Wolverine-like skeleton. Well, you may not be challenging Logan to a fight after pumping iron, but your skeleton will be significantly stronger. Research at Indiana University (Warden and Fuchs, 2007) found that exercising while you're younger makes you less likely to fracture anything when you're older. You might not appreciate this every day, but you will be thankful if you ever fall off your bicycle and come away with no broken bones.

8. More Energy

Spending energy to get more energy. It's a funny little conundrum. You'd like to tell yourself, 'I don't have the energy to exercise,' but it really doesn't work that way. Exercise will give you more energy than a coal mine. Regular exercise plays a consistent role in reducing fatigue and improving energy. Even if you work a 10-hour day and come home too tired to kick off your shoes, regular training will give you the oomph to tackle your job, health and private life with more vigour.

9. Better Sleep

Few things will ruin your day more than a terrible night's sleep. Lack of sleep can make you feel as though you've got the weight of the world on your shoulders and can affect your performance at work, costing you cold hard cash. A study at Oregon State University (Loprinzi and Cardinal, 2011) found that people sleep significantly better and feel more alert during the day if they get at least 150 minutes of exercise a week. Consider a better relationship with the sandman to be a big reward for only a smidgen of effort.

10. Improved Sex Life

There's a reason the gossip magazines feature the scandals of your favourite professional athletes: Being fit bolsters sex drive. (Hopefully this newfound drive won't create the same trouble for you that came to your athlete.) A body that looks better will attract more attention, and if you're in a relationship your partner will benefit from the added hormonal improvements that exercise creates. Regular sweating increases testosterone—your sex drive hormone—by dramatic amounts, found research in *European Journal of Applied Physiology and Occupational Physiology* (Kindermann et al., 1982). Skipping a workout before a big date could be one of the worst mistakes you ever make.

The biggest kicker is that exercise really is fun. Once you find something you enjoy doing, it won't seem like a chore and will be something that you want to do. The advantages listed here aren't available only to athletes and gym freaks. They're right there waiting for you, even if you put in very little time. In fact, you can reap a host of health benefits in just one exercise session. If you're after instant results with very little effort, keep reading about how to set your feet on the path to becoming a health millionaire.

Assessing Yourself

Why should you bother taking a long, cold look at yourself? Your end game is simply to look amazing, right? And, of course, to reap the rewards of better health, improved athleticism and longevity, to name just a handful of the benefits. It's pretty cut and dry: Take your current reflection and turn it into the after picture. But before you turn to the section of the book you think best fits your goals, consider that the fastest route from one side of the mountain to the other is not around it or even over it but directly through it.

The following section is the drilling tool for getting you through the mountain that is your before photo so you can arrive sooner at the after photo. It might not be a smooth ride but it gets the job done quickly. When you follow the correct technique for your individual body shape and goals, you become your own after picture faster. Expediency is key. To achieve your goals, use the self-assessment tools that follow. They're not the be-all and end-all, but they can be useful for figuring out what condition you're currently in. The starting point is what you'll look back on in a few months to assess the progress you have made, so you want it to be accurate. Smile: You're about to get a snapshot of who you are. Treasure it because it won't be there for long.

Body-Fat Test

A picture phone might have been the height of technology several years ago, but today you wouldn't even consider getting a handset without a camera. Such is also the case with body-fat readings. You used to have to visit a personal trainer to get a test. This could set you back a fair amount, especially if you got tested every few months. Today a body-fat measuring scale costs half of what a personal trainer would charge. It may be worth buying one because you'll certainly get your money's worth. A scale may not be quite as accurate as a personal trainer but it will give you a rough idea of where you stand. Get one, stand on it and get a reading, even if you have to do it on the display model in a store to save yourself the cost of purchasing one. Once you have a reading, use table 1.1 to find out whether you should gain muscle or burn fat.

If you've come in underweight, look to add a bit of muscle to your frame. Conversely, if you're holding onto a bit too much body fat, follow the fat-burning workouts after you've progressed to the workouts for intermediate lifters in chapter 6. Record your body-fat percentage in a diary or on your iPhone; it is part of your before picture.

Strength Test

Whether you're overweight or underweight you should try a test to see how strong you are. Table 1.2 lists the number of push-ups you should be able to complete at one time without

Table 1.1 Body-Fat Percentage and Health for Men

Age (yr)	Underweight (%)	Healthy range (%)	Overweight (%)	Obese (%)
20-40	< 8	8-19	19-25	> 25
41-60	< 11	11-22	22-27	> 27
61-79	< 13	13-25	25-30	> 30

Adapted from D. Gallagher, S.B. Heymsfield, H. Moonseong, et al., 2000, "Healthy percentage body fat ranges: An approach for developing guidelines based on body mass index," *American Journal of Clinical Nutrition* 72(3): 694-704.

Table 1.2 Push-Ups Completed in 1 Minute

Age (years)	Superior	Excellent	Good	Fair	Poor	Very Poor
<20	≥62	47-61	37-46	29-36	22-28	<22
20-29	≥52	39-51	30-38	24-29	17-23	<17
30-39	≥40	30-39	24-29	18-23	11-17	<11
40-49	≥39	25-38	19-24	13-18	9-12	<9
50-59	≥28	23-27	18-22	10-17	6-9	<6

Adapted with permission from The Cooper Institute, Dallas, Texas. From *Physical Fitness Assessments and Norms for Adults and Law Enforcement.* Available at www.CooperInstitute.org.

stopping based on your age (Golding et al., 1986). Simply warm up your body by jogging on the treadmill for 5 to 10 minutes, then have a rest and get into the push-up position. (See chapter 3 for a description of how to do the perfect push-up.) Ready. Set. Go.

Push-ups measure the overall strength and endurance of your entire upper body. If you're weak at push-ups, chances are you'll be weak everywhere else. Fortunately, all the programmes in this book will help strengthen your body from top to toe. Write your score in a training diary that you won't lose.

Cardiovascular Test

Here you'll test your heart, lungs and overall endurance. The most foolproof method is the Cooper 12-minute run test (Cooper, 1968), which tests how far you can run in 12 minutes. All you need are a pair of running shoes and a running track or a treadmill. Free websites such as www.walkjogrun.net and smartphone apps such as www.mapmyrun.com can help track exactly how far you've run if you a prefer a route around your local neighbourhood. Strap on your running shoes, then run as far as you can in 12 minutes. Compare your score with

the scores in table 1.3 to see whether you need to improve in this area.

Use these three tests to figure out where your body currently stands and record your results. Remember that goofy photo of you at your first formal school dinner? Well, the smile that comes across your face when you look at that picture is the same one you'll flash when you look back on these results. Don't be disheartened by your scores if they aren't what you want; at least you took the test and are going to be showing some dramatic improvements. Improvements all start with setting goals that are rewarding to achieve and offer the motivation to keep you going.

Setting Your Goals

Use this step-by-step guide to accurately set your goals so that they start to motivate your efforts.

Step 1: Decide Your Ideal Body Weight

You probably already have a very clear idea of what you'd like to weigh. This may mean

Table 1.3 Distance Run in 12 Minutes

Rating	Distance (m)	Distance (miles)
Excellent	2,700	>1.7
Good	2,300-2,700	1.4-1.7
Average	1,900-2,300	1.2-1.4
Below average	1,500-1,900	.9-1.2
Poor	<1,500	<.9

that you'd like to add muscle mass or lose fat mass. Sometimes this goal can seem completely unattainable—that's fine. Your goals shouldn't be modest or merely what you think you can achieve; they should be what you want to achieve. People who set conservative goals have a harder time achieving satisfaction than those who set ambitious goals. You're stuck with the body you're in for life, so you might as well make the most of it, especially at the goal-setting stage. There is no such thing as aspiring too high.

With this in mind, one of the biggest mistakes an exercise newbie can make is focusing too much on the scale. Your weight can become an obsession and isn't an entirely truthful reflection of the progress you've made. If you're trying to lose weight using weight training, you'll probably add a few kilos of muscle while losing fat. Set your long-term weight goal and check the scale once a month just to see where you're at.

Now that you have your body-weight goal, write it down alongside your ideal body-fat percentage. Weight loss and muscle gains are long-term goals, and everyone loses or gains weight at a very different rate. The winning secret to achieving your goal is how you *feel* about achieving it.

Step 2: Refine Your Goals

Once you have locked in your long-term goal, it's time to add a few bells and whistles to it. Nobody exercises so that they can smile each time they step on a scale. Instead, we exercise for a number of reasons that make us happy. What makes you happy is sure to be vastly different from what makes the next guy happy. You may want a six-pack or a bigger peak to your biceps or to run a 5K race. These are all good goals that will motivate you and help you personalise your programme and efforts.

In your journal, write down 10 things you'd like to get out of exercise. Remember to keep your goals as personalised as possible and don't fall into the trap of writing down the cover lines of your favourite magazine. You are not the masses. You are an individual with a unique personality, and your goals should reflect that. Make your goals as unique as possible so that they fit with who you are and provide specific motivation. Focusing on the *why* rather than the *how* will help you achieve your goals faster and easier. Take the following guidelines on board when you write down your goals.

1. Keep your own well-being close to heart. Don't brush aside the benefits of getting eight hours of unbroken sleep or bounding up a flight of stairs without raising your heart rate. These goals are very achievable and will make you feel incredible.

2. Make your goals realistic. You're not going to be standing on the Mr. Universe stage in a luminescent codpiece by the end of the year, so don't set yourself up to be disappointed. Figure out what you think you can do with the time you have and how you can achieve it.

3. Be specific. Setting a goal of 'Be healthier' is like asking yourself 'How many grains of sand are on the local beach?' It is ambiguous and cannot be quantified, so you'll never know whether you've achieved it. Write that you want to lose five kilograms of fat instead of saying that you want to get leaner.

4. Know that you need down time. Don't try to tell yourself that you're going to train 7 days a week or set a goal that demands that you lose 10 kilograms of fat a month. That would require all-out effort without allowing time for rest and recuperation, mentally and physically. Training 3 to 5 days per week will actually make your workouts more productive.

5. Choose goals that you can track, whether through recording progress in a workout log or ticking boxes off a calendar. If you want more energy, keep a chart where you rate your energy level on a scale of 1 to 10 daily. This will be a built-in motivation source when you look back on how you felt when you first started keeping the records.

TIP Write your goals in a positive light rather than a negative one. 'I want to miss only one workout a week' is bad, but 'I want to enjoy four exercise sessions a week' is positive.

Step 3: Set a Time Frame

Once you have a goal, figure out how quickly you want to achieve it. If the answer is 'right now', you're not alone—we all want instant results. Cut yourself some slack and don't apply too much pressure. Check out your work and family schedule for the next six months and work around your life commitments. But don't give yourself too long either or you'll dampen the spark you have for improvement. Gaining a kilogram of muscle in six months is way too easy; trying to gain it every three weeks

is achievable but also sufficiently challenging. Now go back to your goals and write down the time frame in which you think you can achieve each goal.

Step 4: Keeping Records

You might think an exercise journal is for newbies and people with obsessive–compulsive disorder, but it is actually very important for long-term success. It helps you keep a strict, entirely accurate record. With this information you can figure out what worked for you and what didn't. If you were building a kilogram of muscle each week two months ago, why aren't you now? Flick through the log and you'll be able to see what kind of gains you were making on a particular programme.

Training Log

Date _____   Weight _____

Week number in training cycle _____

Exercise	Sets	Repetitions	Rest (seconds)
1.			
2.			
3.			
4.			
5.			
6.			
7.			
8.			
9.			
10.			

RESTING HEART RATE (BEATS/MINUTE)			SLEEP (HOURS)		
Sleep quality	1	2	3	4	5
Energy level	1	2	3	4	5
Training quality	1	2	3	4	5
Muscle soreness	1	2	3	4	5
Motivation	1	2	3	4	5
Health	1	2	3	4	5
Nutrition	1	2	3	4	5

Scale: 1 excellent; 2 good; 3 OK; 4 poor; 5 awful

From R. Klerck, 2014, *Body Trainer for Men* (Champaign, IL: Human Kinetics).

Figure 1.1   Sample training diary.

Sample Food Diary

Date _____

Time	Meal	Food, fluid, supplement intake	REACTIONS		
			Before eating	Immediately after eating	2 hours after eating
	Breakfast				
	Mid-morning snack				
	Lunch				
	Afternoon snack				
	Dinner				
	Evening snack				
	Training				

From R. Klerck, 2014, *Body Trainer for Men* (Champaign, IL: Human Kinetics).

Figure 1.2 Sample food diary.

A journal is an extremely powerful motivational aid that provides evidence of improvement and that can become a game plan for your long-term success. It doesn't have to be an old-school paper-and-pen log; plenty of free apps for your smartphone, such as IFitness or RunKeeper Pro, will help you record your progress. Figures 1.1 and 1.2 provide sample training and food diaries that you can use if you prefer the reliability and nostalgia of paper.

Step 5: Schedule Rewards for Yourself

You should be the one who decides what milestones and incentives you need in order to succeed. If you want to cut out junk food, that doesn't mean you should swear off burgers forever. Instead, go out for dinner at your favourite restaurant on a Saturday as a reward for cutting out the bad stuff all week. Life works best when it's in balance. Depriving yourself of the things that make life worth living will never work in the long term. The best strategy is to find equilibrium and figure out ways to still do all the things you love while hitting your goals. Chances are you'll enjoy your vices far more when they're done infrequently.

You can reward yourself weekly, monthly or at the attainment of your final goal. Just be sure to keep the rewards in proportion. A weekly reward might be a single outing to a restaurant, a monthly reward might be a weekend trip to Octoberfest with all the trimmings and a final reward could be a holiday to a tropical paradise complete with buffet tables. You can also repay yourself with things that don't relate to your goal. If you want to avoid junk food, reward yourself with flashy new pair of jeans that you wouldn't want to grow out of.

Step 6: Find the Resources You Need to Achieve Your Goals

At this point you'll start putting into play the pieces that will help you achieve the goals you've written down. Scout around for the best gym membership or set yourself up with a home gym. Clear your schedule and start telling people about the new you they can expect. If you regularly sink a few beers after work, tell your drinking buddies that you've decided to use that time to exercise and explain the reasons why. They might give you a hard time initially but will understand in the long term and will soon be asking for your secrets. Get some new workout gear if you have to and pack a gym bag that's ready to go. These actions will reaffirm your goals and slowly gear your brain to accept that the old you is about to get a kick in the pants.

That's not to say that the motivation to get started will come easy. You may find it a little tough to take the final step. The next section, geared towards helping you get motivated, starts off with one man's story for inspiration.

Getting and Staying Motivated

Kickstarting your journey isn't always easy. Hell, you've probably resisted it for so long that doing it a while longer will be second nature. But there are some tricks you can do to convince yourself that taking better care of yourself is the right thing to do.

If you're reading this sentence, deep inside you've subliminally made a small, albeit intangible, commitment to exercise. You might not have firmed it up with actions just yet, but your subconscious has taken the reins and decided that it would like its flesh-bound host to make a change. The trouble is getting your conscious to agree with that decision and serve up the necessary commitment, effort and discipline. When you get those factors working in unison, nothing will stand in the way of your success.

But that's often easier said than done because commitment, effort and discipline work together like a three-man basketball team. When one factor fails, the others have to work harder for you to get points on the board. Getting these traits to team up can feel like herding cats: impossible.

The following easy-to-digest tips and tricks will give you inspiration and help you motivate yourself. You don't have to adhere to them 100 per cent; rather, you can tailor them to your own personality and situation. Think of it as team building that'll make both your brain and body stronger, healthier and fitter.

Mark Whitfield (47 years old) had been slight his whole life and wanted to go from scrawny to brawny before his holidays abroad. He decided on five goals:

1. Add 10 kilograms of muscle mass.
2. Develop arms he could flex with pride.
3. Create abs that looked good on the beach.
4. Find the time to exercise at least every second day.
5. Have the confidence to take off his shirt in public.

The Problems

Mark is one of London's most prominent photographers and is always on the road. Eating a high-protein, high-calorie diet while travelling for work can be difficult. Mark felt self-conscious about going to a gym for the first time, and his age meant he was at a muscle-building disadvantage.

The Solutions

Mark bought a membership to a club that has multiple gyms around the country so that he could find a gym when he travelled. He began using premixed protein shakes and packed a lunch every day to make sure that he always had enough of the correct nutrients to finance his muscle building. Mark, a really friendly guy, grew to know just about everyone at each club, which made exercising seem like more like a social gathering. The fellow gym users eventually thought of him as one of their own and dished out advice and friendship, which made him keener to keep at it. Because Mark was a total novice he added muscle easily, which more than offset any disadvantage from his age.

The Eating Plan

Because Mark has an incredibly fast metabolism, he had to develop a new appetite and make a change from his standard three-meals-a-day routine. When his packed lunches ran dry he filled up on high-protein meals wherever he could and followed the muscle-building nutrition plan in chapter 2. He occasionally paid an odd visit to a coffee shop, but the calories counted towards gaining muscle and bulk. His calorie-burning potential was naturally high so he never let hunger pains take root.

The Training

Mark was a total beginner so pretty much anything would work, but he could risk injury and lack of motivation if the postworkout pain became too great. He followed the plan in chapter 5, which uses high reps and works the entire body in each session, to help his muscles gradually become accustomed to being put through their paces. He felt a little pain for the first two weeks, but after the initial shock wore off he loved the satisfying feeling that his muscles had been worked, and he gradually increased the weight and reduced the reps.

The Drive

Mark's desire to take off his shirt in the summer months fuelled his exercise ambitions. He didn't want to be the only one in his family snaps sporting a yoghurt complexion after a trip to Spain. Enjoying more time with his family became his inspiration, even though the demands of his job were stacked against him. He bought a five-month supply of protein, half of which was premixed, so he could take it with him wherever he went. This outlay may have been hefty but it sent a clear message to his subconscious that he was in it for the long run and that backing out would cost him more than just muscle.

The Results

Mark gained more than 10 kilograms of lean muscle in just two months and maintained a lean waist. After two months his daughter commented that he looked like a model. If that's not motivation enough to stick to it, then nothing is. Time to book another holiday.

- **Combine the things you love.** Take your girl on a run or a cycle around the park followed by a healthy, protein-rich picnic. Get the family to the beach, kick a ball and do sprints chasing after it and your kids. The trick to more fitness is integration. The more you combine fitness with everyday activities, the less exhausting and time consuming it will be.

- **Put your stats in a public place.** Write down this week's body fat, bench press max, body weight or whatever is relevant to you. Put it in a place where everyone can see, such as a small slip of paper on the company notice board, in the office kitchen or on Facebook. Aim to improve those results each week. If you feel especially courageous, write something cheesy on the scrap of paper that has your results. You'll be ridiculed at first, but it will draw attention to your motivational plight and spur people to ask you questions about it. You can turn this to your advantage when your results start to improve.

- **Trick yourself into going for just eight minutes.** On days when you don't feel all that strong, make the only requirement of your exercise session very small and undemanding. Think of doing a single set of your favourite exercise. Once you've started, you'll probably finish. If you still don't feel like training, then go home—you've lost nothing. Using this trick you never actually stop exercising; you just have a few gaps in your training log.

- **Ask a friend to be brutally honest with you.** Swallow your pride and get your training partner to tell you what muscle groups are your weaknesses. You don't have to get naked or anything—just tell him not to hold back then sit back and take it on the chin. This will crack the whip. If you're really brave, ask your missus what she likes and dislikes about you. Make the body part that got the lowest score the focus of your workout for the next two months, then repeat the quiz for more motivation.

- **Sign up for an event.** Signing up for 10K race, cycling meet or fitness challenge is a long-standing and very simple way of kick-starting your motivation and helping you focus your attention towards a definitive goal and date. When the end is in sight, the journey becomes easy.

- **Link exercise to your longevity.** Check your cholesterol. Set a goal of lowering your low-density lipoprotein cholesterol by 20 points and increasing your high-density lipo-protein cholesterol by 5 points. You'll decrease your risk of heart disease and provide yourself with a very important, concrete goal. Ask your doctor to write a prescription for new blood work in a month. You just have to go to the lab and the doctor will call you with the results.

- **Create competition.** Guys are hard-wired for competition, so making a bet can help you improve your performance. Challenge your nemesis, friend, swaggering coworker or noisy neighbour to a contest. The first person to bench 100 kilograms or drop 5 kilograms of fat wins. Add a monetary or physical wager to it, and you'll be keener than a scientologist with a personality test in a schizophrenic asylum. It does work better if it's someone you don't particularly like. It doesn't matter if they don't know you think they're a chump.

- **Schedule a body-fat test every two months.** It's a clear end date for the simple goal of losing body fat and gaining muscle. Tangible results are the best motivator. Almost every gym offers body-fat testing; just make sure the same trainer performs the test each time to get accurate results. Try to do it at the same time of day each time because your body fat can fluctuate according to what how much water you drink, how much you eat and the time of day.

- **Plan all your workouts well in advance.** Schedule all of your workouts at the start of each month and cross them off as you complete them. In an average month you might try for a total of 20 workouts. If any are left undone at the end of the month, tack them on to the following month. Make sure you have a contingency plan for bad weather and unscheduled meetings.

- **Get a hold on yourself.** If you feel unmotivated or tempted, grab a handful of the flab around your belly. Wobble it, then push your index finger into it until you feel something hard—your abs. Do you want to see them? Well, skip the burger and get exercising.

• **Become a member of a new gym.** If you can't be asked to keep going down to the gym then change gyms. Find one that's closer or one that's slightly upmarket if that's your thing. In truth, you're better off downgrading to a no-name basement gym that costs less than the lint in your pocket. These hardcore gyms are full of people who don't care about watching a massive plasma screen while they run or lift weights. They come to the gym with a goal in mind and don't let distractions get in their way. Train there for just one week and you'll be equally inspired.

Case Study: Starting Out and Sticking With It

The fitness ambitions of Adam Pratt (29 years old) come and go with the pace of a flash mob. He's never really stuck to any kind of programme but likes to think he's fit. One month he's keener than a weasel and the next he gets screenburn from his Mac. He's tried his hand at sprint triathlons, rock climbing, gym, running, kite boarding, kayaking, you name it. His approach is actually on the right track because cross-training is the best way to get real-world fitness that gets you ready for anything, including longevity. Unfortunately, cross-training works only if you actually get sweating, and the only thing that he regularly sticks to is his penchant for a postwork pint. Each time he finds a new activity he throws himself into it with gusto: new kit, club memberships, weekends away. A month later his coffee table has all the makings of a climber who has summited Everest but his climbing harness rots away in his cupboard. He has a busy job and thrives in chaos but struggles with direction. His wife recently had their first child, the surest thief there is of free time, which adds another element of disorder. So what inspired him to get a build he can now be proud of?

The first step was admitting to himself that his exercise commitment was lacklustre. I got him to place his sport kit in his driveway. That didn't work so well because there was so much of it that it spilled into the street. But he got the point after I had him put a sticky note on each item with the date he last used it. He could see that he'd thrown money, not effort, at the problem. He made a deal with himself: Anything that doesn't get used at least every six months gets the online-auction cure. That way his wallet gets fatter and his gut gets thinner because he's more likely to use it.

But that's only the stick element in his story. There's also a carrot: a box-fresh son. Although his boy will love him unconditionally, Adam knew that showing a lack of commitment to anything, his health included, was setting a very poor example. He realised that he'd have to be fit to play with his energetic son in the next few years and that he needed to create a commanding physique that showed his family he could look after and protect them. He knew he didn't need to have pecs powerful enough to deflect hollow tips, but he needed to be able to carry his family to safety if there was ever a house fire. After all, it is his—and every father's—duty to be strong enough to keep his loved ones out of harm's way. Overpreparation? Maybe, but if that's not enough motivation then nothing is. With these two elements firmly in mind, all that kit he'd been accruing suddenly got used. He still does a bit of everything (postwork pint included) but is now fit, strong and a master of several sports. All he has to do is wait for his son to get out of diapers and join him.

Ready, Set, Go!

You should now know everything you need to know about yourself. Your starting point is clear and the route to your perfect physique should be taking shape. Don't worry if new goals arise or if problems stand in your way. That happens to everyone. It's just a pesky little thing called life, and it's been known to get messy. We don't live in a world where everything goes according to plan, and if we did life would be pretty damn boring. If you hit an obstacle that seems insurmountable and threatens to derail your progress, remember how easy it was start again.

After just a few months of following the plans in this book you'll be equipped with the physical and mental strength to know you can change anything. Whip out a piece of paper, take the tests (at which you will have improved) and set new goals that take your new situation into account. Even if it feels as though you're back at square one, you're not because you will have made progress. You've taken charge of your problems and slapped a label on them and are in complete charge of your physique. Success is yours. All you have to do is keep reading, because the only muscles that have taken action so far are the ones controlling your eyes. You're about to learn about the inner workings of all your most important muscles, even the ones you're using to hold this book right now.

Eating Right

Lifting weights and possessing good genetics are not the most important things for adding size or burning fat. Your knife and fork are your most powerful body-changing weapons. Read on for the how and why.

You might be doing the absolute best exercise programme known to man. You may push tonnages so big you turn heads or run so hard you win marathons. You could even get the perfect amount of sleep and recovery time. But all of that amounts to nothing if you don't eat the right kinds of nutrients. Muscles grow only when enough nutrients are available to finance their expansion. If you don't have healthy protein, fats and carbohydrate floating around your body, your system won't devote those extra calories to expanding your biceps. Fortunately, the rules of healthy eating apply to both blokes trying to lose weight and those trying to gain it. All you have to do is adjust your portions accordingly. Eat more to get big. Eat less to get small. Simple, eh?

The foods you should eat to get big and those you should eat to trim down are exactly the same. Your body responds to healthy, nutrient-dense foods the fastest, so to achieve results in the shortest time possible you shouldn't be filling up at your local fast food dealer. Excess calories from poor food choices will do the job if you're trying to bulk up but they can cause long-term health problems. Being a good-looking corpse isn't worth it. Every single thing you put into your body has a side effect. Action–reaction. No food is neutral. If it's not doing you good, then it's probably doing harm.

Before you learn about how to eat to bulk up or lose fat you need to embrace the golden rules for staying healthy inside and out. Be warned: These might come as a shock to your established eating patterns. Unfortunately, there's no way to sugar coat the correct way to eat. You can cherry pick what you like from this list and forget the rest, but if you stick to it you'll be sporting abs and growing your guns well into the 22nd century.

Your Healthy Eating Guide

Your body has evolved to eat foods that you'd be able to collect in the wild. If you can't kill it, pick it or grow it then you shouldn't eat too much of it. This is the most important piece of advice. Stick to it religiously, and you'll find yourself in rude health. If you can't pronounce an ingredient or don't keep it in your pantry, simply don't eat it. Because humans haven't been eating these ingredients for very long, there's no way to know what they'll do to you in the long term. To live to old age, eat the way your grandparents ate. A lot of choice exists nowadays, and with so many hidden calories in strange containers there's no telling what you're really putting into your body. Eat like the old folks did and maybe you'll live long enough to ride your own hoverboard.

To make sure you don't feel like you're living a life of deprivation, have one or two cheat meals a week in which you get a fix of all your favourite foods. This is when you can have your burgers, cakes, fizzy drinks and white breads. You need these meals to keep yourself sane. However, try to cook as much of the foods yourself as you can so that they'll still have some nutrients and you'll know exactly what's in them.

Pay attention to how you feel, whether good or bad, after each meal. If a certain food doesn't agree with you, then don't eat it. This includes old favourites such as milk. A lot of people are lactose intolerant but don't know it. If milk agrees with you then drink it all you want—just listen to your body's messages. However, don't misinterpret those messages because sugar can be pretty appealing. Though you should try to limit sugars, you shouldn't use chemical sweeteners as a substitute because they also haven't been around for very long. If you have a sweet tooth, limit your consumption to one to two tablespoons of sugar each day.

Try to eat six to eight meals every day. If you're trying to lose weight, limit portions to one and a half times the size of your fist. If you're trying to gain weight, eat portions that are two or three times the size of your fist. This hikes up your metabolism and makes you burn more calories, but if you're bulking then the extra calories will rush to your muscles.

Never go without food for more than three hours. If you don't get regular fuel injections, your body goes into starvation mode as it would in a time of famine. The next time you eat you'll store nutrients, making you fat. If your body is well fed all the time, you'll steadily lose weight or gain muscle.

Kick off each day with a solid breakfast because the longest you go each day without food is the time you're snoozing. You literally fast at night, hence the name *breakfast*. The problem: While you sleep your body steals amino acids (the building blocks of protein) from your muscle tissue to fuel your brain and nervous system. In this catabolic state your body starts to cannibalise your hard-earned muscles. Ever wake up feeling smaller? That's why. A protein-rich breakfast is the solution.

Don't limit protein intake to the mornings. You should eat two grams of protein per kilogram of body weight per day. For example, if you weigh 93 kilograms, you need to eat 186 grams of protein every day. If your training increases dramatically you can eat three to four grams of protein per kilogram of body weight, but only for a maximum of six weeks.

To make sure you're healthy, always eat five to eight portions of fruit or vegetables each day. Trying to get ripped? Limit the fruit to two portions a day—fruit is often high in calories and natural sugars—and make up the shortfall with more veggies. All vegetables and fruits are important and not one of them is bad for you. Just remember to eat them in moderation depending on your goals.

Finally, drink at least two litres of water each day. Use the following formula to figure out how much of this you should drink before exercising: 65 millilitres of fluid per kilogram of body weight. For example, an 81 kilogram (180 lb) bloke should drink 500 millilitres (18 oz) before he trains.

Pre- and Postworkout Nutrition

The meals you eat before and after your training sessions are some of the most important meals in your diet because they fuel your gym sessions and refuel your body afterwards. If you don't give your body the nutrients it needs to train hard and build muscle (and thus finance fat burning), you'll start yourself off on the wrong foot and won't make much progress. Here's the lowdown on the best eating strategies.

Preworkout Food

The aim of the preworkout meal is to jack up the glycogen (energy) stores in your muscles and liver so that you have plenty of fuel for exercise. Carbohydrate and proteins, such as the ones listed in 'Stock Your Shelves', give your muscles the fuel they need to perform. Eat approximately 60 to 90 minutes before your workout to make sure that the meal is digested and can be used to supply oomph.

Try a whey protein shake with oats or some kind of carbs mixed in. You can take protein shakes all the time. If you can, buy plain, no-name-brand protein with no additives from

Stock Your Shelves

PROTEIN
- Chicken
- Oily and white fish
- Cottage cheese
- Turkey
- Prime cuts of red meat
- Whey protein
- Eggs
- Cheese
- Lentils
- Prawns and shrimp
- Quinoa
- Avocado
- Nuts
- Beans
- Pumpkin seeds
- Chickpeas
- Seeds

CARBOHYDRATE
- Brown rice
- Basmati rice
- Sweet potato
- Squash
- Pumpkin
- Parsnips
- Lentils
- Beans
- Root vegetables
- Quinoa
- Steel-cut oats

your local health store. Flavour it yourself with a banana and a cup full of frozen berries. Now, hit your training session and keep reading to find out what you should eat afterwards.

Postworkout Food

Move over, breakfast: The postworkout meal is the most important of the day. Make sure to include plenty of protein, the nutrient that is responsible for tissue repair and the growth and formation of new tissue (in other words, muscle building). Take advantage of the one-hour window after exercising to restock your protein and carbohydrate levels. Eat three grams of carbohydrate to one gram of protein to achieve optimum gains from your training sessions. The best option is to take a protein shake as soon as you put down the last dumbbell and then have a healthy meal about an hour afterwards.

Great Pre- and Postworkout Smoothies and Fast Food

When pressed for time, filling your belly can take longer than the average exercise session. If you're on the street, you have to wait for someone to prepare your food for you and you take the risk that the food isn't going to match up with your training goals. If you're at home, you have think what you can eat, prepare it, eat it and clean up.

Fortunately, there is a way to streamline your healthy dietary habits: Drink your food. Smoothies are one of the quickest stealth-health meals you can make. You can drink them in seconds, and clean-up consists of swishing a little water over your blender. The nutrients support your goals and leave you feeling full for hours afterwards, and prep takes just three to five minutes. Here are some of the best recipes to help you hit your goals in the tastiest way possible.

Ache-Fixing Shake

4 thick slices fresh pineapple
1 stick celery
2.5 cm (1 in.) piece ginger
200 ml (6.8 oz) water

Pineapple contains a compound known as bromelain, which is a painkiller and natural anti-inflammatory agent. Celery is used to fight pain associated with arthritis and gout, and ginger contains chemicals that have anti-inflammatory and painkilling properties.

Immune Booster

1/2 to 1 can (450 ml) coconut milk
2 raw eggs
1 scoop whey protein
1 handful berries (strawberries, raspberries, blueberries) or 1/2 to 1 banana
2 tbsp ground almonds
1 tsp honey
1 tbsp flaxseed oil

The fats in coconut are not stored as fat. They are easily digested and pass straight to the liver, which improves energy levels and assists the digestive system by reducing stress on the pancreas. The fats are similar to those in mother's milk and help support the immune system. People with chronic fatigue can really benefit from consuming coconut milk as it helps increase metabolism, thereby assisting in weight loss. It is also antibacterial, antimicrobial and antifungal and can benefit those with candida (yeast and fungal) infections or digestive problems and those who regularly suffer colds. The berries are a great source of vitamins, minerals, antioxidants and enzymes. Nuts provide essential fats and protein. Honey is the best thing to use as a sweetener because it is a natural product. The flaxseed oil is a great source of omega-3 fatty acids, which help electrical impulses move from the brain to muscles across the membranes around all the cells in the body and prevent heart disease.

Super-Cheap Preworkout Shake

1/2 cup oats

1 banana

1 small (50 g) yoghurt

3 tbsp powdered milk

400 ml (13.5 oz) water

The best preworkout eating strategy is to keep things simple. The ingredients should be minimal and you shouldn't eat anything too acidic that might repeat on you during exercise. This shake has the perfect mix of fast- and slow-digesting carbs, protein and fats for fueling any exercise session and it won't come back to haunt you while you train.

Super-Cheap Postworkout Shake

2 or 3 slices canned pineapple rings

1 diced apple

1 peeled, piped satsuma

Ginger to taste

3 or 4 heaped tbsp almond meal

1/4 cup semolina

450 ml (15 oz) water

Ginger and bromelain-rich pineapple reduce inflammation. The fruits, which are high in vitamin C, help further boost your recovery from exercise. The semolina replaces the carbs you'll lose during training and helps get the protein from the almond meal to your muscles.

The Energiser

75 g (2.6 oz) frozen strawberries

115 g (4 oz) mango

125 ml (4 oz) orange juice

250 ml (8 oz) fat-free milk

2 tbsp honey

1/8 cup whey protein

Powdered eggs or 4 raw egg whites

Honey is an antioxidant and provides 17 grams of carbohydrate per tablespoon, making it a great booster as part of your postworkout and preworkout meals. The mango contains potassium that helps create a healthier nervous system and releases energy from the rest of the protein, fat and carbohydrate in the shake.

Poor Man's Protein Shake

1/2 cup semolina

1/2 cup raw oats

1 banana

1 whole egg

3 or 4 tbsp powdered milk

6 drops vanilla essence

118 ml (3.9 oz) goat milk

118 ml (3.9 oz) water

The carbohydrate-rich semolina, proteins from the eggs, milk powder and milk and fats make this the perfect combination of calories for consistently adding mass to any frame.

Metabolism Accelerator

1 scoop vanilla-flavoured protein
4 small chunks pineapple
1/2 peach
Juice of 1/2 lime
450 ml (15 oz) cold water
1 handful crushed ice

Pineapple and peaches are high in fibre. When combined with the protein, they take longer to leave your stomach and leave you feeling full for a longer period of time. You won't feel the need to sneak in extra snacks.

Best Overall Protein for All Workouts

1 banana
2 apricots
236 ml (8 oz) full-fat milk
1 scoop whey protein
2 tbsp flaxseed flakes
1/2 cup raw oats
120 g (4 oz) plain yoghurt
2 tsp honey

The oats and flaxseed provide carbs and omega-3 fatty acids that replace lost energy and add muscle. Yoghurt and milk provide natural fats and protein, and the fruits are rich in antioxidants that'll boost your recovery.

Big Bertha Bulking Shake

2 heaped scoops strawberry protein shake

1 small scoop chocolate protein shake

3 fresh strawberries

1 banana

1 scoop vanilla ice cream

100 ml (3.4 oz) goat milk

1/4 cup oats

1/8 cup semolina powder

400 ml (13.5 oz) water

This liquid lunch packs in a huge amount of natural calories and protein. The potassium in the banana and strawberries helps you absorb these proteins and calories. This smoothie is a delicious source of fodder that will help you fuel and recover from your exercise.

Muscle Power Shake

1 cup strawberries

1 cup sliced mango

118 ml (3.9 oz) orange juice

236 ml (8 oz) water

1 tbsp honey

1/8 cup whey protein powder or 4 raw egg whites

The eggs in this smoothie help ramp up your supply of fat, which in turn creates the testosterone you need to increase strength. These little orbs also provide enough protein to help your muscles grow and recover as quickly as possible.

Dieter's Breakfast Shake

2 tbsp ground flaxseed

2 or 3 tbsp coffee

4 tbsp powdered milk

1 small (50 g) plain yoghurt

400 ml (13.5 oz) ice-cold water

Flaxseed, caffeine (from the coffee), milk protein and yoghurt are all proven weight-loss aides. Drinking cold water has been shown to increase metabolism by up to 30 per cent.

Bulking-Up Breakfast Shake

1/3 cup raw oats

1 banana

1 cup frozen mixed berries

1 tbsp omega-3 oil or olive oil

1 egg

2 tbsp powdered milk

1 small (50 g) plain yoghurt

350 ml (11.8 oz) water

Oats and oil keep you feeling full for several hours, and the banana gives you instant energy to start your day. The egg, yoghurt and powdered milk dish up the fast-digesting protein your muscles crave after several hours with no food.

Where to Next?

Now that you have a good idea of how to eat to be healthy, you can tailor your eating towards your goal of either building muscle or burning fat. This chapter first discusses the ways to build muscle because these ways lay the foundation for eating when you're training. You can then tweak this foundation based on your goal of losing fat. Lick your chops because you're about to tuck in.

Eat to Upsize Your Muscles

Lifting, pushing, pulling or throwing weights does not, and will never, build muscle. Recovery from this pushing, pulling and throwing is what builds hard-won muscle. The biggest part of recovery is rest. That's the time when you're sleeping, working at your desk or watching the latest box set. Resting is pretty easy, unless you're plagued with hyperactivity.

When you're done carving your imprint on your couch, the next—and equally important—step of muscle building is approaching your fridge. Food is to muscle what a lie is to a politician: Essential to power and success. You need to flood your body with excess calories so that it uses them to repair the damage you do to your muscles when you spend time beneath the bench press.

Your body's way of storing these extra calories? Muscle. But you don't need to be big to be strong. Watch an Olympic weightlifting contest and you'll see slightly-built men and women hoisting inhuman quantities of steel. They're still able to get strong from iron mongering, but they limit their calories so that they don't store them as overblown slabs of muscle or fat. To build muscle without gaining fat, all you need to do is eat plenty of the right kind of calories. This is where the approaches differ.

The first approach is best summed up by a single word: *more*. This approach involves consuming a mix of high protein and high carbohydrate. The second approach ropes in a well-known dietary foe: fat. The high calorie demands of both approaches are responsible for the guns of just about every bodybuilder who has squeezed into a tiny Speedo. Results do vary slightly, so keep reading for the skinny on getting big.

High-Carb, High-Protein Approach

The high-carb, high-protein approach is the easiest method to follow and is the approach used most often by blokes trying to get stacked quickly. It's bound by a single rule: Eat plenty of protein and carbs with every meal. Using this method you'll eat five to eight meals a day. Make sure to consume one of these before training and one directly after exercise. (Protein shakes count as a meal.)

The reason the approach works is simple: Eat more calories than you burn and your body will store them as muscle. Unfortunately, a certain portion of these calories will also settle as fat. It's a small price to pay. You can diet afterwards if you want to get ripped.

When you go out for dinner, simply eat more. No specific food is off limits. You effectively go on a seafood diet, as the joke says: When you see food, you eat it. It's dead easy, can be healthy (if you make the right food choices) and works very quickly. The diet plan that follows is a working example of the kinds of foods you should eat to start tightening your sleeves. Bon appétit, big fella.

High-Carb, High-Protein Sample Week

Monday

Breakfast: 3 whole eggs scrambled with 50 g (1.8 oz) mozzarella or cheddar cheese and 2 handfuls baby spinach, 250 ml (8.5 oz) fruit juice

Snack: 100 g (3.5 oz) almonds and dried fruit, 1 apple, 1 orange

Lunch: 200 g (7 oz) grilled sirloin steak, 1 cup brown rice, mixed vegetables

Snack: 150 g (5.3 oz) plain, sugar-free yoghurt with 1 handful blueberries, ground mixed seeds and nuts and manuka honey; 1 diced banana

Dinner: 300 g (10.6 oz) salmon fillet, mashed potato with the skin, mixed vegetables

Tuesday

Breakfast: 3-egg omelette with sliced mushrooms, olive oil, 1/2 diced onion, 1 diced bell pepper and 2 handfuls baby spinach

Snack: 200 g (7 oz) plain, sugar-free yoghurt with 1 handful berries and 200 g (7 oz) mixed seeds and nuts; 1 apple

Lunch: Chinese-style beef stir-fry with veggies, brown rice

Snack: 200 g (7 oz) cottage cheese with mixed seeds, dried fruits and nuts

Dinner: 2 grilled chicken breasts, 1 sweet potato, mixed vegetables

Wednesday

Breakfast: 2 large handfuls oats cooked in 250 ml (8.5 oz) skim milk with 2 tsp honey and whey protein

Snack: Canned salmon, cream cheese, dill and black pepper (mixed together); sliced carrots

Lunch: Small baked potato with baked beans, chillies, cheese and sliced pork sausages

Snack: 1 grilled seasoned chicken breast, 2 small beets

Dinner: 250 g (8.8 oz) lean minced beef chilli with corn, mashed sweet potato

Thursday

Breakfast: Smoothie containing whey concentrate powder, 1 handful blueberries and raspberries, 40 g (1.5 oz) plain yoghurt, 2 tbsp ground flaxseed, 1 tbsp rolled oats and 1 banana

Snack: Antipasta (bought or homemade) containing diced olives, mozzarella balls and peppers with olive oil; 2 apples; 1 banana

Lunch: 400 g (14 oz) sushi, brown rice

Snack: Canned mussels or oysters on sliced carrots, 1 small basket cranberries, 1 orange

Dinner: 2 roasted turkey or chicken breasts with lemon, garlic and herb sauce; stir-fried vegetables

Friday

Breakfast: 3 whole eggs scrambled with 3 egg whites, 2 large mushrooms and cheese; rye bread

Snack: Canned sardines on oatcakes, 2 apples, 1 banana

Lunch: 2 grilled chicken breasts, 1 sweet potato, salad with olive oil dressing

Snack: Avocado, mayo and prawn salad dressed with olive oil; 1 banana; 1 apple

Dinner: 2 grilled whitefish fillets, 1 cup brown rice with light gravy, mixed vegetables

Saturday

Breakfast: 2 kippers, 3 poached eggs, 1 sliced and fried pepper, 1 slice rye bread

Snack: 200 g (7 oz) plain yoghurt, 1 handful mixed nuts, 2 apples, 1 banana

Lunch: 4 thick-cut slices roast beef, mustard, lettuce and tomato on 2 slices rye bread

Snack: 200 g (7 oz) hummus, 3 large carrots, 1 orange, 1 apple

Dinner: 2 or 3 whole-wheat pitas filled with 350 g (12.3 oz) steak and mixed salad

Sunday

Breakfast: 2 cups muesli; 473 ml (16 oz) low-fat milk; 200 g (7 oz) plain, sugar-free yoghurt; 2 boiled eggs

Snack: 125 g (4.4 oz) cottage cheese on oatcakes, 50 g (1.8 oz) almonds, 1 apple, 1 orange

Lunch: 200 g (7 oz) lean minced beef burger and 1 slice cheese on whole-wheat burger bun, mixed salad

Snack: Tuna salad with olive oil dressing, 1 large mango

Dinner: 3 or 4 grilled lamb chops, 1 cup couscous, dark-green vegetables, salad with olive oil dressing

High-Fat, High-Protein Approach

If you ask the average mouth-breather to name the nutrient he thinks is worst for him, the first word to leave his mouth will likely be *fat*. Fat is synonymous with poor health. Unfortunately, nobody could think of a better word for the wobble in your gut, so the fat on your plate got saddled with the same name as the fat on your body. Fat got its bad rep during the Jane Fonda era, but things have changed since then, and new research has offered fat an official pardon. Fat recently got a reprieve when a review of 21 studies (including a total of almost 20,000 people) showed that fat is not linked to any cardiovascular disease (Siri-Tarino et al., 2010). It doesn't clog your arteries or stop your ticker from beating its tune. Funnily, obesity began to take off right when fat was considered public enemy number one. This happened largely because people substituted fats with sugars and carbs, which are far worse for the state of your six-pack.

Fat may offer nine calories per gram, which is more than any other nutrient, but the ways fat calories work are different than the ways calories from other nutrients work. Dr. Mauro Di Pasquale, a former world champion powerlifter and author of *The Anabolic Diet* (www.anabolicdietblog.com), became suspicious of the way fat was being perceived. He did research and found that people on a high-fat, high-protein diet gained more muscle and had higher testosterone levels. Protein is the stuff that fuels muscle growth, and testosterone is the man-hormone behind bedroom mojo and brawn building. But Pasquale's system wasn't all bacon and eggs. He recommends following a high-protein, high-fat plan all week and then following a high-carb, high-protein plan on weekends. This means you can gorge on all your favourite junk foods on Saturdays and Sundays. This system works on the rationale that when your body is flooded with so much fat that it believes it has enough, it stops storing the fat and begins to burn it as fuel. Pasquale even suggests that lifters following this system lose less muscle when they get lean and gain more muscle when they bulk up. However, his plan is somewhat restrictive in that you have to drastically alter your eating habits during the week. You're allowed to eat only 30 grams of carbohydrate each day; these are best reserved for low-carb veggies such as those listed in the diet plan that follows. After all, you do need to keep yourself healthy. This system is similar to the Atkins diet because you're not eating many carbs. The flip side is that you're encouraged

to gorge yourself on the weekends, which is a time when you're away from your routine and often eating out at restaurants. How regimented your week is will likely determine your level of success. All you have to do is choose one of the plans.

Aside from bigger biceps and abs that show, you should expect to experience the following.

The good: More energy and reduced hunger. Fat is energy dense, so your oomph levels won't yo-yo. This means you won't feel heavy after a meal and you'll wake up with the battery power of a five-year-old.

The bad: A tough first week. Your body will be adjusting to your new fuel sources, so you might feel a little off. Give it time and you'll be on track to hit your goals.

The ugly: Erratic bowel movements. It will take your guts a little time to get used to the new regimen. Take a fibre supplement to help you along.

The money: Carbs are cheap; healthy protein isn't. You'll find yourself eating more animal products that are more expensive, so buy in bulk to save yourself a few pineapples.

High-Fat, High-Protein Sample Week

Monday

Breakfast: 4 fried eggs, 4 to 6 pieces nitrate-free bacon

Snack: Beef jerky, apple

Lunch: Sliced lamb kebab with extra meat (eat half the wrap)

Snack: 100 g (3.5 oz) cottage cheese on crackers

Dinner: 400 g (14 oz) salmon steak, Brussels sprouts, leeks, mushrooms

Tuesday

Breakfast: 4 poached eggs on bed of smoked salmon

Snack: 1 tin oysters in oil

Lunch: Beef chilli with beans (no rice or pasta)

Snack: Avocado and tuna mixed with olive oil

Dinner: 4 pork chops, cauliflower, broccoli, asparagus

Wednesday

Breakfast: 3 scrambled eggs, cheddar cheese

Snack: 100 g (3.5 oz) mixed nuts

Lunch: Sashimi, dried beans

Snack: Avocado and cooked prawns dressed with olive oil

Dinner: Chicken stir-fry with asparagus, celery, spinach, onion and peppers

Thursday

Breakfast: 3 boiled eggs with 2 or 3 kippers

Snack: 25 g (.9 oz) dry-roasted peanuts, 1 glass milk, 100 g (3.5 oz) cottage cheese

Lunch: 200 to 300 g (7-10.6 oz) sliced beef in wrap with avocado, mustard, onion and spinach

Snack: Beef jerky, apple

Dinner: Sirloin steak strips (marinate in soy sauce and pepper), broccoli and cauliflower drizzled with garlic and olive oil

Friday

Breakfast: 4 fried eggs in butter, 4 slices nitrate-free bacon

Snack: 1 bag salami, 1 handful pecans

Lunch: Avocado, tuna, spinach salad

Snack: 1 packet beef jerky, few slices cheese

Dinner: Rack of lamb, broccoli, corn, cabbage

Saturday

Breakfast: Pancakes with bananas and Nutella

Snack: Several slices toast with almond butter, apple, banana

Lunch: Grilled fish, sweet potatoes, salad

Snack: Banana, yoghurt, cereal

Dinner: Your favourite cheat meal (e.g., pizza, burger)

Sunday

Breakfast: 3 or 4 English muffins with eggs or jam

Snack: Pate, carrots

Lunch: Pasta (your choice)

Snack: Cheese, crackers

Dinner: Your favourite cheat meal (e.g., creamy pasta, chips)

Big Questions About Muscle Food

Here are the answers to the questions most commonly asked about muscle building.

Q: **Will vitamin and mineral drinks help me bulk up?**

A: To answer this yourself, take a glance at the calorie content of your vitamin drink. Chances are you never knew how energy rich water could be. Plain water has no calories, which means you're actually drinking flavoured water. Yes, you'll get some vitamins, but you'll also swig more kilos onto your frame. Some vitamin drinks contain as many calories as a soft drink and are sweetened with sugar or aspartame. This makes them nothing but glorified soft drinks and puts you in danger of being duped out of your water habit. In fact, Coca-Cola filed a lawsuit against Vitamin Water over the claims that Vitamin Water is good for you. If you're looking for vitamins, you're better off taking a multivitamin and sticking with plain water, especially if you're trying to lose weight. If you're trying to bulk up, drink plenty of plain water and have the odd vitamin drink when you're away from your kitchen.

Q: **Are organic foods really worth the extra coin if I'm trying to build muscle?**

A: That depends who you believe: the hippies or the suits. A study by the suits at Stanford University (Smith-Spangler et al., 2012) found that no nutritional difference exists between organic and conventionally produced food. The levels of protein, fats and carbs were the same between foods; however, the study didn't measure the taste of the foods. Price is a big factor because eating healthy is more expensive than eating junk food. A good ploy is to always buy seasonal, locally produced grub because fresh food is the best for you. Both genetically modified (GM) and organic food from abroad have to travel, which depletes their nutrients. If you can't be bothered to get to a market, visit online market sites and be a suit-wearing hippie who gets his food delivered to his door.

Q: **If I'm trying to bulk and be healthy, should I choose soy over diary?**

A: First up, milk is for babies. You're not a baby, are you? Soy can be useful in the odd bowl of cereal. For people who are lactose intolerant, calcium-fortified soy milk is an alternative source of protein and calcium. However, the calcium in milk is absorbed better than that in soy milk, and milk has vitamin D, which is necessary for your bones. Low-fat milk has been linked to healthy blood pressure, colon and prostate health and even fat loss. The proponents of soy say that it can prevent prostate cancer and lower the risk of heart disease. However, it's often recommended to menopausal women. As a red-blooded male, you should probably avoid anything that helps your mom balance her hormones.

Q: **Is the hype about omega-3 fatty acids all it's cracked up to be?**

A: In a word, yes. Omega-3 fatty acids have been proven to—deep breath—boost memory, improve aerobic capacity, reduce chances of a heart attack, beat inflammation, decrease joint pain, help reduce body fat and bolster muscle size. Try saying that fast. Look for a supplement with at least 1,000 milligrams of docosahexaenoic acid, the stuff that gives this fatty acid its potency, and drop two or three doses a day. If you have problems with aftertaste, stash the tablets in the freezer to put an end to fish burps. If better health, a longer life and abs that show are on your agenda, be sure to get fishy every day.

Q: **Why do meats such as salami and bacon take such a beating in the press?**

A: Just about every nutritionist will tell you that these meats wreak havoc on your insides. Sodium nitrate is added to cured meats to preserve taste and freshness. If it wasn't added, your bacon would be gray rather than pink, and nobody would buy dead-looking food. Your digestive system converts nitrates into nitrosamines, which have been linked to cancer in animals and humans. Despite all the damning studies, however, a lot of food boards say that this additive is safe, mostly because a worthy alternative isn't available. The scientific jury's still in session on this one so you'll have to make up your own mind, but it's best to be safe rather than sorry. Fortunately, you should be able to find freshly carved meats at your deli if you don't want to give up your ham sandwiches.

Q: **What should I do if I'm starving and not near any eateries that serve healthy food?**

A: If you're in a restaurant, there's not a chef in the world who won't make a steak with some blanched veggies. All you have to do is ask. That's a pretty healthy option for anyone looking to lose weight or gain muscle. But if you're dead set on gaining muscle even if it means adding a little fat, eat whatever you like. You're better off filling the gap with something high in protein such as a kebab or a burger than anything sugary or sweet. There's nothing worse for your muscle-building ambitions than a grumbling stomach.

Q: **How important are 'use by' dates?**

A: Not wasting food is sure to keep your wallet healthy, but food that is past its prime tends to be lower in flavour and nutritional value. It is more than possible that the food won't actually harm you, but be careful about eating meat, especially chicken and fish, more than three days after its sell-by date because meat picks up bacteria easily. A quick smell test often will tell your body whether you can stomach the food.

Q: **Is the batter on fish really that bad?**

A: Batter is usually made from cheap, GM ingredients such as battery hen eggs and white flour. These ingredients can overrule the goodness in fish once it's deep fried. But if takeaway is on the menu, fish is the best option because it is still a good source of healthy protein. Ask for it grilled and you should have no problems at all.

Q: **Is fresh or dried pasta better for building muscle?**

A: Nutritionally, no difference exists between the two. The fresh variety has more water to start with, but both types are the same once cooked. Most blokes generally eat too many carbs and not enough protein, so if you want to be ripped start by cutting these out at night.

Q: **What's the healthiest kind of concentrated fruit juice: with pulp or without?**

A: Juice concentrate is made when water is removed from fresh juice so that the juice can be transported easily. After transportation, water is added to the concentrate and—presto—you can drink it as fruit juice. The flavour of concentrated juice is approximate to that of the fresh kind but the nutritional content is the same. The pulp is rich in flavonoids, which are antioxidants that work in the same way as vitamin C. Pulp also contains fibre, which aids digestion and weight loss. Washing down your creatine with concentrated juice helps the creatine absorb into your muscles faster.

Now that you know how to build muscle with food, the next step is to learn how to use food to lose fat. The final section in this chapter teaches you how to get leaner in the fastest and healthiest way possible, without even having to sweat.

Eat to Lose Fat

If you can do basic math, you can burn fat. No magic bullet, no secret, zero-calorie food, and no supplement—legal or illegal—works

better, faster, cheaper or healthier than good, old-fashioned food.

If you eat more calories than you burn you'll start to store said calories. They have to go somewhere, don't they? Usually that place is your gut. Fortunately, the same mechanisms that made you a little more man than you'd perhaps like can also help you achieve your perfect weight. You just have to adjust the content and portions that you consume.

Nutrition alone will not make you lose fat or boost your performance. Rather, the lack of nutrition kickstarts your fat-burning journey. Nutrition is the biggest player you can adjust if you want to get leaner and perform better. That's because food gives you energy. Even those evil carbs everyone harks about are useful for giving you the energy you need to exercise. To lose fat through eating, all you have to do is follow these simple rules. No diet. No rapid-weight-loss programme that has you abusing your soup pot. And definitely no avoiding your favourite foods. The secret is to create a new you using these easy-to-follow rules.

Rule 1: Eat Little and Often

Even if your primary information source is the newspaper you find in the toilet at work, you've probably heard that you need to eat upwards of six small meals a day to lose weight. This strategy makes your body constantly burn fuel and ensures that you're always eating and never hungry. It's akin to the way our ancestors ate: by popping food into their bearded mouths as they hunted or collected it. However, you shouldn't eat six huge meals a day. Rather, stick to palm-sized servings for snacks and servings the size of two fists for main meals. Alternatively, you can keep all your meals more or less the same size. Keeping all portion sizes the same tells your body that food is abundant and that it doesn't need to store any as fat.

The 'eat six small meals a day' mantra works well in a perfect world in which we all work from home and are two steps away from the kitchen. It's not always practical, however, if you work in an office, are on the road or are just plain busy. Fortunately, a recent study at Purdue University (Leidy et al., 2010) found that eating three normal-size meals that contain high amounts of lean protein can make you feel fuller than eating smaller, more frequent meals. In the study the three larger meals contained less than 750 calories each and were carefully portioned to encourage weight loss. The researchers found that eating protein during breakfast and lunch—meals one might not normally include protein in—made the system work and that proteins such as meat, eggs and legumes were good choices. That's a pretty good excuse to order a tasty 250-gram steak on your lunch hour.

Rule 2: Fill Up on Fibre and Protein

These two nutrients are the champion weight-loss tag team. They both slow the rate of digestion so you feel full longer and can reduce sugar cravings. What's more, fibre also helps hustle calories out of your body and helps get rid of your lunch quicker. A diet rich in fibre helps people keep weight off in the long run. How much is enough? The current recommended daily allowance for fibre is about 25 grams, but don't stop there. Eat as much as you can. It won't harm you as long as you drink plenty of water with it. The same goes for protein; make sure you get plenty in every meal. If you're trying to add muscle—and you should be to maximise fat burning—eat about two grams of protein per kilogram of body weight. If you were in Australia, that would mean throwing another shrimp on the barbie.

Rule 3: Ration Carbs

Since 1980 the food intake of the average bloke has grown by 500 calories a day, and nearly 80 per cent of this increase can be attributed to carbohydrate. In that time, the prevalence of obesity has become a pretty big burden on the world economy. Carbs are dense in calories, which your body uses very quickly. This can often make you feel full to capacity after a meal and then hungry enough to eat a low-flying pigeon less than an hour later. What can you do to keep yourself at your fighting weight? Cap your intake of the most carbohydrate-dense foods, such as grains and spuds, at just a couple of servings a day. Eat them before

or after training or any time before lunch. This ensures that you put these energy-rich foods to use in either fuelling or recovering from an exercise session. You can go one better by always eating high-fibre, minimally processed versions of these foods. That way, you'll be leaner as well as healthier.

Rule 4: Leave the Counting to Accountants

Losing weight should never feel like you're actually doing it. It should feel natural and instinctive. Cravings for poor foods are often caused by a lack of proper nutrients. By regularly snacking on the right foods, you'll eliminate hunger and control your calorie intake. That will not happen if you try to tally every calorie that crosses your lips.

That doesn't mean you can smash as many healthy, all-natural foods as you like. Natural foods such as fruit are often loaded with calories and are rich in fructose. These can be as dangerous as sugar to the size of your gut. Limit yourself to a few portions of fruit a day and choose to have more vegetables. You can check out the calorie counts (www. nutritiondata.com) of your favourite foods to get a feel for how energy dense they are.

Most important: Don't avoid fat. Fat might be rich in calories but it is essential to life because it increases your immunity and metabolism, boosts brain function and helps you absorb vitamins A, D, E and K and antioxidants. However, you need to discriminate between good and bad fats. There is just as much place for unsaturated fat (olive oils and omega-3) as there is for saturated fats (the white stuff hanging off the end of your steak). Both kinds help produce muscle-building and fat-burning hormones, keep joints healthy and protect your innards against a host of diseases. However, there is absolutely no place for trans fats. You're better off taking up smoking. Trans fats, which can be found in most fried-food eateries, clog your arteries and stack on weight. Junk food might make life worth living but it's not worth dying for. Limit yourself to one or two cheat meals a week from your favourite fast-food pedlar. You'll feel like you still get to eat your favourite cuisine and it'll taste twice as nice because you've had to abstain from it.

Rule 5: Watch What You Drink

Gone are the days when drinking something meant quenching your thirst. Nowadays the variety of drinks to choose from makes water look pretty average. Fact is, you do not need any of them. Most of them will do you no good from a health perspective and almost all of them—barring H_2O—will boost your overall calorie intake. Sugary sodas, fruit drinks, alcohol and other high-calorie beverages such as coffee drinks are all adding to the obesity crisis. With all we sip, we are getting far more calories from beverages than we used to.

Thirsty? Simply adopt a water habit and you'll be leaner. Water is an appetite suppressant, and thirst often masquerades as hunger. Most importantly, water helps your body metabolise lard. Placing your body into an arid state stresses your kidneys and stops them from functioning properly. Ever felt a little lower-back pain after a night on the razz? That's your kidneys biting back. If your kidneys aren't working properly, the workload shifts to your liver. This old workhorse converts stored fat to energy and can't do its job efficiently if it has to pick up slack because you're dehydrated and your kidneys are overworked. In short, put down the fizzy drink and stick your facehole under a tap. They're not hard to find.

Rule 6: Eat Your Breakfast

The morning rush means that breakfast is the easiest meal to skip, but forgoing these valuable calories puts you at a disadvantage if you want to shift your paunch. According to a recent study in *American Journal of Epidemiology* (Purslow et al., 2008), men who got 22 to 50 per cent of their daily calories from breakfast gained only .7 kilogram over 4 years whereas those who ate only 11 per cent of their daily calories in the morning gained 1.4 kilograms. The very best kind of breakfast? Foods with a low glycemic index, such as beans on toast or a big bowl of muesli, that digest slowly and make you feel fuller for the rest of the day. Set your alarm eight minutes early and gorge on this banquet. You'll soon be saying good morning to your abs.

Fat-Burning Eating Plan

Using your knife and fork to lose weight should never be a flavour-free affair. Nor should your belly grumble for more. Why? You'll never stick to a plan that leaves you hankering to fill your hunger gap. For that reason, the sample meals that follow are all rich in fibre and protein that'll leave you feeling fuller than Rupert Murdoch's wallet. This plan works on the simple premise that if you're not hungry you won't overeat or be tempted by the wafts coming from your local chippie. Research in *American Journal of Clinical Nutrition* (Johnstone et al., 2008) found that a high-protein, low-carbohydrate diet is most effective for reducing hunger and promoting weight loss in the short term but that a healthy, balanced diet is more successful at keeping the weight off in the long term.

This diet combines both the long-term and short-term approaches to give you a sustainable eating plan that will get and keep you ripped for the rest of your life. It will also quell the urge to fall back into your old habits. Prepping the meals is quick and simple, and you can buy the ingredients from your local supermarket or eatery. If you can't be bothered to cook and prefer going to restaurants that don't serve these dishes, simply ask the chef to cook you something rich in protein and vegetables; a steak and veggies will do. This sample menu is a working example of the kinds of foods that are perfect for weight loss. You don't have to follow it bite for bite, although you can. Repeat this week, then add your own variations and a few different recipes to spice it up. Dig in. The lighter you is less than a month away.

Fat-Burning Sample Week

Monday

Breakfast: 3 whole eggs scrambled with 50 g (1.8 oz) mozzarella or cheddar cheese and 2 handfuls baby spinach, 250 ml (8.5 oz) fruit juice

Snack: 200 g (7 oz) almonds and dried fruit

Lunch: 200 g (7 oz) grilled sirloin steak, 2 to 3 cups mixed vegetables

Snack: 100 g (3.5 oz) plain, sugar-free yoghurt with 1 handful blueberries and manuka honey, ground mixed seeds and nuts, diced banana

Dinner: 300 g (10.6 oz) salmon fillet, mashed sweet potato with skin, mixed vegetables

Tuesday

Breakfast: 3-egg omelette with sliced mushrooms, olive oil, 1/2 diced onion, diced bell pepper and 2 handfuls baby spinach

Snack: 200 g (7 oz) plain, sugar-free yoghurt; 100 g (3.5 oz) mixed seeds and nuts; 1 apple

Lunch: Chinese-style beef stir-fry with veggies, 1/2 cup brown rice

Snack: 200 g (7 oz) cottage cheese with mixed seeds, dried fruits and nuts

Dinner: 2 grilled chicken breasts, 1 sweet potato, mixed vegetables

Wednesday

Breakfast: 2 large handfuls oats cooked in 250 ml (8.5 oz) skim milk with 2 tsp honey and whey protein

Snack: Canned salmon, cream cheese, dill and black pepper (mixed together); sliced carrots

Lunch: Small sweet potato with baked beans, chillies, cheese and sliced pork sausages

Snack: 1 grilled seasoned chicken breast, 2 small beetroot bulbs

Dinner: 250 g (8.8 oz) lean minced beef chilli with corn, mashed sweet potato

Thursday

Breakfast: Smoothie containing whey concentrate or isolate powder, 1 handful each blueberries and raspberries, 40 g (1.4 oz) plain yoghurt, 2 tbsp ground flaxseed, 1 tbsp rolled oats and 1 banana

Snack: Antipasta (bought or homemade) containing diced olives, mozzarella balls, tomatoes and peppers with olive oil

Lunch: 200 to 300 g (7-10.6 oz) sushi or sashimi, seaweed or brown rice

Snack: Canned muscles or oysters on sliced carrots, 1 small basket cranberries, 1 orange

Dinner: 2 roasted turkey or chicken breasts in lemon, garlic and herb sauce; stir-fried vegetables

Friday

Breakfast: 3 whole eggs scrambled with 3 egg whites, 2 large mushrooms and cheese

Snack: Canned sardines with celery or carrot sticks, 1 apple

Lunch: 2 grilled chicken breasts, 1 sweet potato, 300 g (10.6 oz) salad with olive oil dressing

Snack: Avocado, mayo and prawn salad dressed with olive oil; 1 banana

Dinner: 2 grilled whitefish fillets, 1 cup brown rice with light gravy, mixed vegetables

Saturday

Breakfast: 2 kippers, 3 poached eggs, 1 sliced and fried pepper, 1 slice rye bread

Snack: 200 g (7 oz) plain yoghurt, 1 handful mixed nuts, 2 apples, 1 banana

Lunch: 4 thick-cut slices roast beef, mustard, lettuce and tomato on 2 slices rye bread

Snack: 200 g (7 oz) hummus, 3 large carrots, 1 orange

Dinner: 2 or 3 extra-large lettuce leaves filled with 350 g (12.3 oz) steak, mixed salad

Sunday

Breakfast: 2 cups muesli; 473 ml (16 oz) low-fat milk; 200 g (7 oz) plain, sugar-free yoghurt; 2 boiled eggs

Snack: 125 g (4.4 oz) cottage cheese, carrot sticks, 50 g (1.8 oz) almonds

Lunch: 200 g (7 oz) lean minced beef burger and 1 slice cheese on whole-wheat burger bun, mixed salad

Snack: Tuna salad with olive oil dressing, 1 large mango

Dinner: 3 grilled lamb chops, 1 cup couscous, dark-green vegetables, salad with olive oil dressing

Burning Questions

Here are the answers to the questions most commonly asked about fat burning and food.

Q: **I work the night shift. How should I change my diet?**

A: That's simple. Nothing changes; it just gets delayed by a couple hours. If you snooze when you get home from work, then train just before you go to work the way a nine-to-fiver would cram in an early-morning session before work. If you mince about when you get home and get on the nod around noon, then go to the gym at 7 or 8 a.m. the way most blokes train after work. Regardless of when you train, your muscles will always need the same balance of nutrients to fuel your sweat sessions. Eat a high-protein, high-carb meal 45 minutes before exercise. A protein shake is first prize, but you can also have a couple of carrots dipped in hummus or a sweet potato and tuna or chicken. Plan ahead and you'll be rewarded with a queue-free gym thanks to training during the off-peak hours.

Q: **Every time I hit a restaurant I want to flatten the bread basket. Why?**

A: There's a support group for that. It's called *everyone*. You're not addicted, you're just hungry, which is why you went to a restaurant in the first place. Curb the impulse by snacking two hours before going out. Necking a protein shake works well and will probably halve your dinner bill. When you get to the restaurant, order a salad or shrimp cocktail as soon as you sit down. If the waiter brings the bread, simply tell him you don't want it.

Q: **How bad are hot drinks for my six-pack quest?**

A: They're pretty good, actually. You don't even have to skip the sugar. Consuming a 5-gram portion of sugar, which contains 16 to 20 calories, every day isn't going to bolster your waistline. Skipping the sugar would save you less than one kilogram of calories per year. But if you're a sugar junkie, find small ways to reel in the sweetness quotient in everything you eat, including that first cuppa. If you skip all sugar, including sugar-rich foods such as yoghurt, fizzy drinks and cereals, you'll be on the fast track to losing your body fat. Be vigilant and check the labels because sugars are hiding in all sorts of foods you'd never expect, such as tomato sauce. In short, give sugar the boot. You really are sweet enough.

Q: **Will my wife's diet programme work for me?**

A: Yes, but you don't have tell your buddies about it. If something gets you to eat less it will work. The real issue is how healthy the diet is, how active you are and how well you can stick to it. You'll be more successful at sticking to your diet if you and your wife diet as a team. You can motivate each other and cook joint meals, and you can use some of your male competitiveness to lose weight. To succeed you need a goal, some structure, some accountability and some exercise. Oh yeah—try eating a little less, too.

Q: **When I first started dieting the weight dropped off me, but now it's coming off slowly. Why? I still eat healthy and exercise.**

A: Most blokes reach a tabletop thanks to problems on top of the table. If you eat too little, your body think it's starving and stores fat as an emergency measure. The problem could also be excessive tension; this makes your body release the stress hormone cortisol, which inhibits fat loss. You could also eat a little more before your workouts so you can hit them harder. Adaptability is the key to long-term success. Changing your exercise routine and then changing the foods you eat while still eating a low-calorie diet will help you bust out of that rut.

Q: **After a tough day at the office all I want to do is eat all night. How can I stop this?**

A: Witching-hour munchies can quickly conjure a cauldron-sized belly. Regardless of how much you toss and turn in the sack, you simply aren't going to burn off the calories like you do when you're awake. That's not to say you need to starve. You should eat something to reduce the nighttime wave of low blood sugar. Go for healthy, appetite-curbing oats, an apple and cheese or a thin turkey sandwich on rye. If you crave sweets, try fruit yoghurt, cereal with a little brown sugar on top or berries with a drizzle of chocolate sauce. Cottage cheese is also a good option because it digests slowly. Avoid spicy or high-fat foods, which can make it harder for you to fall asleep. If you must reach for the unhealthy stuff, try to pair it with something healthy. Your belly will be gone in a poof.

Q: **What's the deal with cheat days? How much can I cheat?**

A: Think of cheat days as your reward for sticking to your programme. You need to enjoy life and, more importantly, food. Weight gain isn't the only issue here. It takes a 3,500-calorie surplus to pack on .45 kilogram of fat, so you'd really have to chow down to notice an effect. The real worry is that even one high-fat, high-carbohydrate load can boost the amount of stress on your organs and make it harder for your brain to resist new temptations. The bottom line: Cheating on your diet doesn't mean abandoning it entirely. Limit your splurge to a few of your favourite forbidden snacks. Once you've stuck to a healthy eating plan long enough to see a difference in how you look and feel, you'll find that those greasy old favourites aren't as seductive anymore.

Q: **I train late at night. What should I eat afterwards? A big dinner?**

A: Chug a protein shake after your workout, then cook up a small meal of meat and vegetables sans carbs such as pasta and spuds. No studies show that eating before bed makes you put on weight; rather, the total number of calories you eat throughout the day determines your waist size. However, to be safe, allow an hour between your last bite and bedtime. Your metabolism slows down a little at night and you won't easily digest the contents of a stuffed gut. More importantly, having a large meal before dozing off can interfere with your sleep. But so can going to bed hungry. Don't deny yourself a light snack if you had an early dinner or feel hunger pangs. Satiate cravings with the food groups you skipped during the day. If you missed out on dairy or fruit, grab some yoghurt and berries, a smoothie or an apple and some cheese. If you're hanging for starch, a bowl of oats is a safe bet. Never go to bed with a stomach howling for food because a good night's sleep will serve you better in your quest to get lean.

Q: **I love sandwiches, but are the carbs bad for my six-pack?**

A: Not if you choose wisely. Start with the solid foundation of rye bread, which is rich in fibre and will keep you full for ages. Lay out the inside with solid walls of whole protein such as sliced chicken breast or a bit of meat. Decorate with at least three fruits and vegetables of different colours and you have the perfect meal to make a body worth building.

Q: **Is it true that celery has negative calories?**

A: This is a pack of hocus pocus. Celery has 10 calories per 100 grams. You cannot lose weight by eating a food that takes more energy to absorb than you get from it. To conjure a six-pack you need a balanced diet, not calorie sleight-of-hand tricks.

Where Next?

Now that you have a basic idea of how to eat you can get started with the training plans. Your new diet will give you the energy you need to complete your new workouts, and the postworkout nutritional strategies will help you feel less stiff the following day. If you already eat the way described in this chapter, stick with it. If you don't, change your diet a week or two before you launch into the workouts. Instituting two big changes, such as taking up both exercise and a new way of eating, can confront your comfort zone. It may be too overwhelming and can make you more likely to throw in the towel. Ease yourself into your new routine with little steps and don't try to completely revamp your diet. When you start to exercise, add or subtract certain foods based on your goals. As time progresses you'll find yourself interacting with food in a different way. Use this approach and you'll be rewarded with a body that acts and looks very different from what it once was. Eat strong and stay strong.

Site-Specific Gains

Training all your muscles can be like a *Big Brother* series with each contestant battling to give the dumbbells airtime. And it's no mean feat, splitting your time equally among each body part. A touch of sickness here, an all-weekend wedding there or an extended business trip can easily derail your burly balancing act. And if you don't show a muscle group quite enough love, it may lag behind the rest.

To make sure you're aware of what you've got, this chapter breaks your body down into the major muscle groups: arms, shoulders, chest, back, abs and legs (figure 3.1). It also gives

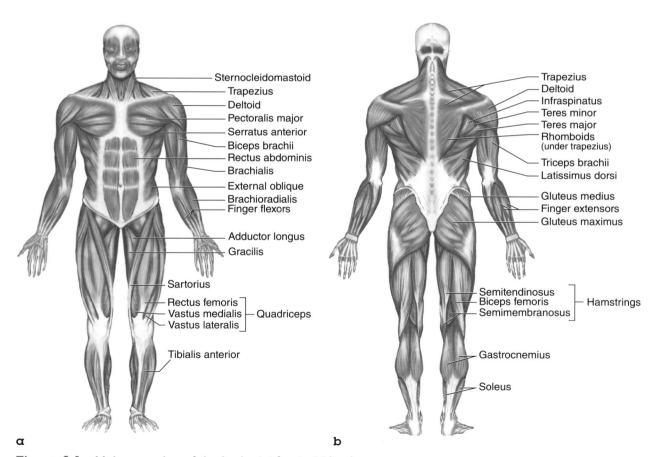

Figure 3.1 Major muscles of the body: *(a)* front; *(b)* back.

you the blueprints to make each of these muscles perform and look impressive. You don't have to commit all of it to memory. Just have a casual read and come back to it when you've started working each body part and want a bit more in-depth detail. The info will be somewhere in your brain, and exercise is sure to jog your memory about what you've read. Continue to take a leisurely look through the chapter to find out exactly what you're made of.

The first step in this excursion educates you about why lifting heavy things grows muscles whereas running road races seems to cannibalise them. Here's the anatomy of you along with an explanation of how and why you are built with the capacity for limitless upgrades.

Why Your Muscles Grow

Knowing why your muscles grow will help you gain more size and strength. But leave your thinking cap behind: It's all too simple.

Improving your body by building muscle is rugged, brutal and demanding. It's a far cry from the glitz and glamour the Nike-clad gym membership consultant tells you it is. The story of why your guns get bigger when you pump out curls is best told by the dark side of yesteryear's Hollywood. Consider the legend of the most cinematically famous muscle man, Conan, originally played by a young Arnold Schwarzenegger.

Conan is thrust into gothic slavery at an early age. He and his cronies are stacked in the desert and whipped into pushing a heavy wagon-wheel shrine in circles. As the years pass, members of the wheel-pushing team drop off from exhaustion, making more work for the rest of the pushers. By the end Conan is the last man standing and is pushing the wheel by himself; this furnishes him with more surplus muscle than the Russian mafia. His brawn helps him escape. The following lessons tell you how he gained his strength, size and freedom. These tales are worth understanding so you can create a legendary physique of your own.

Lesson 1: A Snail's Pace Wins the Race

Conan didn't begin pushing the load by himself. His fellow slaves were there to help, which made the weight lighter. Had he tried to push the wheel by himself it wouldn't have moved and he would've become frustrated and possibly injured.

You shouldn't get other exercisers to help you push your weights, but you should begin slowly and gradually work your way up to more challenging workouts. Establish a reasonable goal and keep progressing towards it at a pace you can handle. Haste leads to injury.

Lesson 2: Test Your Mettle

Conan became steadily stronger because he lifted progressively heavier weights each day and year. Had the weaker slaves not dropped out of their pushing duties he would've used the same size of weights every day. He wouldn't have become more powerful because his muscles wouldn't need to adapt, grow and become stronger.

To grow you need to gradually overload your muscles with more weight. Likewise, if you've stopped getting results from your training, your muscles need a new stimulus in the form of more reps, sets, weights or exercises to change things up and create a new challenge.

Lesson 3: Become a Control Freak

Conan was not allowed to push the religious shrine in a disrespectful or erratic fashion. He pushed it slowly and with control and the same way experienced lifters like to murder their weights up: bit by bit. The same holds true for your training. Lifting carefully and deliberately places your muscles under tension for longer. Never use momentum to swing the weights. If you can't control them, they're too heavy and you're letting gravity steal effort from your muscles. You're also more likely to injure yourself, which means you won't be able to lift again until you've healed. Luckily, the consequences of injury don't mean becoming lion fodder like in *Conan the Barbarian*.

Lesson 4: Be Consistent

The legend of Conan illustrates the need for consistency in an exercise programme. If Conan had been allowed a few months off or pushed the wheel only on good hair days, his strength would have floundered, and he may never have caught up. By sticking with it day after day Conan proved how important a consistent routine is to adding power and muscle. Every day is a step towards your goal. Never be afraid to take a bigger step today than you did yesterday.

Lesson 5: Question Yourself After Every Workout

Eventually Conan questioned why he was pushing the wheel, fought and escaped. You too must question your actions. What are you doing today? Is it challenging enough to prepare you for tomorrow's goals? How does this affect you? Increasing the amount you can squat today will give you tree-trunk legs because, like Conan, you're placing a new stress on your quads, glutes and hamstrings. They respond by getting bigger to deal with the new load.

Always work towards the future. You might think that this is all you need to know: Push weights, get big. However, understanding how it works will help you train better, schedule rest cycles and improve gains. Keep reading to learn what happens under your skin.

First Type of Fitness Gain: Neurological

For a total novice, strength gains made in the first six weeks of a programme come from improved communications between the brain and muscles. The brain of a veteran lifter is more accustomed to telling his muscles, 'Yes, I can do this.' In a sense, the brain holds back the muscles of a novice lifter purely in the interest of protecting him from injury. With training, the body develops a can-do attitude that helps the lifter push more weights or run farther. This gradually dissolves the natural self-defence mechanism.

Without this mechanism you would be able to bench perhaps 100 kilograms on your first trip to the gym. Your brain allows you to bench only 60 kilograms because it is kind enough to protect you. As you lift more frequently, your nerves become more efficient and accustomed to pushing weights. Most importantly, they understand that the crazy pursuit of iron mongering is actually safe. They are no longer suspicious of the poundage you're lifting or distances you're running and allow your muscles to work to their full capacity. Your subconscious eventually yields to your conscious. For this reason, you'll make improvements very quickly at the beginning of a strength- or fitness-training programme. Keep reading to find out why it can take up to two months to start adding serious size and fitness.

Second Type of Fitness Gain: Myological

That's *myological*, not *mythological*. Once you have maximised neurological gains it's time to kickstart your next set of gains. It works like this: Brains first, then brawn.

You have two types of muscle fibres. Type I, or slow twitch, fibres help you in endurance exercise such as running. Type II, or fast twitch, fibres are the large fibres responsible for strength and size when you weight train. To damage type II fibres enough to make them grow you have to keep your muscles under enough tension to recruit satellite cells, which help grow, maintain and repair your muscles. These cells often lie dormant until you do heavy lifting. The heavy lifting causes microtears in the muscle fibres, which makes your satellite cells multiply and move towards the areas you've damaged, such as your triceps after a heavy set of dips. They rope in the proteins from the food you eat to thicken and strengthen your muscles and—voila—you have tighter sleeves.

Unfortunately, this is not as cut and dry as it might sound. Debate exists about whether muscles get bigger because more muscle fibres are added or because the existing fibres get thicker. Some studies support the former and discredit the latter. The most important thing you can do is understand the best practises before you start. Many of the best practises are limits that you should impose on yourself; others simply give you the latest research that'll hasten your results. These are throughout this chapter. Look them over and you'll know more than most exercisers before you even pick up a weight or lace up your running shoes.

Now that you know the basic principles for success, here are the rules for building muscle. Break them and you'll end up taking two steps forward and three steps back. Front foot moving forward now.

Five Muscle-Building Rules

It's damn tough balancing work, play, family time and exercise that will give you the muscles and health to get through it all. If you're making a comeback to sweating or just want a new way to train, let out a sigh of relief because right now you're holding the rules to both. Before you bolt out of the blocks, get clued up on the very basics. Warning: Some of this may challenge every bit of exercise dogma you've ever heard, so prepare to be amazed. Remember these simple truths and you'll endow yourself with a lifetime of muscle.

Rule 1: For Fast Results, Treat Your Body as a Whole

You are not the sum of your parts. Despite what the juggernaut in your gym tells you, your muscles work best if you train them all in the same workout. Strictly speaking, it's impossible to isolate muscles. They're woven together with facia, tendons and ligaments. Yes, it is possible to emphasise a muscle group, but it's tough to isolate it. Think of a pull-up. It may work the back but it also works the biceps, forearms and abs.

A landmark study (McLester, Bishop and Guilliams, 1999) has proven this. The labcoats at the University of Alabama found that full-body regimens led to an average of 2.27 kilograms more muscle gain per month than did sessions that focused on single muscle groups.

Don't get confused: Training one or two muscle groups in a workout the way bodybuilders do will work. Check out chapter 7 to see how to do it. However, this strategy can backfire if you skip a few training days.

Full-body workouts spread the muscle-building stimulus for every muscle over the entire week. Instead of growing only on the days after your chest workout, your chest will grow all week. Think of full-body regimens as the low-hanging fruit of the muscle-building world. When life throws up a business meeting, no muscle is ignored. You simply train three days a week instead of four and continue to grow in perfect proportions and keep yourself injury free. For the fastest muscle growth, treat your muscles as a team that performs best when all players graft together.

Rule 2: The Starting Point is the Number of Days You Can Train a Week

As you learned in chapter 1, setting exercise goals is the easy part. The hard part is finding the time to reach those goals. The first step: Click your diary and decide how many days a week you can train. Be realistic. An accurate prediction will make or break your muscle growth.

Everyone's enthusiasm is rock solid at the start of a programme. Optimistically assuming that you'll do six sessions a week often ends in disappointment. It may go well in week 1, but your life might get busy in week 2 and your priorities may change. Be conservative when you map out how many sessions you can make each week because time is sure to bring justice to your estimations and uncover the truth, leaving you either scrawny or brawny.

Of course, the number of days you are able to exercise each week will change from month to month and often depends on the sunshine, your next fishing trip or when Santa imposes on you. This isn't a disadvantage; it's life. The trick to achieving continued growth is to mix things up. Train five days a week for six to eight weeks and then try three days a week for two months. Life is change, and growth is optional.

Choose wisely. The variety will spark new gains in size and strength year after year.

Rule 3: Variety is Key

It's easy to find a groove and stick to it. Just look at the rest of the dudes in your gym. They look comfortable with the poundage they're shifting and that's probably part of the reason they have cushy-looking physiques. That's not what you want.

You don't need all sorts of fancy exercises to build muscle for years to come, but you do need to change up your reps, sets, rest periods and the intensity at which you exercise. Your body will stop getting results from a training routine in about 4 to 8 weeks. An athlete's gains taper after about 4 weeks, whereas beginners can soldier on for up to 12 weeks. Your muscles are brilliant at adapting to the stress you make them suffer through. The trick is to keep challenging them. Change your programme the second you find yourself not pushing heavier weights.

The golden rule? Listen to what your body is telling you. If you're not making progress each week, your muscles are bored and it's time to try something new. Refer to 'Refresh Your Workout' in chapter 6 to learn how to manipulate your training using the same exercises so that you're constantly progressing towards achieving your goals.

Rule 4: Understand the Basics

This Muscle 101 class explains the brawn-building basics.

- Repetition (rep): Doing an exercise, such as a push-up, just once.
- Set: Doing a group of reps without a break. For example, completing five push-ups.
- Lifting speed: How long you take to lower and raise a weight.
- Rest: The length of a break you take between sets.
- Frequency: How often you train, usually each week.

- Order: How you arrange the exercises.

By tweaking these variables you can create thousands of workouts that'll keep you muscled well into old age.

Rule 5: Settling the Intensity and Volume Debate

Ask 10 trainers whether a volume- or intensity-based routine creates the best results and you'll get 10 different answers. But what does each approach mean? If you follow a volume routine, you'll bombard your muscles with a massive quantity of sets and reps (several times a week in 60- to 90-minute sessions) so that they have no choice but to adapt and grow. If you follow an intensity routine, you'll do brief and intense workouts (two or three times a week in 30- to 60-minute sessions) with extremely heavy weights and then take a few days' rest to recover, which is when you grow.

Both types of routines have their merits. The former is based on work and the latter is based on rest. The solution? Raise your right foot and stamp it firmly on the fence. Try a mix of both approaches. Do a volume routine for a few months and then try an intensity-based approach for a while. You'll soon see which approach gives you the best results.

For beginners, it is best to start with a volume-based routine like the first beginners workout in chapter 5. A volume-based routine teaches you good exercise technique because it doesn't demand that you lift relentlessly heavy weights that can compromise form.

By now you understand the ground rules of exercise and how to put them into practise. The next step is to acquire the building materials that take the plan off the drawing board. The remainder of this chapter includes guidelines for working each of your key body parts and descriptions of the exercises that are included in the workouts and programmes throughout this book. Load your armoury because here's the lowdown on the site-specific brawn every man wants more of. Let's start with the muscle group that's most on display: arms.

Arms: Immersing Yourself in Gun Culture

Your upper arms are made up of two muscles: triceps and biceps. The biggest cause of spaghetti arms is putting too much effort into the biceps at the front of the arm and not enough into the triceps. Triceps make up 66 per cent of your arm muscle, so even though they face away from you they add crucial mass to your guns.

Want more ammunition? Train the muscles around your arms. But first heed this warning: These aren't routines filled with hours of mind-numbing biceps curls. Biceps account for just 3 per cent of your total-body muscle mass, so spending an hour on them can be a little wasteful.

The best way to work your biceps is to team them with the triceps. Your biceps flex as your triceps relax and vice versa, so your triceps will warm up in any case. Many trainers pair biceps workouts with legs, chest or back workouts and pair triceps workouts with chest or shoulders workouts. Before you get started you need to know the underlying rules for getting arms so big you look like you're always carrying watermelons.

Strengthen the Supporting Cast

For superior arm growth, work the muscles that support your arms, which means everything—including legs. If you try to lift a weight that's too heavy for your supporting muscles, your form will suffer and the tension from that weight won't fall on your biceps. Most likely your body will shift the load to your lower back. Although you may be curling 50-kilogram dumbbells, your lower back is doing all the work. Few people will comment on how great your lower back looks.

Muscle Growth Isn't Localised

In a study at Ball State University (Rogers et al., 2000), guys did full-body workouts that included compound exercises such as squats and bench presses. One half of the group also performed biceps curls and triceps extensions. The participants' arms grew in precisely the same proportions in both groups, proving that you don't need hours of curls and extensions to get big arms. Take-home message: Work your entire body and your arms will grow.

Big Arms Require More Muscle Everywhere

Many famous trainers and bodybuilders believe that to add 2 to 3 centimetres to your arm you need to add at least 5 to 10 kilograms to your overall weight. This backs up the previous two points: It's easier to add that kind of muscle mass using compound moves such as pull-ups than it is to add it with biceps curls. If you have a headache you don't crush a painkiller into your forehead; you swallow it so that it goes to your entire body. Do the same for your arms and they'll grow to pharmaceutical proportions.

Form is Crucial

Opening and closing your elbow joint may seem like a tough thing to get wrong. It works as simple as a door hinge, right? But you'll get it horribly wrong if you use the rest of your body to create momentum. Do whatever it takes to keep super-strict form. Bend your knees a little here or bob your back there and you won't feel the burn in your biceps. To keep strict form, do your arm exercises while looking in a mirror, have a friend critique you or lean up against a wall to keep your back straight. Most importantly, leave your ego with the gym receptionist and use weights that are light enough to enable you to keep strict form.

Use Isolation Moves Sparingly

Some isolation work for your arms is no problem, but think of it as the icing on the cake. When isolation moves such as biceps curls and triceps push-downs are teamed up with heavy dips and rows, your arms will quickly explode with size.

Get Unstable

Don't read this heading and head for the nearest Swiss ball, BOSU or Indo Board. The effectiveness of these items is limited for all training, especially if muscle building is your goal. Rather, grab a pair of dumbbells and take a slow walk while you curl. Muscles fibres will fire in your arms to stabilise you during even a very slow walk.

Watch Out for That Pest Called Gravity

When you're training biceps and do a curl, the top 7 to 20 centimetres of the movement is assisted by a reliable friend: gravity. To stop this, lie back on an incline bench while you do your curls. For standing curls you can lean forward at the end of the movement to counteract gravity. Fortunately, this force doesn't blight your triceps training.

Slow Down, Sonny

For all arm exercises, concentrate heavily on slowing down repetitions. Opening and closing your elbow joints takes a very short time—probably the shortest time of all the joints because the weights travel such a small distance. Pay attention when you bang out your curls and extensions. Hopefully you're brave enough to use big weights that force you to slow down, especially during the lowering phase.

Test Your Waters

Because arms are such a localised body part, you can easily test them with different protocols. Some blokes report huge growth from doing heavy exercises only whereas others report getting huge gains from 15 to 20 reps with light weights. It all depends on genetics, so take the time to figure out which way yours bend. The same goes for frequency. If you're not gaining fast, try training your arms twice a week, such as on Monday and Friday.

Look After Your Elbows

If you feel a tweak in your elbows while you're lifting, especially during triceps exercises such as skull crushers, stop immediately. Do not try to go heavy—this will only inflame the area more. Rather, grab some massage oil and give your biceps, triceps and elbow joints a rubdown. They're in an accessible spot, so there's no reason you can't self-heal.

Now that you have all the tricks up your sleeve, here are the exercises you'll do to put them into practise. Remember to recruit the services of a spotter when you're doing your heaviest lifts. There's nothing manly or safe about getting pinned underneath the steel.

Hammer Curl

Prepare to get the arm strength to rip phone books in half.

Muscles

Biceps, abs

Execution

1. Stand with your feet hip-width apart and hold a dumbbell in each hand (figure 3.2a). Your palms are turned out.
2. Bend your elbows and curl the weights to your shoulders (figure 3.2b).
3. Squeeze your biceps at the top of the movement, then slowly lower the dumbbells to the starting position.

VARIATION: Seated Hammer Curl

Sit on a sturdy weight bench. Perform the hammer curl.

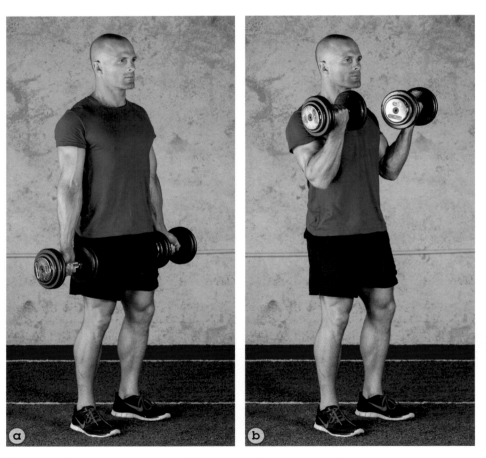

Figure 3.2 Hammer curl. *(a)* Starting position. *(b)* Curl the weights.

EZ-Bar Curl

Here's your surefire remedy for spaghetti-sized guns. This exercise will help you win your next arm-wrestling match so quickly the crowd won't have time to spur you on. The uniquely manoeuvrable axis of the EZ-bar allows your wrists to turn and focuses the tension more on your biceps.

Muscles

Biceps

Execution

1. Stand and hold an EZ-bar using an underhand grip (figure 3.3a).
2. Bend your elbows and curl the weight up to your shoulders (figure 3.3b).
3. Pause for a second, then take two to three seconds to lower the weight to the starting position.

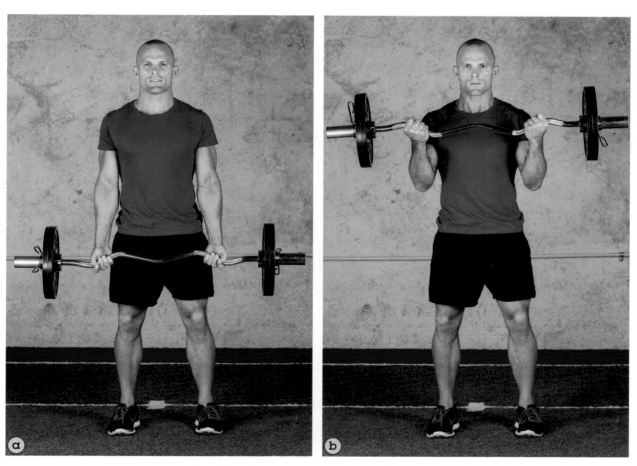

Figure 3.3   EZ-bar curl. *(a)* Starting position. *(b)* Curl the weight.

Underhand-Grip Pull-Up

Some trainers believe that you shouldn't even touch a dumbbell to do curls if you can't do at least six pull-ups. You don't have to listen to what they say. But, in case you encounter any of these folks, learn to do these.

Muscles

Lats, biceps, forearms, abs

Execution

1. Grab a pull-up bar with an underhand grip and place your hands shoulder-width apart. Hang from the bar with your elbows straight.
2. Bend your elbows and pull your chest to the bar (figure 3.4).
3. Peer over the bar for a second, then slowly lower yourself to the starting position.

NOTE   Take care not to wobble or sway back and forth. Keeping steady ropes in more of your abs.

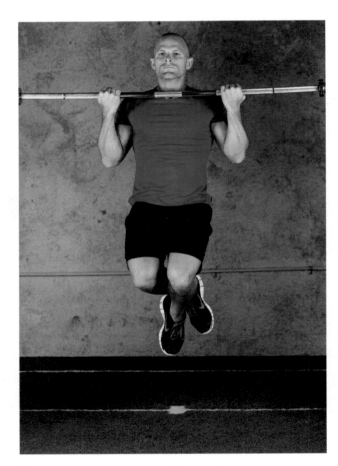

Figure 3.4   Underhand-grip pull-up.

Cable Rope Curl

You're about to win your tug-of-war against your T-shirt sleeves.

Muscles

Biceps

Execution

1. Stand with your legs shoulder-width apart in front of a cable crossover machine. Attach the rope to the lowest notch on the pulley. Grab one end of the rope in each hand and hold your arms straight (figure 3.5a).

2. Bend your elbows and curl the rope towards your shoulders (figure 3.5b).

3. Take two to three seconds to lower your arms to the starting position for the power to open the tightest jam jar.

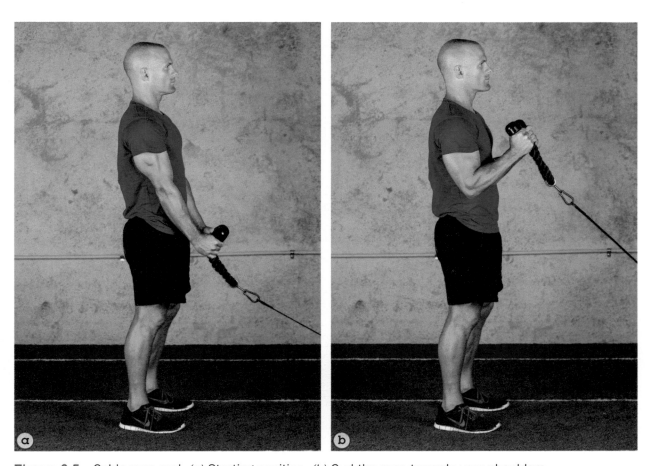

Figure 3.5 Cable rope curl. *(a)* Starting position. *(b)* Curl the rope towards your shoulders.

Barbell Biceps Curl

This biceps builder has been inflating arms since the sand-kicking days that were made famous in black-and-white comics. Get ready for some old skool brawn.

Muscles

Biceps

Execution

1. Stand with your feet shoulder-width apart and hold a barbell in an underhand grip (figure 3.6a).
2. Keeping your upper arms tucked against your sides and your shoulder blades pulled together, curl the weight up until it reaches your shoulders (figure 3.6b).
3. Contract your biceps, then reverse the motion and slowly return to the starting position.

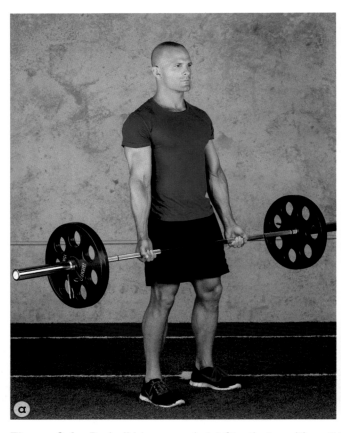 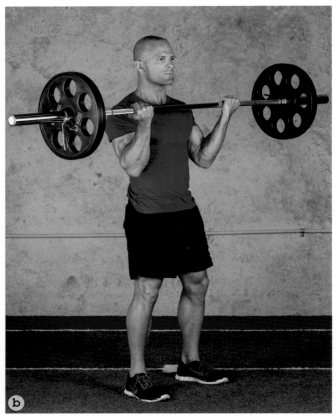

Figure 3.6 Barbell biceps curl. *(a)* Starting position. *(b)* Curl the weight.

Barbell Biceps Throw

Throwing your weight around can build serious arms.

Muscles

Biceps

Execution

1. Stand with your feet shoulder-width apart and hold a barbell in an underhand grip (figure 3.7a).
2. Keeping your upper arms tucked against your sides and your shoulder blades pulled together, explosively curl the weight up, throw it a small way into the air (figure 3.7b) and then catch it.
3. Slowly return to the starting position and then go again.

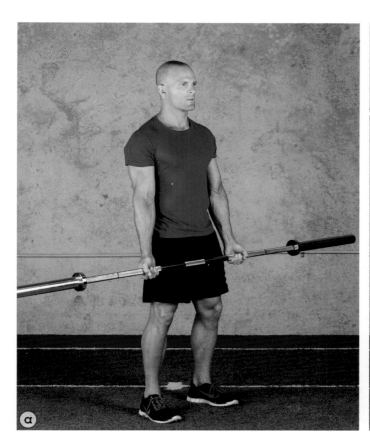 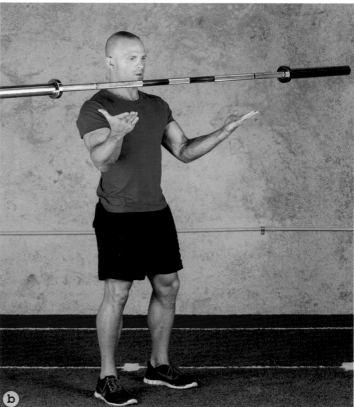

Figure 3.7 Barbell biceps throw. *(a)* Starting position. *(b)* Curl the weight up and throw it.

Triceps Push-Down

If the cable machine was in *The Jetsons*, the straight-bar attachment would have a 'push down for bigger arms' button.

Muscles

Triceps

Execution

1. Attach a straight bar to the high pulley of a cable crossover machine and position the bar so that it is just below chest level. Hold the bar with an overhand grip and place your hands shoulder-width apart (figure 3.8a).

2. Tuck your elbows to your sides and push the bar towards the floor until your arms are completely straight (figure 3.8b).

3. Tense your triceps, then slowly release the bar and move back to the starting position for arms that'll raise you out of your chair with ease no matter how tired your legs are.

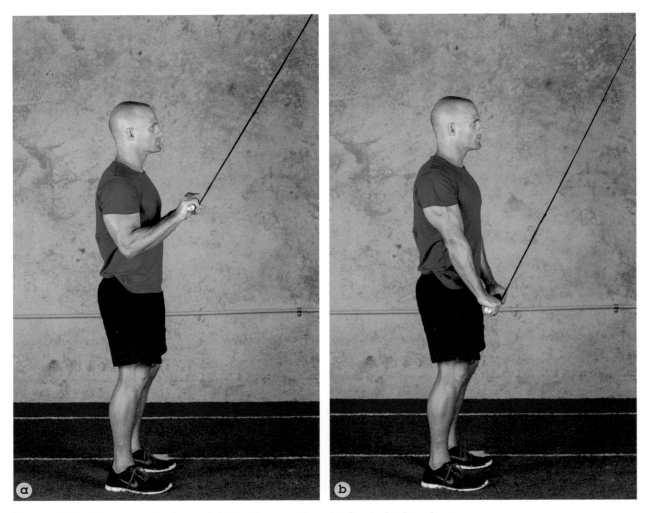

Figure 3.8 Triceps push-down. *(a)* Starting position. *(b)* Push the bar down.

Standing Triceps Extension

If the fronts of your sleeves are sizzling with bigger biceps, it's time to take the welding iron to the backs.

Muscles

Triceps, abs, shoulders

Execution

1. Stand and hold a dumbbell in each hand. Raise your arms above your head so your elbows are next to your ears (figure 3.9a).
2. Bend your elbows and lower the weights behind your head (figure 3.9b). Straighten your arms and raise the weights back above your head.
3. Take two to three seconds to lower the weights. If this doesn't make you the man who takes all your team's soccer throw-ins, nothing will.

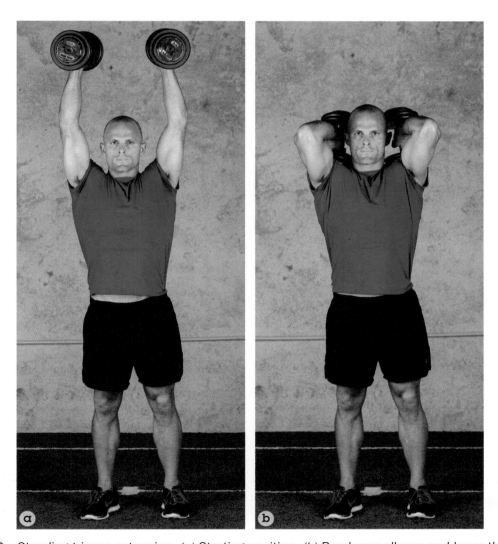

Figure 3.9 Standing triceps extension. (a) Starting position. (b) Bend your elbows and lower the weights.

Close-Grip Bench Press

This move is ideal for pumping up your strength and slapping mass onto the backs of your arms. Don't wimp out. If you want to earn tickets to the gun show, load that barbell until you're too scared to look at it. Use a spotter if you have one at hand.

Muscles

Triceps, shoulders, chest

Execution

1. Lie on a flat bench-press station with your knees bent and your feet flat on the floor. Grab a barbell with an overhand grip and place your hands about fist-width apart (figure 3.10a).
2. Slowly lower the bar until it reaches your chest (figure 3.10b).
3. Pause, then press the weight back overhead until your arms are extended, but do not lock your elbows.

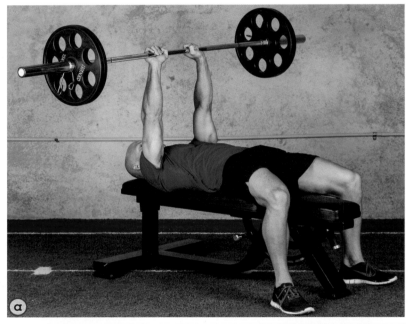

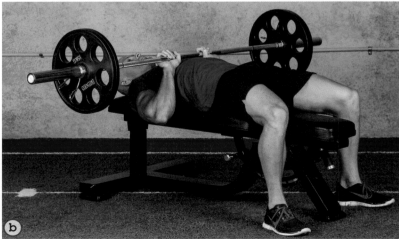

Figure 3.10 Close-grip bench press. *(a)* Starting position. *(b)* Lower the bar to your chest.

Rope Push-Down

This exercise will give you the power to push people—something your new oversized arms probably will attract—away from you.

Muscles

Triceps, abs, shoulders

Execution

1. Fix the rope attachment to the top notch of the cable crossover machine. Grab one end of the rope in each hand and bend your arms (figure 3.11a).
2. Straighten your elbows and pull the rope down, keeping your elbows tucked to your sides (figure 3.11b).
3. Take two to three seconds to release the weight to the starting position.

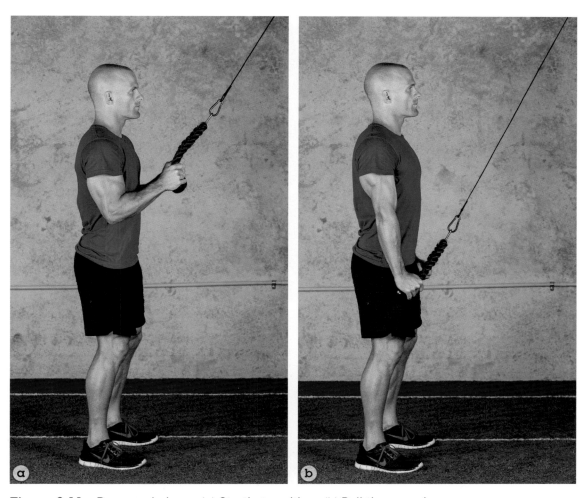

Figure 3.11 Rope push-down. *(a)* Starting position. *(b)* Pull the rope down.

EZ-Bar Skull Crusher

It may be EZ in name, but it's far from easy by nature. This is good—*hard* means that it works.

Muscles

Triceps, shoulders

Execution

1. Lie on your back on a weight bench and hold an EZ-bar with a shoulder-width grip (figure 3.12a).
2. Bend your elbows and lower the weight behind you (figure 3.12b). Keep your elbows tucked to the sides of your head.
3. Straighten your arms and return to the starting position.

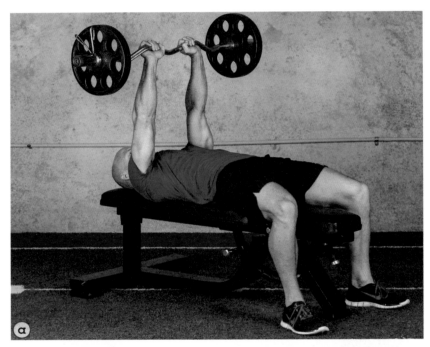

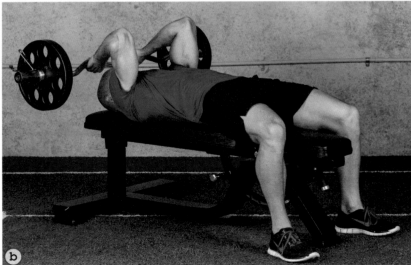

Figure 3.1
EZ-bar skull crusher.
(a) Starting position.
(b) Lower the weight.

Chair Dip

In this exercise, the end of your bed or the seat of a sturdy chair will help you reach your goal of bigger arms. Keeping your back straight flexes your abs the same way the plank exercise does. It's a two-for-one arms and abs move.

Muscles

Triceps, abs

Execution

1. Hold onto the seat of a sturdy chair or bench placed behind you. Slightly bend your knees in front of you and plant your feet flat on the floor. Lock your elbows (figure 3.13a).
2. Bend your elbows and lower your body, keeping your back as straight as possible (figure 3.13b).
3. Straighten your arms and push yourself back to the starting position.

NOTE   Using higher surfaces makes this move easier and using low surfaces makes it harder.

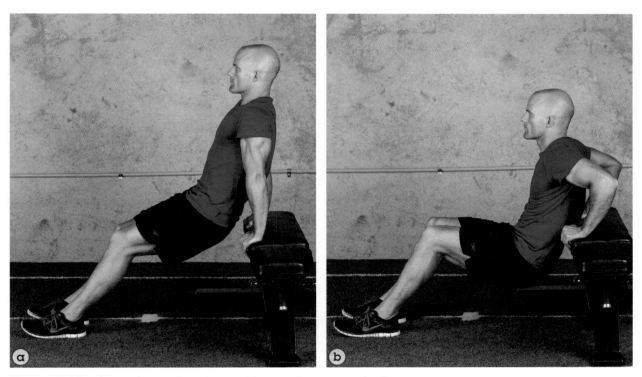

Figure 3.13   Chair dip. *(a)* Starting position. *(b)* Lower your body.

Shoulders:
Worth Resting the World on

Shoulders are made up of three muscles: the front, middle and rear deltoids. They also hold the least fat of all muscle, so you can clearly admire them. You can also consider your trapezius, which stretches down from your neck, to be one of the shoulder muscles, although some people think of it as a back muscle.

If you want to maximise the width of your V-shape and be your absolute strongest in lifts for your arms, back and chest, shoulders are your go-to muscle. They get pulled into play almost every time you touch a weight. Yes, even during a legs workout when you're loading up that barbell. That makes them incredibly important for rounding off your physique and helping the rest of your body get stronger and larger. What's more, they help you decelerate your arms after a throw, hold perfect posture and excel in just about every sport. They're a bit like the coach of a winning football team: The players may get all the glory, but behind the scenes the coach is the one holding it all together and making it look good for the fans. Pay attention to these key points.

Protect Them With Your Life

Holding a book, lifting a coffee mug or opening a door to leave a room. All of these strength-free everyday activities demand a little work from your shoulders. You can only imagine what happens to all the muscles the shoulder supports if you get injured. Your chest, back and arms are likely to wilt away, undoing countless hours of hard work. The take-home message: If you feel a ping in your shoulders while lifting, immediately stop what you're doing. If you think pain is a badge of honour, you've been watching too many action flicks.

Lift What You Can Lower

Almost every free-weight shoulder exercise involves lifting a weight above your head, to the side of your body or in front of your body. That means you're always going to be lifting against the force of gravity and then letting gravity wield its sword when the lift is over. But you put your shoulders at risk when you drop the weights to the starting position because the jerking movement can damage your ligaments. To cut out this risk, always take two to four seconds to lower the weights. Limit the size of the weights to those you can lower with control.

Pair Them Wisely

Shoulders are the socialites of the muscle party circuit: They're roped in when you train your chest, back, arms and even legs. Because their schedules can get packed pretty quickly, be careful not to overtrain them. Try to leave at least one or two days of rest between your chest and shoulder workouts because those muscles are big players in your bench presses. The same goes for your back workouts. The best strategy is to do chest or back on Monday or Tuesday, rest on Wednesday, do legs or arms on Thursday and do shoulders on Friday or Saturday. This allows your shoulder muscles to rest their weary fibres and not get partied out.

Stick to Dumbbells

Almost every exercise you can do with a barbell or a machine can be done with dumbbells, and it's best to roll in this substitution as much as possible. Barbells create strength imbalances in the shoulders very quickly. These imbalances come to light when you train your chest and back with dumbbells. What's more, barbells and machines can cause injury and mess with your symmetry. Machines are set to a fixed range of motion and your shoulders may not respond to such rigid guidelines. After all, the shoulders are the most versatile joints in the body. Keep them healthy and keep yourself happy by using dumbbells and you'll be rewarded with an athletic-looking frame.

Look Behind You

It's easy to get caught up with the front and side shoulder muscles. These are the muscles that glare at you in the mirror and add size and width to your frame. They are also the muscles that get worked when you train other muscles. Your rear shoulders, which are more often ignored, are, in part, responsible for keeping your shoulders back and making your chest look bigger. They also bulk up the width of your side profile so that anyone looking at you down the bar will have a little more to size up.

Be Mindful of Your Cardio

Legs muscles are big and ugly enough to take on a serious gym session and then hammer a cardio session on the stationary bike. Shoulders, on the other hand, are more delicate and can be put under too much stress if they're roped in during cardio activities such as swimming, elliptical training and rowing. These activities can be good for a cool-down or warm-up, but be sure to pay attention to how your shoulders feel while you're sweating buckets in the pool.

Don't Skimp on the Presses

As a rule, the backbone of your shoulder-training regimen should be pressing exercises. That means you have to lift something heavy above your head. You can accomplish this by performing full-body muscle makers such as the squat press and power clean. Other options include the Arnold press and dumbbell seated shoulder press. As you can see, a lot of variations exist. Most of them work all three muscles of your shoulders, giving you more muscle for your time. Keep trying all of them and boulder shoulders will soon be yours.

Watch the Intensity

Chapter 6 describes techniques for increasing intensity such as drop sets, supersets and cheat reps. Although these techniques work fantastically well with shoulder training, limit their use because they can be very taxing on the nervous system. Of all your muscles, your shoulders are at the most risk of becoming overstressed because the shoulder joints are so fragile. Keep training sessions straight and simple and you'll be rewarded with plain increases in width and size.

Standing or Seated?

You can perform almost all shoulder moves while standing or sitting. The main difference is that you're more likely to be able to use bigger weights on the seated versions of the exercises, provided you use perfect form. Standing versions burn more calories and rope in your abs more because you have to tense to keep upright. However, standing also makes it easier to cheat thanks to even a slight bend of the knees. The best strategy is to alternate between the two positions. Be sure to increase the size of the weights you use when you take a seat.

Get Explosive

The occasional explosive exercise will boost your overall upper-body strength and athleticism. You'll get an extra snap of power in just about every sporting discipline and increase the size of the weights you push when you strength train. In one set a week, throw a medicine ball or sandbag above your head or in front of you. Do it often enough and the Frisbees you throw might get reported in *The National Enquirer.* To get the kind of power that'll perform as well as show, use these exercises.

Lateral Raise

You're about to experience a little hurt, so mentally tell yourself to toughen up. Pain is your body releasing its weakness.

Muscles

Shoulders

Execution

1. Stand with your feet shoulder-width apart and hold a dumbbell in each hand. Let the weights hang and keep a slight bend in your elbows. Your palms should face each other (figure 3.14a).
2. Raise your arms straight out to your sides to shoulder height (figure 3.14b).
3. Slowly lower your arms back to the starting position.

NOTE Some debate exists about whether one should stop raising the arms when the weights are level with the shoulders. If you don't have shoulder problems and you can move through that range of motion, then you can build muscle through it.

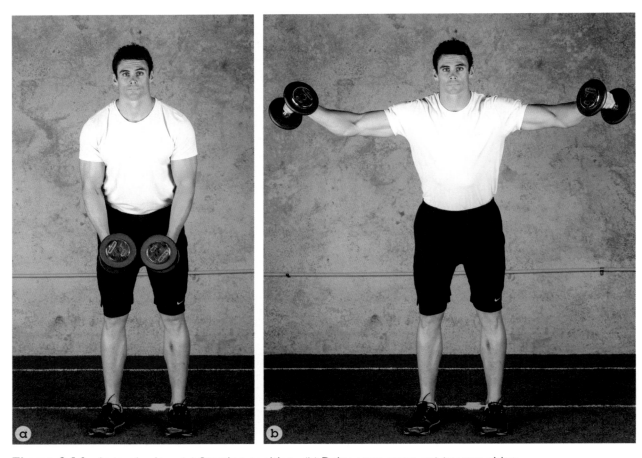

Figure 3.14 Lateral raise. *(a)* Starting position. *(b)* Raise your arms out to your sides.

Dumbbell Seated Shoulder Press

For perfectly proportioned shoulders of fortune, look no further than this move.

Muscles

Shoulders, abs

Execution

1. Sit on the edge of a seated bench. Set the back pad to vertical or just below.
2. Hold a dumbbell in each hand and hoist them up so that they're on either side of your head (figure 3.15a). Straighten your arms and push the weights above your head (figure 3.15b). Do not lock your elbows at the top of the movement.
3. Slowly lower the weights to the starting position.

VARIATION: Dumbbell Standing Shoulder Press

Do this exercise while standing with your feet shoulder-width apart.

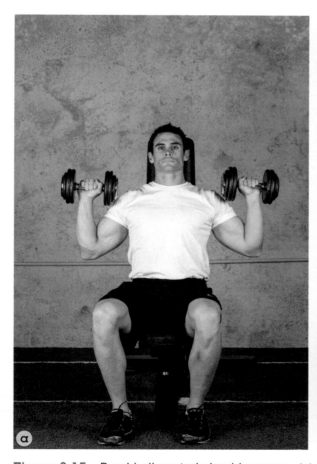 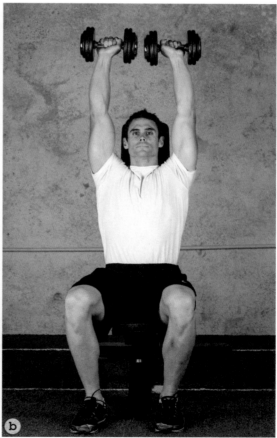

Figure 3.15   Dumbbell seated shoulder press. *(a)* Starting position. *(b)* Lift weights above head.

Cable Lateral Raise

This exercise will make your suits seem like they're straight out of the 1980s: stacked full of shoulder pads.

Muscles

Shoulders

Execution

1. Attach two D handles to the cable crossover machine's lowest setting. Stand in the middle of the cable crossover station and hold the left D handle in your right hand and the right D handle in your left hand (figure 3.15a). Keep a slight arch in your elbows.
2. Simultaneously pull your hands out to your sides. Stop when your hands are level with the tops of your shoulders (figure 3.16b).
3. Pause, then lower your hands along the same path.

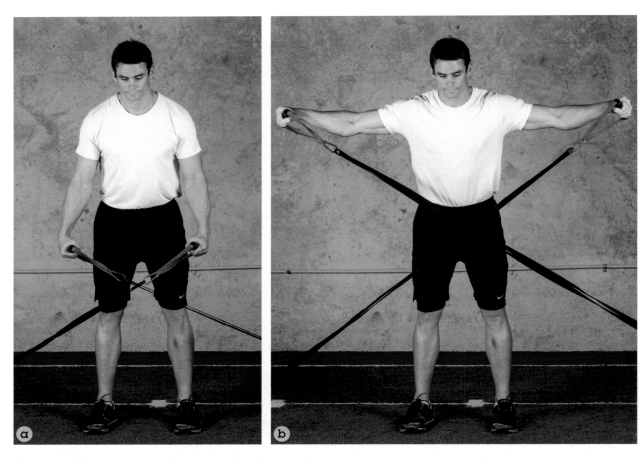

Figure 3.16 Cable lateral raise. *(a)* Starting position. *(b)* Raise hands out to sides.

Power Clean

Just like it says on the tin, this move will add sparkling strength to your shoulders, lower back and legs.

Muscles

Quads, hamstrings, glutes, lower back, shoulders, traps, abs

Execution

1. Stand with your feet shoulder-width apart and position your toes beneath a barbell. Bend at the knees, fully extend your arms and grab the bar with an overhand grip. Keep your back straight.

2. Yank the bar by quickly straightening your back and knees (figure 3.17a). Pull with your arms and keep the bar as close to your body as possible. When the bar is just below your chin, dip underneath it and rotate your elbows around the bar (figure 3.17b).

3. Pause, rotate your elbows back and slowly lower to the starting position. There you go: You'll be ready for the Olympics in no time at all.

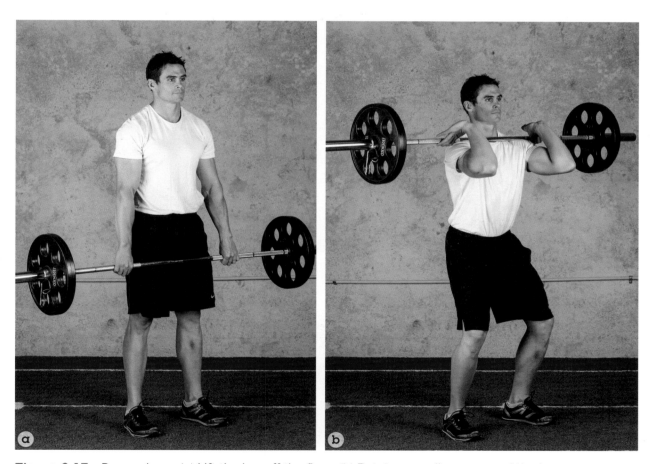

Figure 3.17 Power clean. *(a)* Lift the bar off the floor. *(b)* Rotate your elbows around the bar.

Incline Reverse Fly

This exercise works the shoulder muscles that decelerate the arms every time you throw or swing. Not being able to slow down your arms stresses your elbow joints and can cause an injury that can dampen your muscle growth.

Muscles

Shoulders

Execution

1. Lie facedown on an incline bench set to 45 degrees so that you can see over the top. Hold a dumbbell in each hand with your palms facing each other (figure 3.18a).
2. Keep a slight arc in your elbows and raise the dumbbells until they are level with your shoulders (figure 3.18b).
3. Hold for a second, then slowly lower to the starting position. Maintain a straight back throughout the movement. You'll soon have shoulders that pull back effortlessly and appear wider.

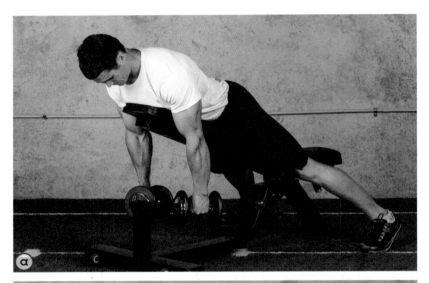

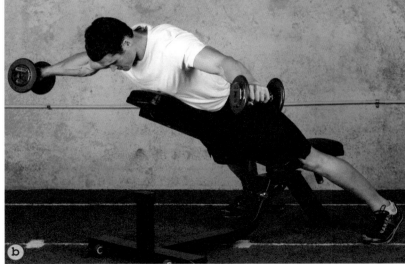

Figure 3.18 Incline reverse fly. (a) Starting position. (b) Raise the dumbbells until they are level with your shoulders.

Dumbbell Upright Row

Imagine you're standing up to sing the national anthem and rowing for the national team at the same time, and you have an upright row.

Muscles

Traps, shoulders, upper back

Execution

1. Stand with your feet shoulder-width apart and hold a dumbbell in each hand in front of you.
2. With your palms facing your body, raise the weights straight up until they're in line with the base of your chest and just below your chin (figure 3.19).
3. Pause, then slowly lower the weight.

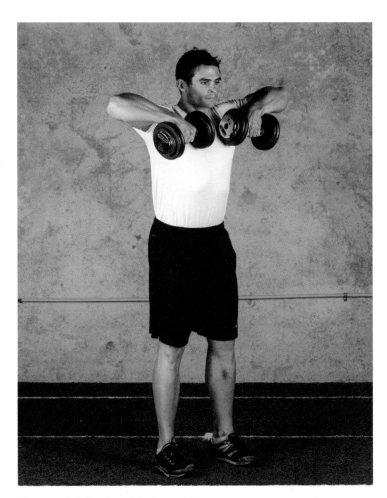

Figure 3.19   Dumbbell upright row.

Arnold Press

Arnold created these—hence the name—and he sported some of the widest shoulders known to man.

Muscles

Front deltoids, middle deltoids, triceps, upper trapezius

Execution

1. Stand and hold a pair of dumbbells at chest height with your palms facing you (figure 3.20a).
2. Push the weights overhead. At the same time, rotate your wrists so that your palms face forward at the top of the move (figure 3.20b).
3. Pause, then take two to four full seconds to lower the weights back down. Rotate your wrists as you go so that your palms face you again. Don't be surprised if your broader frame forces you into Saville Row for a new suit jacket.

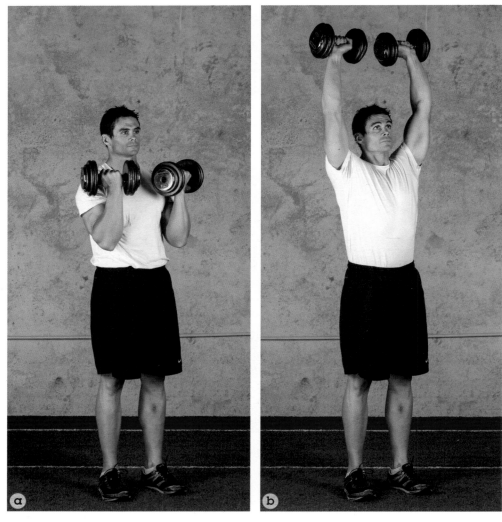

Figure 3.20 Arnold press. *(a)* Starting position. *(b)* Push the weights overhead.

Dumbbell Front Raise

Few moves are simpler than raising some big ol' heavy thing in front of you. Luckily, simplicity creates muscles better than anything else.

Muscles

Shoulders, traps

Execution

1. Stand with your feet shoulder-width apart and hold a dumbbell in each hand (figure 3.21a).
2. Raise the weights directly in front of you until they're in line with your shoulders (figure 3.21b).
3. Take two to three seconds to lower the weights to the starting position.

NOTE   Some trainers suggest stopping when the weights are level with the shoulders. If you have no injuries, lift through your full range of motion for more muscle and a stronger delta force.

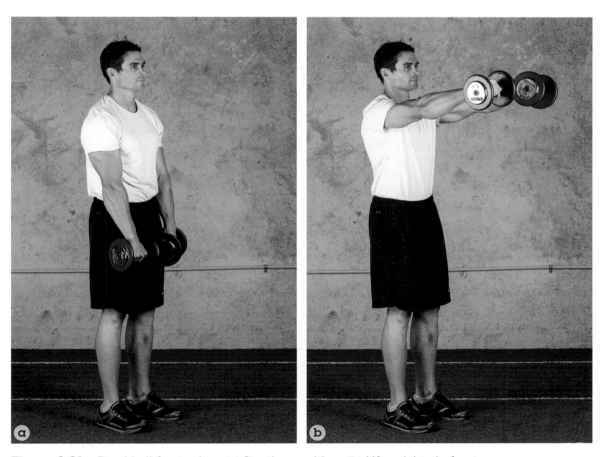

Figure 3.21   Dumbbell front raise. (a) Starting position. (b) Lift weights in front.

Pecs: Developing a Chest You Will Treasure

Your pecs are made up of two muscles: the pectoralis major (the bigger of the two) and the pectoralis minor. The latter sits under the former and is used mainly to pull up your ribs when you breathe. It's pretty useful.

A big chest is probably one of your main goals. A solid chest enters every room before you do and makes a more muscular first impression. If you happen to have a decent rack, it's likely you'll field the question 'waddaya bench?' But don't be fooled into thinking bench pressing is the sole exercise responsible for creating a noteworthy chest. Yes, it's a great exercise for building strength, but a huge catalogue of exercises are better at carving out concrete slabs of muscle frontage and don't carry the danger of trying to press loads of steel away from your heart. Here are the most important rules you should follow to get barrel chested.

Stick to Dumbbells

Over time, training with barbells will make your strength and muscular imbalances more pronounced. This is because your dominant side steals a fraction of the effort from the weaker side. If you're right handed, your right side often becomes stronger and more muscular than the left. You'll look less symmetrical and eventually accrue an injury. Training with dumbbells eliminates this problem and may be just as effective as training with a barbell. If you train strictly for strength, hit the barbell with all your might. But if you want a bit of everything, alternate between the bar and dumbbells.

Take It Slow

Lowering the bar at a slow pace (two to four seconds) is excellent for building strength in your chest. Get a partner to help you lift the weights while you lower them. Mix it into your chest programme whenever you need a strength or power boost.

Watch Your Shoulders

Most people stick to big pressing moves such as bench presses and dips to build their chests.

Rightly so, given that these exercises let you use the most weight and build the most muscle. But they also use a lot of your shoulder muscles, so pay attention to how you're feeling. Tweaks or grinding noises in your shoulders mean that you need to take a two-week rest from chest training. If you consistently damage your shoulders you won't be able to train anything but legs. You are not Rambo, and this kind of pain is not to be pushed through.

Form is Imperative

Even if you aren't benching truckloads of steel, chances are you want to answer the 'waddaya bench' question with a smile. You might be inclined to load up the plates or bells and push yourself the hardest on your chest exercises. This can lead to form errors and serious injury. Wearing a barbell as a necklace is not good fashion. Increase the weight only when you can do the moves with excellent form, and always use a spotter. Your lower back and shoulders will thank you by becoming bulletproof.

Don't Always Go Heavy

Big weights look impressive, but this kind of puffery is limited to the gym. A big chest is something you can take out the door. An ego can limit your range of motion because you're trying to work weights that are too heavy. A light, full-range-of-motion chest movement is a great complement to your heavy lifting. Just be sure to include a mix of exercises rather than spending all your time doing isolation exercises. So ditch the cartoonishly big weights and the ego and occasionally grab the small weights (not the pink ones) to feel the stretch.

Wear Belts Outside the Gym, Not Inside

Do not wear a weightlifting belt on the bench-press machine. Olympic lifters and powerlifters wear belts at two times: when they lift their competition weights and when they need to keep their trousers up. They need to develop core strength first by not using a belt, and the same holds true for you. Aim to improve stability in your shoulders, torso and hips in your workouts. None of this will happen if you belt up on chest day.

Keep Off Swiss Balls

You may want to combine your chest and abs workouts by using a Swiss ball. However, the wobbling about will make it impossible for you to use weights that are heavy enough to build muscle. A study in *Journal of Strength and Conditioning Research* (Uribie et al., 2010) found that doing dumbbell chest presses on a Swiss ball resulted in a decrease in chest strength compared with doing the same exercise on a bench. Never turn your workouts into a ball game. Use big weights on a stable, flat bench for a big, stable chest.

Challenge Your Chest With Push-Ups

Although push-ups may seem vanilla, they're chocolate in chest-building results. Many muscle-building pundits applaud the chest-buffing benefits of the humble push-up. You can do a few push-ups every day without risking over-training. Try setting a target to do 100 each day. By the time you reach that goal your chest will be impressively bigger.

Don't Forget Your Upper Chest

The most overlooked part of the average lifter's physique is the upper chest. This is the part that sticks out when you wear V-neck shirts. Working this area will make your chest look bigger from every angle. One week start with flat benching and the next week start with incline-bench movements, which work your upper chest.

Clench Your Teeth

If you want to grow your chest muscles the most, you'll probably work your chest until it completely gives into your demands. Here's a tip to maximise your power: Clench you jaw when you bench press or do any other heavy exercise. It helps your muscles go from 0 to 100 faster, so you'll lift significantly more weight. You may want to wear a mouth guard. A broken-glass smile isn't going to help your chest grow. Check out the following set of exercises to find out how to make your chest grow while brandishing a winning smile.

Dumbbell Incline Chest Press

Here's how to add a steeper slope to your frontage. This move will give you the upper-chest muscles that, when you wear an open-neck shirt, will make her want to see more.

Muscles

Upper chest, triceps, shoulders

Execution

1. Lie on an incline bench set to 30 to 45 degrees. Place your feet flat on the floor and hold a dumbbell in each hand above your chest.
2. Keep your head, torso and hips pressed onto the bench. Lower the weights to your sides (figure 3.22a).
3. Straighten your arms and press the weights up so that they are above your chin at the end of the movement (figure 3.22b).

NOTE Do not completely lock your elbows at the end of the movement.

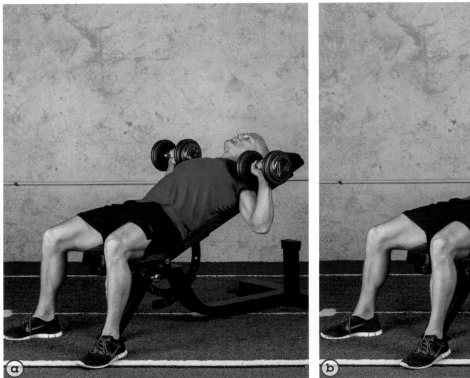

Figure 3.22 Dumbbell incline chest press. *(a)* Starting position. *(b)* Press the weights up.

Dumbbell Flat Chest Press

This chest carpenter will give you more frontage than Harrods, so make sure you do it right.

Muscles

Chest, triceps, shoulders

Execution

1. Lie on a flat bench and hold a dumbbell in each hand above you at arm's length.
2. Keep your head, torso and hips pressed onto the bench. Bend your elbows and take two to three seconds to lower the dumbbells to either side of your chest (figure 3.23a).
3. Pause, then straighten your elbows and press the weights up (figure 3.23b). You'll now have the power to pop her heavy suitcase on the top shelf of your wardrobe.

NOTE   Do not completely lock your elbows at the end of the movement.

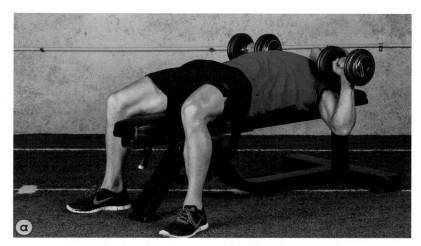

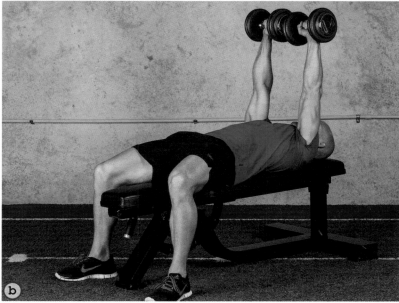

Figure 3.23   Dumbbell flat chest press. (a) Starting position. (b) Press the weights up.

Parallel Bar Dip

You've watched the muscled gymnasts toy with this machine. Here's your chance to develop their kind of Olympic strength and power.

Muscles

Chest, triceps, shoulders

Execution

1. Grab the parallel bars of a dip station and lift yourself so that your body weight rests on your hands.
2. Keep your arms straight but not locked. Bend your knees and cross your ankles (figure 3.24a).
3. Keeping your elbows close to your sides, lower your body for a count of three seconds until your upper arms are parallel to the floor (figure 3.24b). Take one second to press yourself back up. Keep your elbows unlocked at the top of the move to work a whopping two-thirds of the muscle in your upper arm and carve out a chest worthy of a gymnast.

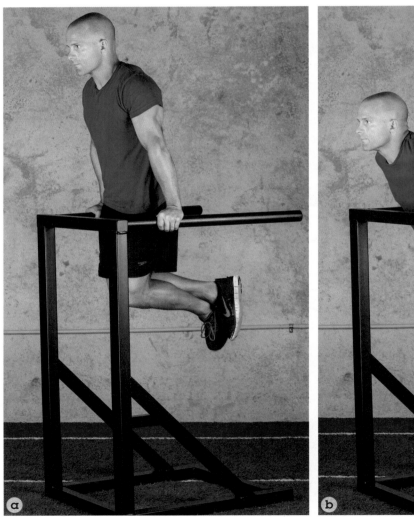
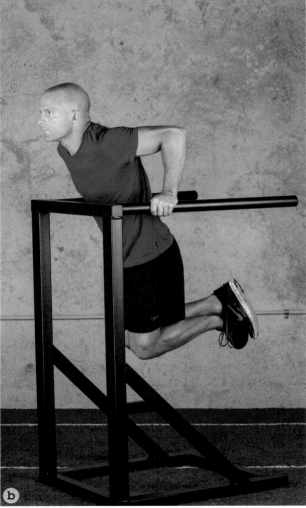

Figure 3.24 Parallel bar dip. (a) Starting position. (b) Lower yourself until your upper arms are parallel to the floor.

Dumbbell Chest Fly

Get ready to bear hug an imaginary friend. In the name of a bigger chest, of course.

Muscles

Chest, shoulders, triceps

Execution

1. Lie on your back on a flat bench. Hold a dumbbell in each hand and raise them directly above your chest (figure 3.25a).
2. Arc your elbows and slowly lower the weights as far as you can out to your sides. Keep your back flat on the bench (figure 3.25b).
3. Raise the weights to the starting position. The result? A treasure chest is yours for the taking.

VARIATION: Dumbbell Incline Chest Fly

For a variation, do the same movement while lying on an incline bench set to 30 to 45 degrees.

NOTE Try to keep the same angle in your elbow joints when you lower and raise the weights.

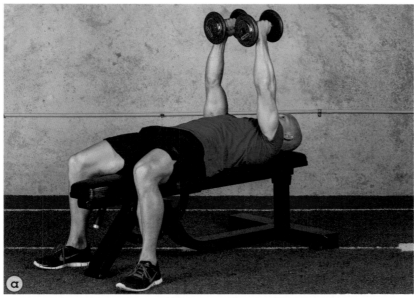

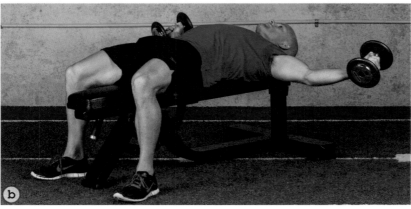

Figure 3.25
Dumbbell chest fly.
(a) Starting position.
(b) Lower the weights
to your sides.

Dumbbell Flat Pullover

You'll zip a Frisbee harder, lift luggage easier and punch that tosser out faster, all with one move. This exercise carves out the brawn in the middle of your chest, making it look deep with muscle from every angle. It also adds definition to the often hard-to-work lower abs.

Muscles

Chest, triceps, shoulders, abs, lats, forearms

Execution

1. Grab a light dumbbell in each hand and lie back on a flat bench. Place your feet flat on the floor.
2. Bring the dumbbells together so that they touch one another (figure 3.26a). Bend your elbows to about 30 degrees, then lower the weights as far behind your head as you can (figure 3.26b). Keep your upper arms as close to your ears as possible.
3. Raise the weights along the same path.

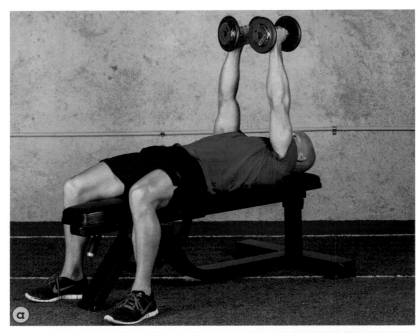

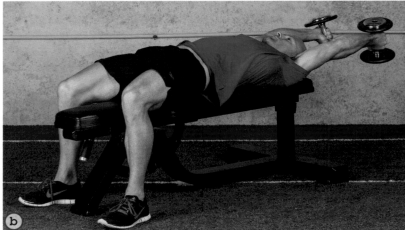

Figure 3.26
Dumbbell flat pullover.
(a) Starting position.
(b) Lower the weights behind your head.

Cable Crossover

The adjustability and constant resistance of cables will challenge your physique in new ways. Here's one of the best chest moves you can use.

Muscles

Chest, shoulders, abs, triceps

Execution

1. Stand with your feet staggered between the towers of the cable crossover machine. Set the D-handles to a level higher than chest height. Grab a handle with each hand.
2. Draw your arms behind you (figure 3.27a). Pull the handles across each other at a point in front of your chest (figure 3.27b). Your arms should form a cross in front of your body. You're permitted to feel a bit gangster at this point.
3. Flex your chest and slowly release to the starting position for a divide between your pecs so pronounced you could clasp a coin between them.

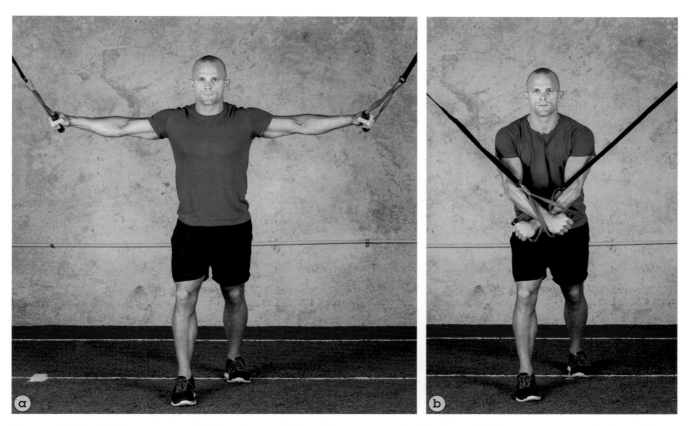

Figure 3.27 Cable crossover. *(a)* Starting position with your arms behind you. *(b)* Cross your arms in front of your chest.

Medicine Ball Lying Throw

Time to find a place with a high ceiling. Users of dungeon gyms may have difficulty. This move works best if you do it outside.

Muscles

Chest, shoulders, abs, triceps

Execution

1. Lie on a flat bench. Position a medicine ball on your chest and hold it with both hands (figure 3.28a).
2. Push the ball into the air (figure 3.28b), then catch it and return it to the starting position.

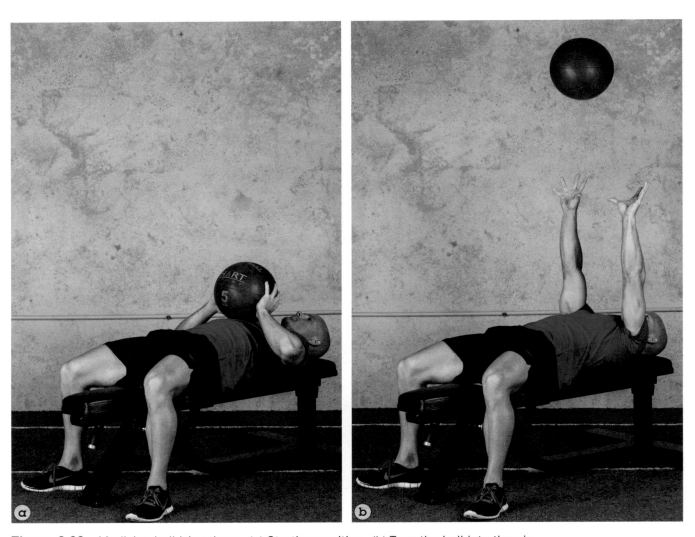

Figure 3.28 Medicine ball lying throw. (a) Starting position. (b) Toss the ball into the air.

Explosive Push-Up

You don't need fancy equipment to accelerate the speed of your punches and serves. All you need is good old gravity and this exercise.

Muscles

Chest, triceps

Execution

1. Get into a push-up position and place your hands slightly wider than your shoulders. Your body should form a straight line from your shoulders to your ankles.

2. Keep your back flat and lower your body until your upper arms are lower than your elbows (figure 3.29a). Pause and hold this position for a second.

3. Forcefully thrust yourself upwards as high as you can so that your hands leave the ground (figure 3.29b). Clap your hands while airborne, if you can.

NOTE   Keep your back straight throughout the exercise.

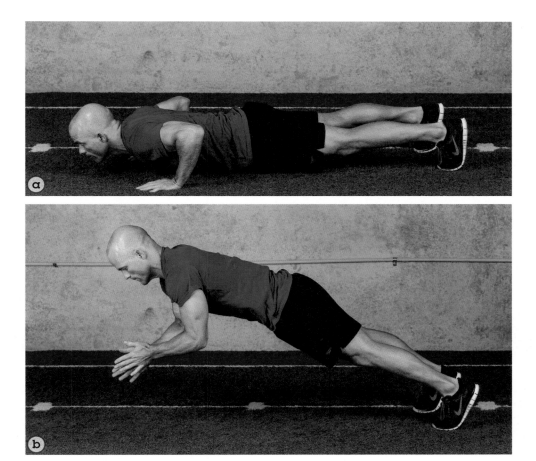

Figure 3.29   Explosive push-up. *(a)* Down position. *(b)* Hands off the ground.

Medicine Ball Slam

Get ready to make noise with this explosive exercise that'll nail your entire upper body.

Muscles

Shoulders, abs, chest

Execution

1. Stand with your feet hip-width apart. Hold a medicine ball at arm's length above your head like you're hoisting a winner's trophy (figure 3.30a). Imagine a crowd cheering.
2. Quickly bend your torso over and slam the ball onto the ground in front of you (figure 3.30b). Mind your toes.
3. Catch the ball as it bounces back up—mind your face—and lift it up to the starting position. Take a quick bask in the glory of your newfound speed and explosiveness.

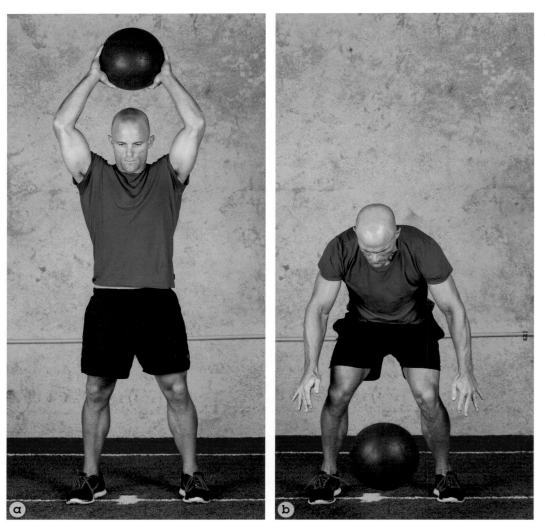

Figure 3.30 Medicine ball slam. *(a)* Starting position. *(b)* Slam the ball to the ground.

Push-Up

For a weapons-grade chest, get your nose in the dirt, soldier.

Muscles

Shoulders, chest, triceps, abs

Execution

1. Lie facedown on the ground. Support your body on the balls of your feet and place your hands shoulder-width apart (figure 3.31a). Keep your arms straight but not locked.
2. Bend your elbows and lower yourself to the floor (figure 3.31b). Keep your elbows tucked to your sides.
3. When your chest touches the floor, straighten your elbows and push back up to the starting position.

VARIATION: Incline Push-Up

Place your feet on a raised object such as a park bench or weight bench and rest your hands on the ground. Perform the push-up.

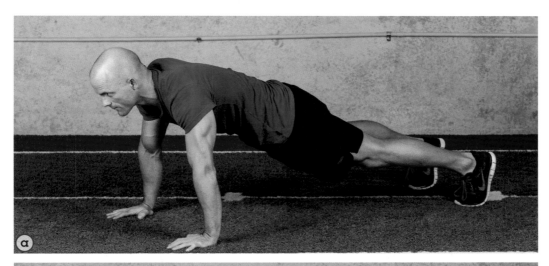

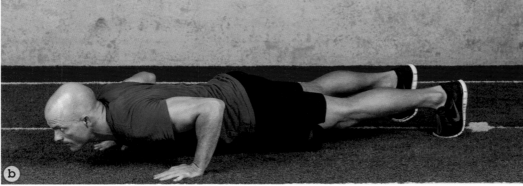

Figure 3.31   Push-up. *(a)* Starting position. *(b)* Lower your chest to the floor.

Back:
Get a V-Shaped Torso

If you're looking for big muscles, none are larger in total surface area than the ones in your upper back, called your lats. They have a few helpers—your biceps and shoulders—that can steal the effort during some back exercises and thereby narrow your V-shape potential. But there are ways to take these thieves out of the equation.

A wide, cobra-shaped back is a symbol of power on the sport pitch and in the boardroom. For your frame to look athletic and imposing, your shoulders and upper back need to be wider than your waist. Whereas the fat-burning sections in chapters 8 and 9 will help narrow your waist, the rules and workouts here will widen your V-shape, instantly making your waist seem slimmer. A strong upper back also helps keep your shoulders back and holds your posture in place. And if you're a sportsman, it will help you in just about every athletic pursuit be it swimming, surfing, climbing or just whipping a ball to your mate so hard he has to blow on his fingers. Keep reading to make your silhouette a peace sign.

Grip Strength is Vital

If you're a creationist your lats are leftover angel wings, and if you're an evolutionist they're old monkey muscles that your forefathers used to swing from trees. Almost every back exercise involves holding onto something: a weight, a pull-up bar, whatever. The goal is to hang onto it long enough to stress your back muscles with tension. But if your grip gives out before your back muscles do, you're doomed to a U-shape instead of a V-shape. If you find this happening, take the time to strengthen your grip or wear straps. After enough back moves your hands will strengthen up and give you a deal-sealing handshake.

Squeeze After You Pull

Almost every back exercise has you pulling something heavy towards your chest or face. Your shoulder blades will be pursed together at the end of the movements, and it's vital to make conscious effort to squeeze them and hold the end of each rep. This adds tension to every exercise and helps keep your shoulders pulled back and your chest pumped out when you stand normally.

Think About It

Because your back muscles don't normally glare at you in the mirror unless you're checking out your glute development, your brain can feel removed from their existence. To maximise your growth, create a mind–muscle link by imagining your back muscles flexing and relaxing while shifting the weights back and forth. Many Mr. Olympias swear by this technique. Trying to convince a man whose arms are bigger than his head that it doesn't work might be a little difficult.

Vary Your Grip

When doing moves such as rows, pull-ups and lat pull-downs, make sure to vary your grip. The wider the grip, the harder the exercise and the more muscle worked. Narrower grips tend to work the muscles in the middle of your back, making you appear thicker, whereas wider grips work the outer edges of your lats, making you appear wider. Mix it up as much as possible and you'll soon have a back that looks good from every angle.

Level Your Back With Your Chest

For an injury-free physique, your back should be as strong as your chest. This means that you should be able to pull as much as you can push. Your pecs are bound to get a thorough workout every week, so make sure your back keeps the pace in both strength and endurance. You can even superset back exercises with chest exercises for a muscle-building fiesta.

Chin Up

When training your back you'll be tempted to bring your head towards the weight you're pulling. It's human nature to keep an eye on things that are coming closer to us. But this often makes lifters pull their chins down, which throws the spine out of whack. Here is an easy solution: Keep looking straight ahead and keep your chin up. This, incidentally, is a very good move for your back development.

Stretch Out

If you've ever tweaked your back, you know it doesn't always manifest in meagre discomfort that you feel when you move in a certain way. It can leave you bedridden for days on end until you find a back cracker to fix you up. The solution? On the days you're not training your back, hang from a pull-up bar for 30 seconds. It'll build grip strength, which is useful in back training, and stretch out your back, which will keep knots from getting a foothold. When you train your back, throw in a few chest stretches to keep both sides limber and injury free.

Go Heavy, Lift Slow

When you train your back, the distance the weight has to travel is short. Each rep of a back exercise (other than the pull-up) can take half the time of a normal rep for another body part such as the legs or chest. Slow it down and stack on enough weight to force yourself to ease up the pace during the pulling and lowering phases of each move.

Hand Out

You'll have to grip and squeeze back-bending loads of steel when you're working your lats; this can batter your hands. Wear gloves on back days only or let your calluses form up. Your hands will soon get tough enough. However, if you let the calluses get too big you risk a weight pulling them off. Blood usually brings a session to an abrupt halt. Every few months trim your calluses down using your fingernail kit. You can bet she'll appreciate the effort.

Master Your Body Weight

The pull-up cycle goes like this: You can't do very many pull-ups. You don't want to look weak, so you hit the lat pull-downs to get strong enough to do pull-ups. A few months later you can rack the lat pull-down machine but you still can't do a pull-up, so you go back to what you know. To break the loop and build that strength, do one or two reps on the assisted pull-up machine. Pull-ups are the gold standard for just about every military, fire department or job that demands physicality because they create strength relative to body weight. Plus, they recruit the arms, forearms, abs and even chest. It's the best move you can do for your back and your entire body. Don't give in until you've mastered the pull-up and the essential back exercises that follow.

Overhand-Grip Pull-Up

Aside from giving you upper-back strength that'll put your chiropractor out of business, this move gives you that extra snap of power whenever you punch or throw.

Muscles

Back, biceps, abs, forearms

Execution

1. Grab the pull-up bar with an overhand grip and place your hands shoulder-width apart. If you're advanced, attach a lifting belt around your waist and hang weights on it. (See the weighted overhand-grip pull-up in chapter 11.) If you're not strong enough for that, use the assisted pull-up machine. Hang so that your elbows are completely extended.
2. Bend your elbows and pull yourself up until your chin crosses the plane of the bar (figure 3.32).
3. Pause, then slowly lower yourself to the starting position without allowing your body to sway.

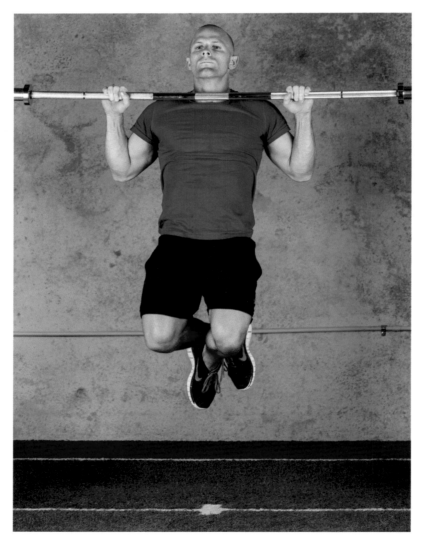

Figure 3.32   Overhand-grip pull-up.

Dumbbell Bent-Over Row

This move will help you stand tall with a wide, V-shaped torso.

Muscles

Lats, biceps, shoulders

Execution

1. Stand with your feet flat on the floor. Hold a dumbbell in each hand.
2. Keeping your back flat, bend forward at the hips until your back is almost parallel to the floor. Keep your legs straight but unlocked, your arms straight under your shoulders and your palms facing each other.
3. Slowly draw the weights up towards the sides of your chest (figure 3.33). Pause, then slowly lower the weights. Repeat to get your back on track.

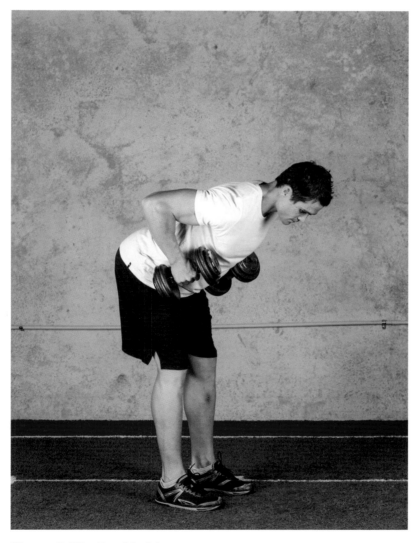

Figure 3.33   Dumbbell bent-over row.

Single-Arm Dumbbell Row

For more pulling power in the gym, this move is a must.

Muscles

Lats, biceps

Execution

1. Place one knee on a bench and balance yourself with your free arm, palm down, in front you. Place your other leg on the floor behind you so that your body forms a tripod shape. Keep your back flat and grasp a dumbbell with your free hand. Let this hand hang at arm's length beneath your shoulder (figure 3.34a).
2. Draw your elbow up past your torso by pinching your shoulder blade in towards your spine (figure 3.34b).
3. Take three seconds to lower the weight to the starting position for lats so big they'll wing their way into any lady's heart.

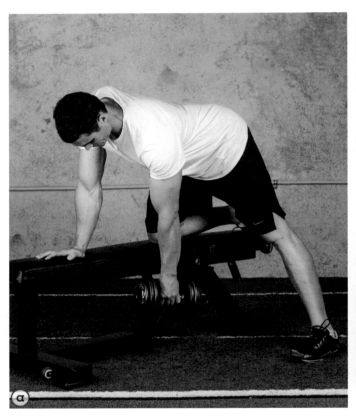 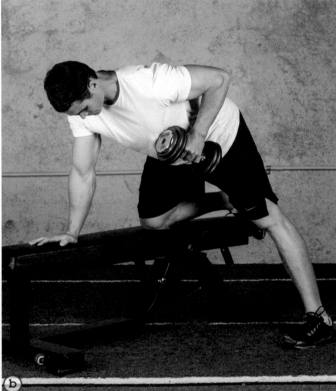

Figure 3.34 Single-arm dumbbell row. *(a)* Starting position. *(b)* Lift the weight.

Dumbbell Incline Row

This exercise will give you a back that makes an impression every time you leave a room.

Muscles

Lats, biceps, forearms

Execution

1. Lie facedown on an incline bench set to 45 degrees so that your eyes can see over the top. Hold a dumbbell in each hand with your palms facing each other (figure 3.35a). Keep your hands below your shoulders.
2. Bend your elbows and pull the weights towards you (figure 3.35b).
3. Hold the top of the movement for a second, then take two to three seconds to release the weights to the starting position.

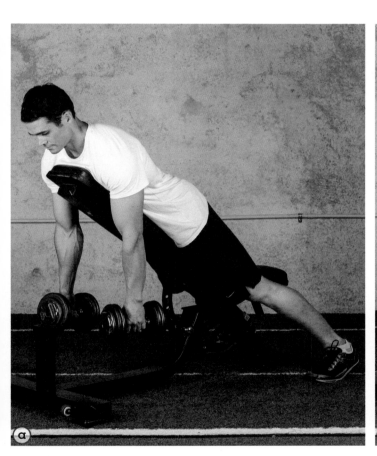 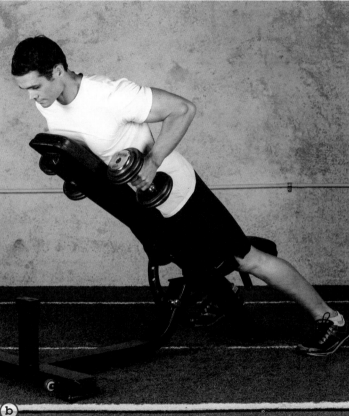

Figure 3.35 Dumbbell incline row. *(a)* Starting position. *(b)* Pull the weights.

Inverted Row

Get good at these and you'll soon be able to yank open that rusty attic door with no trouble at all.

Muscles

Back, biceps, abs

Execution

1. Lie under a barbell that is secured slightly higher than arm's length above the floor. (Imagine you're hanging on to a windsurfing pole, if it helps.) Grab the bar and hang from it. Your body should form a straight line from ankles to shoulders (figure 3.36a).
2. Pull your chest to the bar and pause (figure 3.36b).
3. Straighten your elbows and lower yourself until your elbows are locked. Your chest must touch the bar for a rep to count.

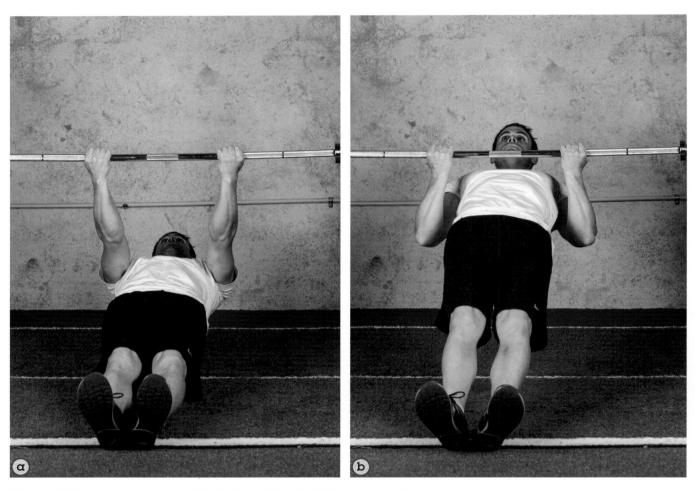

Figure 3.36 Inverted row. (a) Starting position. (b) Pull your chest to the bar.

Cable Face Pull

This is not your chance to present your favourite scowl, although you probably will anyway.

Muscles

Lats, biceps, forearms, abs

Execution

1. Fix the rope attachment of a cable crossover machine to a height that's at eye level. Stand facing the machine. Grab one end of the rope in each hand and step back so that your arms are straight in front of you and parallel to the floor (figure 3.37a).

2. Bend your elbows and bring the middle of the rope attachment as close to your face as possible (figure 3.37b).

3. Take two to three seconds to straighten your arms and return to the starting position.

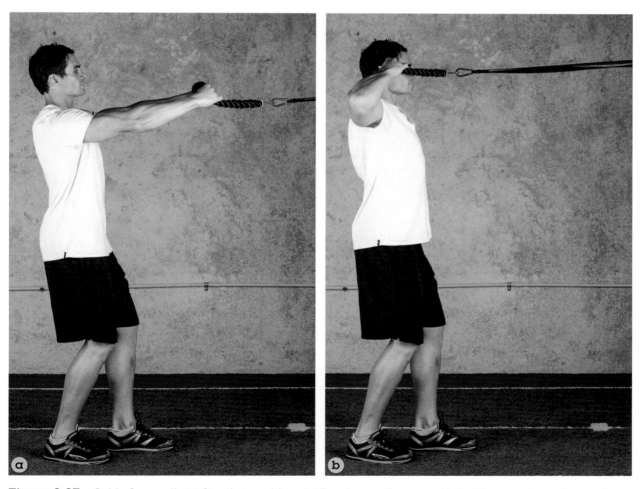

Figure 3.37 Cable face pull. (a) Starting position. (b) Bend your elbows and bring the rope towards your face.

Dumbbell Deadlift

For wholesale muscle at a bulk price, this Eastern bloc move is on the money.

Muscles

Quads, glutes, hamstrings, lower back, abs

Execution

1. Place two dumbbells on the ground in front of you. Stand with your feet together. Bend at your knees and hips and bring your upper body towards the weights. Grab the weights with an overhand grip (figure 3.38a).
2. Use your thighs to straighten your legs and raise the weights (figure 3.38b).
3. Take two to four seconds to lower the weights back to the starting position. Keep your back straight throughout the movement.

VARIATION: Single-Leg Dumbbell Deadlift

For more of a challenge, balance on one foot as you perform the deadlift. After completing all reps on one foot, switch feet and perform reps on the other foot.

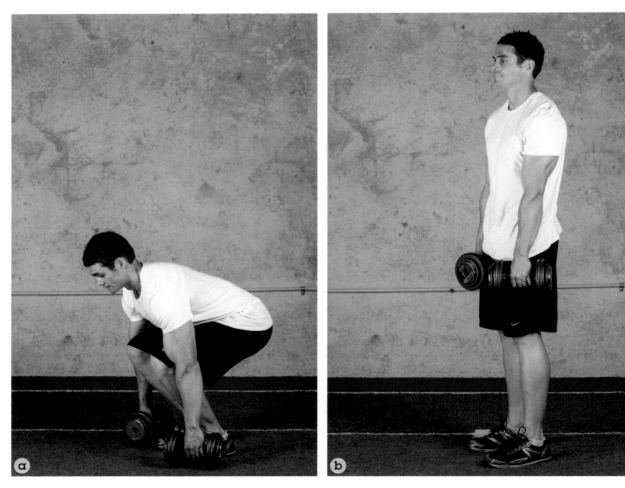

Figure 3.38 Dumbbell deadlift. (a) Starting position. (b) Lift the weights and straighten your legs.

Good Morning

The lower back may not have showy muscles, but you'll wish you worked it if and when you tweak it.

Muscles

Lower back, hamstrings, abs, glutes

Execution

1. Rest a barbell across the back of your shoulders. Bend your knees slightly and with control (figure 3.39a) and start to bend forward, maintaining the normal curvature of your lower back.

2. Lower your torso until it is parallel to the floor (figure 3.39b), then reverse the direction and raise your torso to the starting position. A strong lower back will help you stand up straight, which will lengthen your abs and instantly deflate your gut. Even if you're not Bruce Lee, it's worth taking a bow.

NOTE As you lower your torso, look straight ahead. This will help keep your back in the proper position.

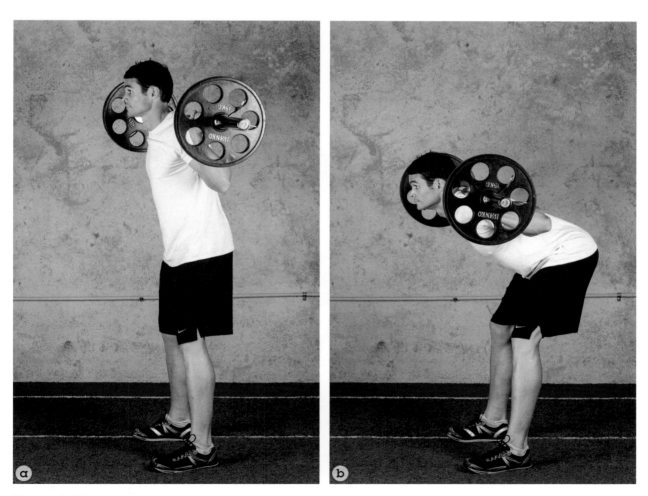

Figure 3.39 Good morning. *(a)* Starting position. *(b)* Lower your torso until it's parallel to the floor.

Back Extension

Strong abs demand a strong counterbalance. That comes in the form of a solid lower back.

Muscles

Lower back, abs

Execution

1. Lie facedown on a back-extension machine. Hook the backs of your ankles under the pads and rest your hips on the pad. Fold your arms across your chest (figure 3.40a) or, if you're strong enough, hold a weight to your chest.
2. Lower your torso towards the ground (figure 3.40b), then rise up to the starting position and hold for one to two seconds.

NOTE   If you don't have a back-extension machine, lie facedown on the ground, interlock your fingers behind your head and raise your torso off the ground for two seconds. Think of them as prisoner-style extensions.

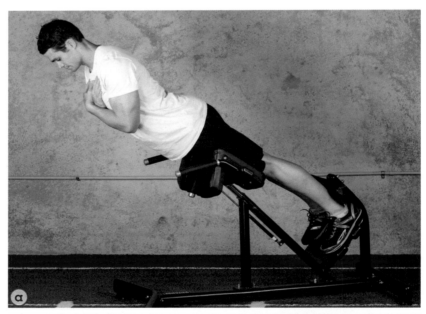

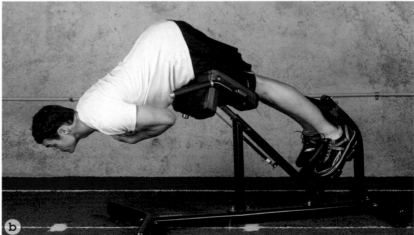

Figure 3.40
Back extension.
(a) Starting position.
(b) Lower your torso towards the ground.

Superman

Here's what to do for a Man of Steel-like lower back and abs.

Muscles

Lower back, abs

Execution

1. Lie on your stomach with your arms stretched out (figure 3.41*a*).
2. Lift your chest off the floor. Keep your hips and legs still (figure 3.41*b*).
3. Hold for two to three seconds, then lower your upper body back to the floor.

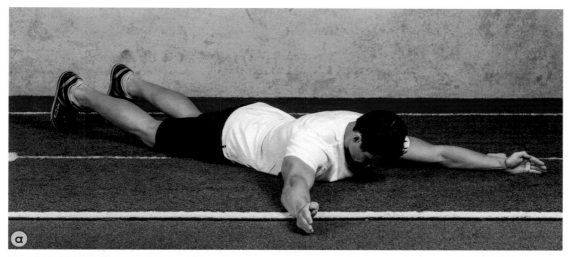

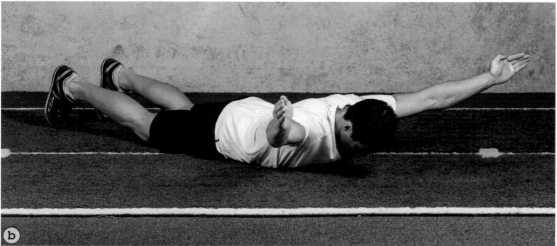

Figure 3.41 Superman. *(a)* Starting position. *(b)* Lift your chest and abs off the floor.

Squat Press

This exercise is the pièce de résistance of muscle building due to its ability to rope in every muscle you own and some you didn't even know you had.

Muscles

Glutes, hamstrings, quads, shoulders, abs, lower back, chest

Execution

1. Position a barbell five centimetres away from your ankles. Stand with your feet shoulder-width apart. Squat down and grip the bar with an overhand grip (figure 3.42a).

2. Use your glutes to push your hips forward and stand up while pulling the bar upwards (figure 3.42b). Keep the bar close to your body and use the momentum from your lower body.

3. Once the bar is at shoulder height, rotate your elbows and hands around it. At the end of this movement the bar should rest across the front of your shoulders and you should be holding it with an underhand grip (figure 3.42c). Bend your knees into a squat.

4. In one quick movement, straighten your knees, rise up onto your toes and drive the weight above your head in the form of a shoulder press (figure 3.42d).

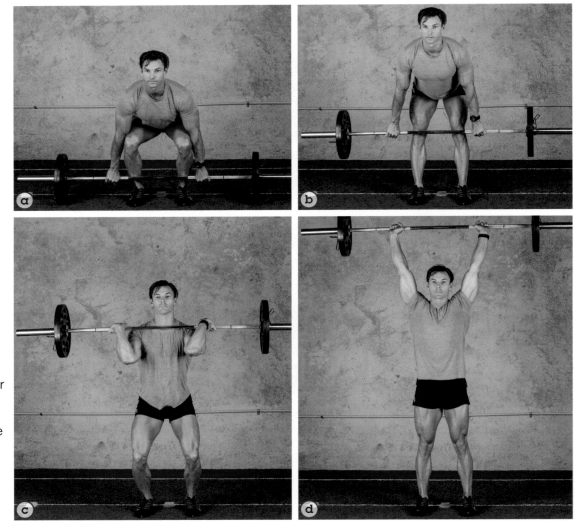

Figure 3.42 Squat press. *(a)* Squat and grip the bar. *(b)* Pull the bar upwards. *(c)* Rest the bar across the front of your shoulders. *(d)* Perform a shoulder press.

Abdominals: Moving Up to Middle Management

The muscles in your midsection are more unified than you may think. The six-pack isn't six or eight separate muscles; it's one band of muscle that is divided by tendons that make it look like a multimuscle washboard. It's then wrapped in supporting muscles such as the obliques and transverse abs that help you twist and turn in every direction.

Undoubtedly, the muscle group that regularly tops all the 'most wanted' lists in girly magazines is abs. Even if you couldn't care less about those manufactured lists, a solid set of abs is bound to get you a little more attention. If aesthetics aren't your style, consider the other benefits: less back pain, improved sport performance, better posture and an iron gut that can easily absorb a sucker punch. Abs are also pretty useful in everyday situations such as staying balanced while carrying a load of boxes when you move house or showing up to the picnic brandishing a few crates of beer without sweating. Thanks to these selling points most blokes would pay any amount to get a stone-carved pack. This means that they often train abs differently than they train other muscles; this is wrong. Here is your guide to avoiding nepotism and getting yourself a pack you've seen only on television—the proper way.

Movement Does Not Equal Abs

Your abs don't work just when your torso or legs go up or down. In fact, some of the most taxing abs moves you can do are those where you don't move at all. The job your abs perform the most is flexing to keep your body upright. When you suspend your body above the ground, such as during a plank exercise, your abs have to work double time to keep it there. Resisting movement is often tougher than creating movement and will produce immovable abs.

Rest is Best

If you crank out your favourite abs moves every day you will be overtraining the muscles and depriving them of the precious recovery time they need to grow. Your abs are already one of the hardest-working muscle groups in your body. You use them to stand upright and walk into the gym and then use them again in almost every weightlifting exercise you perform. Ease off and train them with heavy weights two or three times a week and you'll soon see that warming the sofa in front of the box is just what you need in order to see your six friends again.

Look Forward When Your Back Aches

If you've ever had back problems, stop thinking your back is the problem. Back pain is often related to weak muscles in your trunk. The muscles in your midsection aren't isolated. Rather, they weave through your torso like a web of high-tensile steel—if they're in shape, of course. If your abs are weak, your glutes and hamstrings have to work harder to keep your spine stable; this can lead to back pain. Researchers (Childs et al., 2010) found that U.S. Army recruits who did exercises that worked core muscles had fewer days off as a result of back pain. Hop to it, soldier, and give back pain its marching orders by getting your abs in good shape.

Crunches Are Not the Only Move Worth Doing

If you're not doing squats for your legs, consider using them to build your midsection. Researchers who measured abdominal-muscle activity during several popular exercises determined that squats work the core harder than many abs and lower-back exercises do (Okada, Huxel and Nesser, 2011). Although squatting with the heaviest weights stimulated the most muscle, even light warm-up sets targeted the participants' abs intensely. Get squatting if you want the muscles above your legs to look good.

You Cannot Spot Reduce Your Gut

This isn't news to anyone who has managed to accrue even a single bead of sweat in a gym. But, for proof, take a look at the guy pumping out hundreds of sit-ups and crunches—there's always one. How does his gut look? Chances are it's wobblier than a bowl of unset trifle. Sit-ups are not an efficient use of your time; you'd have to do around 20,000 to burn a pound of fat. Stick to using heavy weights and doing only a few reps and you'll stress your abs enough for them to grow.

Out of Sight Should Not Mean Out of Mind

Just because you can't see your abs doesn't mean they're not there. Your abs could be making unparalleled progress but you'll never know it until you remove the covering layer of fat. If you're in need of some motivation, jab your fingers into your belly fat and feel about. Those hard slabs of muscle you feel are your abs. All you need to do is burn off the fat (see chapters 8 and 9) to reveal their true form. When you get to 10 to 12 per cent body fat, your abs will be poking people's eyes out.

You Cannot Target Your Upper and Lower Abs

Your abs connect to your rib cage and pelvis bones and are one large muscle. You cannot do one exercise for the upper abs and one for the lower abs. When you work your abs, you work the entire length of the muscle. This is pretty handy: It actually saves you time and means that your abs will always grow in perfect proportions. If your lower abs aren't as developed as your upper abs, it's because you're most likely to store your excess blubber in the spot that covers the lower abs. Sad but true. And it means that fat burning is the order of the day.

Swiss Balls Are Not the Answer to Abs

Plenty of men and women build eye-catching abs without the aid of these oversized balloons. In some cases, exercises on a Swiss ball actually recruit fewer muscles than exercises done without a ball. Swiss balls do have their place and are useful for a few exercises, but do not try to do an entire routine of bench presses and every other kind of exercise on them because you'll be weaker than if you did the exercises on a more stable platform. You'll sacrifice muscle everywhere else and your abs won't look any different.

Get a Feel for Your Abs

Tons of studies outline which abs exercise is superior to the next, but the funny thing about abs is that certain exercises work better for different people. What built your mate's six-pack may not have as pronounced an effect on your pack because the mechanics of your physique are unique. The trick is not to limit yourself to the exercises in this book. Go search and observe all abs moves and give them crack yourself. You'll know by the second set whether a move works your midsection the way you want it to. After you've found what works for you, you'll see how quickly your abs will join the party.

Suck In Your Stomach

The action of sucking in your gut, the way you would when someone attractive walks past you on the beach, is worth practising in the gym. When doing abs moves, try to draw your belly button in towards your spine while keeping your ribcage up. This is a Pilates technique that involves your transverse abdominals, which is a deep ab muscle that helps you breathe. Why should you bother? Training the transverse abdominals to stay flexed will help you keep your gut pulled in without having to think about it, making your abs look more pronounced. If a blonde in a bikini surprises you, your gut will look as though you've just finished 100 sit-ups and you can talk to her without holding your breath. For more ways to achieve that look, check out the exercises that follow. They'll help you do it better than any others.

Bicycle Crunch

On your bike, son. This move will help get your abs in the saddle as quickly as possible.

Muscles

Abs, core

Execution

1. Lie on your back with your feet in the air and your knees bent 90 degrees. Lace your fingers behind your head.
2. Bring your knees in towards your chest and lift your shoulder blades off the ground without pulling on your neck.
3. Straighten your left leg so that it is 45 degrees to the floor. At the same time, turn your upper body to the right and bring your left elbow towards your right knee. Switch sides and bring your right elbow towards your left knee (figure 3.43). Continue to alternate sides while pumping your legs back and forth in a cycling motion and you'll wheel a set of roadworthy abs in no time.

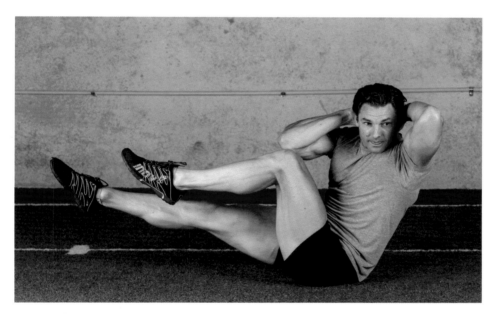

Figure 3.43   Bicycle crunch. Bring your right elbow to your left knee.

Plank and Single-Leg Plank

Preventing your crotch from sagging to the floor is instinctive. Here's how to use it to your advantage.

Muscles

Abs

Execution

1. Lie facedown on the floor with your legs straight and together. Place your hands beneath your chest and rest your body weight on your forearms.

2. Raise onto your elbows and toes so that your body forms a straight line from ankles to shoulders (figure 3.44a). Hold this position for the appropriate amount of time for your specific workout.

3. As a variation, raise one of your feet (figure 3.44b).

VARIATION: Push-Up Plank

Get into the plank position. Place your right hand where your right elbow was resting and straighten both arms to get into a push-up starting position. Return to the plank position and then repeat starting with your left arm.

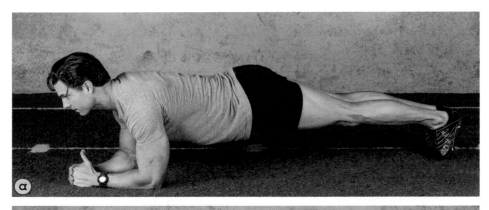

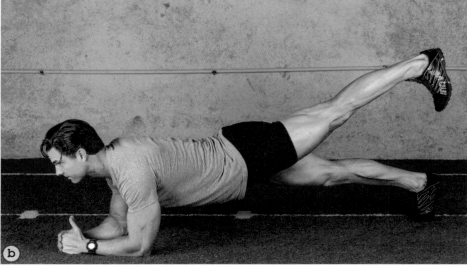

Figure 3.44 *(a)* Plank. *(b)* Single-leg plank.

Lying Leg Raise

Go on, take a load off. You deserve it.

Muscles

Abs, obliques

Execution

1. Stretch out on the floor with your legs completely straight. Rest your hands at your sides (figure 3.45a). If you're strong and brave, hold a dumbbell between your feet.
2. Keeping your knees straight but not locked, raise your legs until they're 90 degrees to the ground (figure 3.45b). Take two to three seconds to lower your legs to the floor. A gut that can take a sucker punch from an Ultimate Fighting Championship fighter is now yours for the packing.

VARIATION: Lying Leg Raise With Pike

As a variation, when your legs are 90 degrees to the floor, slightly lift your lower back off the floor and hold the position for two to three seconds. Lower your lower back and then your legs (don't let them touch the ground) and repeat.

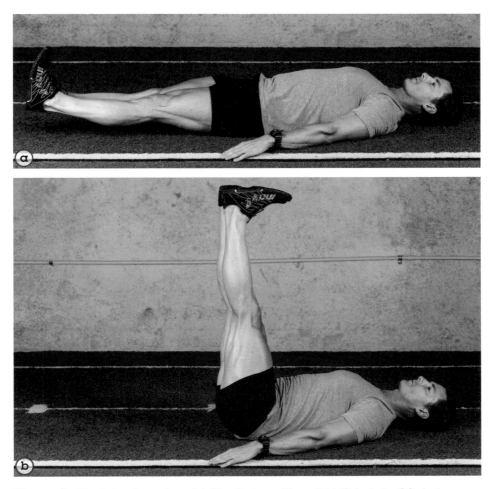

Figure 3.45 Lying leg raise. (a) Starting position. (b) Lift legs to 90 degrees.

Hanging Leg Raise

This move will put a noose around your abs and choke them into growing.

Muscles

Abs

Execution

1. Position yourself in the captain's chair machine and grip the handles. Press your back against the pad and tense your abs.
2. Raise your feet and bend your knees until your knees are level with your chest (figure 3.46).
3. Take two to three seconds to lower your legs and one second to raise them. That'll place your gut muscles under enough tension to build a six-pack of steel.

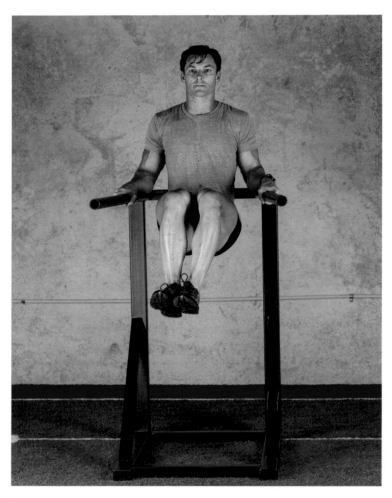

Figure 3.46   Hanging leg raise.

Barbell Rollout

Think of this move as the limbo dance in reverse. After performing this exercise, lowering yourself to see whether your missing keys have worked their way under the bed will require only a smidgen of effort.

Muscles

Abs, shoulders, lower back

Execution

1. Load a barbell with 5- to 10-kilogram plates and stick on some collars. Kneel on the floor and grab the bar with an overhand grip with your hands shoulder-width apart. Position your shoulders directly over the barbell and keep your lower back naturally arched (figure 3.47*a*).
2. Slowly roll the bar forward and extend your body as far as you can without letting your hips sag (figure 3.47*b*).
3. Pause for two seconds and then reverse the movement to return to the start. Your abs have to tense to stop your torso and hips from falling onto the ground.

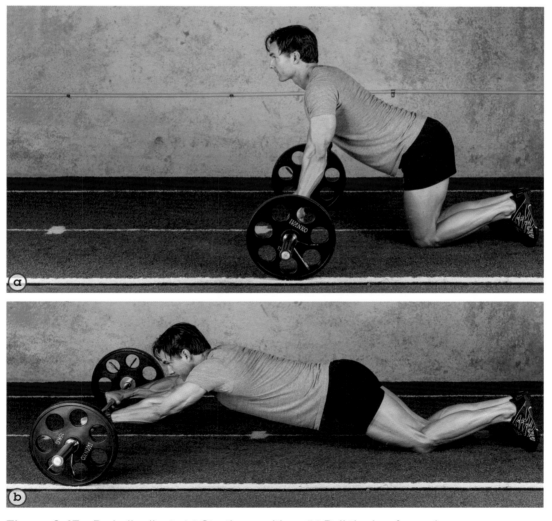

Figure 3.47 Barbell rollout. *(a)* Starting position. *(b)* Roll the bar forward.

Side Plank

Just because you do it on your side doesn't mean it's easy.

Muscles

Abs, obliques

Execution

1. Get into a plank position. Shift your body weight onto your left arm as you roll onto the outside of your left foot.
2. Lift your body off the ground. Balance on your left forearm and place your right foot on top of the left (figure 3.48). Keep your legs straight so that your body is diagonal to the floor. Don't let your hips dip downwards.
3. Hold that position and repeat on the other side. This builds abs without stressing your spine and gives you the endurance to flex your pelvis all night. Resourceful on the dance floor; essential in the bedroom.

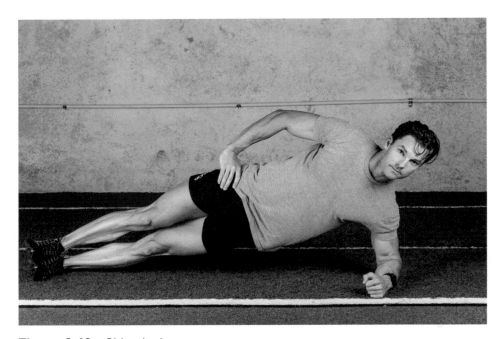

Figure 3.48   Side plank.

Wrestles

Get to grips with one of the most powerful total-body exercises you can do for your midsection.

Muscles

Core

Execution

1. Place a weight on one end of a barbell and wedge the other end into a corner or into the hole of another weight plate. Stand with your feet shoulder-width apart and clasp the end of the barbell (figure 3.49a).

2. Bend your upper body and knees towards the ground and lower the weight to your left in a wide-arcing movement (figure 3.49b). Keep a constant arc in your elbows throughout the motion.

3. Start to pivot your feet in the direction you are lowering the bar. Keep your knees over your toes. Rise onto the ball of your left foot to make the pivoting motion easier.

4. Stop just before the weight reaches the floor. It should end up slightly behind the outside of your left foot. Explosively raise the weight up and along the same arching path that you lowered it on. Use the power in your core and legs to drive it back to the starting position.

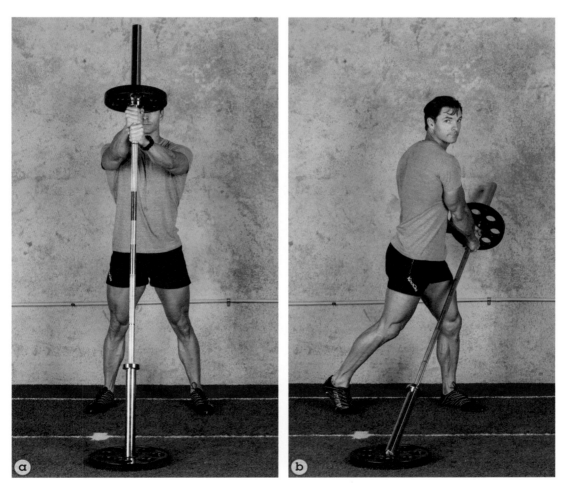

Figure 3.49   Wrestles. *(a)* Starting position. *(b)* Lower the weight to the left.

Pendulum

This exercise will have you doing your best impression of a windscreen wiper. You will drive away with a roadworthy set of abs.

Muscles

Abs, obliques

Execution

1. Lie flat on your back with your arms out to your sides and your legs together. Slowly raise your legs until your feet are perpendicular to your hips (figure 3.50a). Keep your legs together.

2. Contract your abs like a crunch. Slowly roll your legs to the left as far as you comfortably can while keeping a slight bend in your knees (figure 3.50b).

3. Pause, return your legs to the centre and repeat to the right.

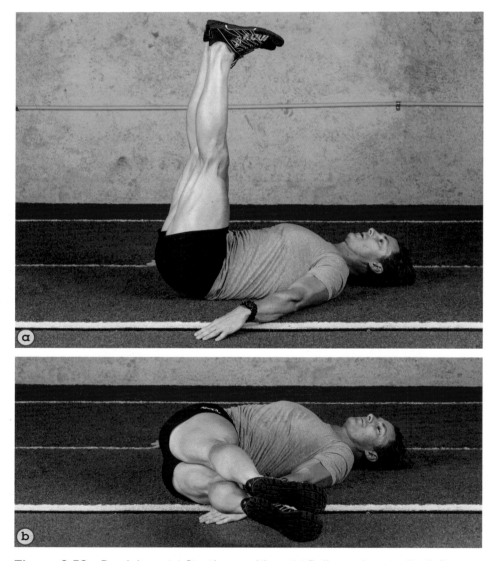

Figure 3.50 Pendulum. *(a)* Starting position. *(b)* Roll your legs to the left.

V-Knee Tuck

The power to spring up off the ground will be yours to flaunt after you get good at this up-and-at-'em move.

Muscles

Abs

Execution

1. Lie faceup on the floor with your knees bent at 90 degrees and your feet raised so that your thighs are perpendicular to the floor. Your arms should be straight at your sides and your palms should face in.

2. Slowly extend your legs so they're 45 degrees from the floor. At the same time, raise your upper body so your torso is also 45 degrees from the floor. Extend your arms (figure 3.51a). Holding this position, slowly draw your right knee in to your chest (figure 3.51b), then extend it back out.

3. Repeat the motion with your left leg. Continue to alternate legs. Go slowly. To keep your pace slow enough to be effective, imagine that each foot is resisting something heavy.

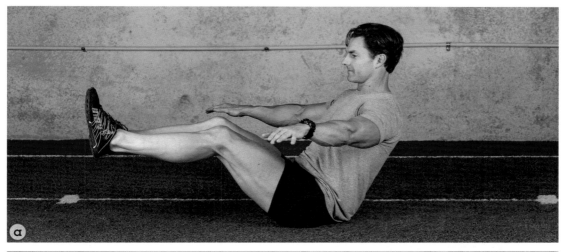

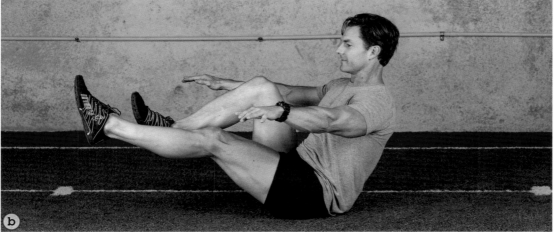

Figure 3.51   V-knee tuck. (a) Extend your legs and arms. (b) Bring your knee in to your chest.

Become a Leg Man

Your thighs are made up of three major muscle groups: quadriceps, which run down the front of your legs; hamstrings, which run down the back of your legs; and glutes, which are the muscles you're sitting on right now. You can isolate them, but they work best when trained as a team.

Your calves are made up of two major muscles: the soleus and the gastrocnemius. Seated calf exercises work the former and standing calf exercises work the latter.

Powerful Thighs

Legs may not top your hit list but they're crucial to looking symmetrical and propping up a muscular upper body. More importantly, they determine how fast you run, how far you jump and how powerful your entire body is. Big exercises, such as the squat, work so many muscles that they force your body to release testosterone, which makes all your muscles—yes, even your arms—grow. When your pins are strong they'll support all your favourite muscles, thereby shoring you against injury and providing stamina and balance. Even if you don't play sports, strong and muscular legs will come in use every day. Here are the golden rules for upgrading your twigs to trunks.

Vary Your Repetitions

Your upper thighs work very hard and are one of your body's biggest muscle groups. They're called into play every time you take a step and are capable of handling huge volumes of work. If you're fast at sprinting, chances are your upper-thigh muscles will grow with low reps (six to eight), but if you're a bit slower they're probably more suited to endurance and will grow with sets of 12 to 20 reps. Whether you're fast or slow, mix it up and even bash out a drop set at the end of your heavy sets to make sure.

Keep Your Back Straight

All leg exercises—on a machine or not—require that you keep your back straight. Fail to do this at the cost of your spine, which is a pretty important asset if you enjoy taking a walk. If you bend or round your back while training your legs, your lower back will start to raise the weights and you'll make more trips to the chiropractor than to the boardshorts store. It took a few million years to straighten your spine, so don't make Darwin roll in his grave.

Go Low

It's universally accepted that the squat is the very best leg exercise. With this in mind, a lot of trainers say you should bend your knees only until the bottoms of your thighs are parallel to the ground. The strange thing is that your legs can bend until your hamstrings touch your calves. Your body can and should be able to move through its fullest range of motion, so train it through that range of motion to maximise your muscle gains. It's different if you have injuries. But if you don't, remind yourself that a five-year-old can do a full squat and that if he can do it without weights, you should start trying it with weights.

Give Them Rest

Make sure you don't overtrain your legs. If you're doing a leg day, think about when you're going to do cardio. Running, riding, rowing and cross-training all demand huge effort from your legs. Regularly putting them to work on cardio machines and a steady diet of weight training can hedge you towards overtraining. The least offensive is rowing, where your upper body does the work, and swimming laps, which is kind on your joints and more focused on your upper body. Mix up your cardio to spare a thought for the muscles that are kind enough to take you everywhere.

Kick Off Your Kicks

When training legs, try to avoid wearing overly cushioned shoes, especially those you run in. This kind of footwear is designed to absorb impact. If you have a weight on your back, your heels will compress into your shoes, which can compromise the strength of your ankles and cause injury. Instead, use weight-lifting or barefoot running shoes when training legs. You'll put your feet in the most natural position, thereby strengthening all your joints and muscles in the right places. Just don't tell Nike.

Use All Angles

Most people train their legs in an up–down (squat) or backward–forward (lunge) motion. However, your body doesn't work exclusively in these planes of movement. Try stepping to the side and then bending your knees when you do your lunges. Side lunges work the muscles responsible for keeping your legs balanced. Apply this knowledge to all your leg exercises and you'll have more rounded legs that'll deliver match-winning performances on the pitch.

Never Lock Out Your Knees

Locking out your knees at the top of any leg exercise immediately steals the tension from the muscles and slaps it onto your kneecaps. Be it on lunges, squats, deadlifts or leg presses, a locked knee is asking for an injury and instantly makes an exercise easier because it creates a moment during which the muscle doesn't have to flex. And, as you know, easier means that less muscle is worked.

Change Your Foot Positions

Your feet don't always need to be parallel to one another or hip-width apart. To add a little variation to your routine, stagger your stance for moves such as the squat and deadlift by putting one foot slightly in front of the other. Or place your feet in an overly wide or very narrow stance. Each variation works new parts of your legs and is a welcome addition to your leg-development routine.

Go One-Legged

Work too much with barbells and you'll create a strength disparity. The problem is that switching a dumbbell for a barbell isn't enough to correct these imbalances because both legs push your body away from the ground. To make yourself more balanced and develop legs that are completely symmetrical, add a single-leg exercise to your routine. Try doing a squat or deadlift one legged and you'll challenge new areas of all your muscles.

Don't Rely Solely on Machines

So many fancy leg machines are out there, but almost all of them require you to work your legs in isolation so that your abs and every other muscle are switched off. This might be great if you're a bodybuilder trying to isolate a very specific muscle. But if you're looking for more muscle everywhere, free-weight exercises will always help you run towards your goal rather than walk there. Machines are useful on occasion, such as when doing drop sets or when injured, so the best plan is a healthy mix of both machines and free-weight exercises. Just don't limit yourself solely to machines. The exercises in this section show you how to put these wheels into motion.

Carved Calves

Of all the muscles in your body, the soleus and gastrocnemius—those resistant little tykes—are the most difficult to grow. Legendary trainer Vince Gironda, an exercise advisor to juggernauts such as Lou 'The Hulk' Ferrigno and Arnold Schwarzenegger, once said, 'The only attributes a person ever needs to look athletic are big calves, wide shoulders and a narrow waist.' When you're in boardshorts, big upper thighs mean diddly but a set of well-defined calves makes you look like a pro sportsman. What's more, genetics play a huge part in how big these muscles will get, so thank grandpa the next time you see him. Fortunately, the tips and tricks that follow will help you defy your DNA.

Do Hamstring Curls

Hamstrings are a supporting muscle of your calves, so it makes sense to rope them into your calf-training routine. Doing hamstring curls with your feet pointing away from your body works your calves much harder than if you point your toes upwards. Mix four sets of hamstring curls into your calf-training routine.

Do 15 to 25 Repetitions Per Set

Every step you take involves your calves, which makes them the hardest-working muscles in your body. To challenge them enough to make them grow, you have to work them with high repetitions. Check out the calves of the next obese person you see; chances are he has enormous calves that any bodybuilder would kill for. Calves respond to high reps (the equivalent of walking) with a heavy load. They also recover fast, so you can train them every day if they're not developing. Just don't try to justify your next trip to McDonald's as a way to build bigger calves.

Work Through the Fullest Range of Motion

When doing raises, lower the weight all the way down until you feel a stretch in your calves. Then raise the weight up, hold it for a second and release. Calves kick into action during the lowest and highest points of each lift. Stretch your calves on rest days to deepen the distance you can dip during each rep.

Kick Off Your Shoes

Trainers and sneakers are designed to help you flex your feet and ankles, but you should force your calves to do all the work without any help from springs and extra cushioning. You can keep your socks on—just make sure they're fresh or you'll stink out the gym. This shoeless technique was pioneered by Schwarzenegger, who had notoriously small calves to start with. He cut the bottom halves of his trousers legs off to draw attention to his calves and force himself to concentrate on growing them. You may not have to go to those extremes, but you might want to make sure you're wearing clean socks.

Rise Onto Your Toes

Do at least four sets of your workout with weights that are light enough to allow you to completely rise up onto your toes like a ballerina and hold the position. This will fully flex your calves at the top of each move. Alternatively, you can hold onto a support, stand on one leg and rise up onto the toes of the leg you're standing on. Do this between sets during your upper-leg workout.

Schedule Calf Training

Give your calves as much attention as you give your biceps. However many sets and exercises you do for arms, do the same amount for calves except do 15 to 25 reps in each set. After all, a man with perfect proportions has arms as big as his calves. This will ensure that you're giving your calves the workload they need to grow. Try to keep them under tension for more than 40 seconds in each set.

Keep Your Feet Straight

Pointing your feet in or out during an exercise doesn't hit your calves from different angles; it merely makes the exercise less effective and can cause injury. You won't work your calves in the direction the muscle inserts into your bones, so the workload will be less. Keep it straight and simple for fast results.

Train Your Shins

Most men train only the backs of their calves by lifting their heels up and down. Training your shins as well can add mass to your lower legs. Lie back on a bench with your lower legs hanging diagonally off the edge. Hold a dumbbell between your feet. Lower and raise the weight to target your shins. Alternatively, do calf pushes on the leg-press machine.

Feel Them Working

Put your mind into the muscle and avoid bouncing the weight. Take two seconds to lift the weight and another two seconds to lower it. Make small adjustments with your feet to keep constant tension on the muscles throughout the set. If you don't feel them working with 15 to 25 reps, do 100-rep sets using only your body weight. This may seem light, but your calves will be stiffer than a corpse the next day. And that means growth.

Grab Them While They Work

Hold onto your calves while you do seated calf raises and push into the muscles. This will help you feel them working, which will strengthen your mind–body connection and help you make minor adjustments to your form in order to make the exercise target the belly of your calf muscle. Doing this during the standing version of the exercise might be a little tough. Check out the following exercises you can use if you were short-changed with flimsy lower-leg genetics.

Squat

People widely agree this is one of the best exercises of all time for all of your muscles. If you can't do it, learn how. This move will give you the leg strength to hold your girl on your shoulders at the next concert—for at least six songs, anyway.

Muscles

Glutes, hamstrings, quads, calves, abs

Execution

1. Stand with your feet shoulder-width apart. Rest a barbell on the back of your shoulders if you're more advanced or hold dumbbells in your hands (figure 3.52a).
2. Bend your hips and knees simultaneously to lower yourself towards the ground (figure 3.52b). Stop when the bottoms of your thighs are parallel to the floor, but lower yourself past this point if it feels comfortable.
3. Straighten your knees and rise to the starting position along the same path.

NOTE   Always keep your back straight and knees in line with your feet.

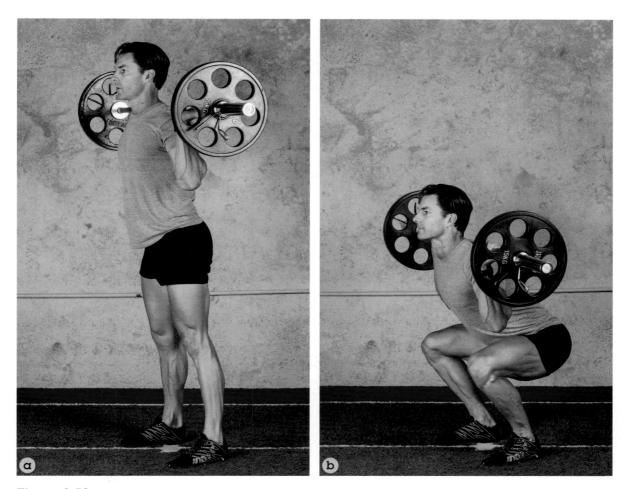

Figure 3.52   Squat. *(a)* Starting position. *(b)* Bend your knees and lower yourself towards the ground.

Step-Up

Get ready to tackle the staircase to muscle heaven.

Muscles

Quads, hamstrings, glutes, shoulders, abs

Execution

1. Stand with your feet shoulder-width apart facing a bench or flat platform that's about .6- to .9-metre high. If you're advanced, hold a dumbbell in each hand and let your palms rest against your sides.

2. Lift your right knee to step up and place your foot on the bench (figure 3.53a). Push down with you right leg to straighten your leg and raise your entire body upwards (figure 3.53b).

3. Step back to the starting position using your opposite leg and repeat the movement using that leg. You've now taken your first steps towards legs that look worthy in the shortest of shorts.

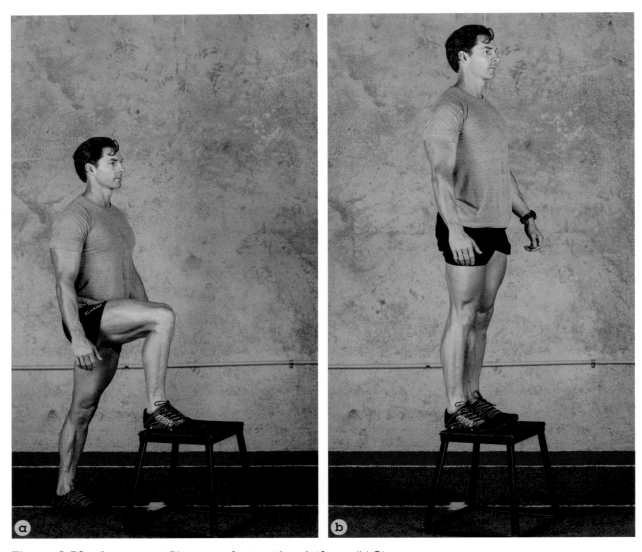

Figure 3.53 Step-up. (a) Place one foot on the platform. (b) Step up.

Lunge

Lunging about like a mad man is probably the sanest way to build insanely large legs.

Muscles

Glutes, hamstrings, quads, calves, abs

Execution

1. Stand with your feet hip-width apart (figure 3.54a). If you're advanced, rest a barbell across the back of your shoulders or hold dumbbells in each hand.

2. Take a giant, John Cleese-style step forward with your right foot and bend your right knee until your right thigh is parallel to the floor and your knee forms a 90-degree angle (figure 3.54b).

3. Reverse the motion and step back into the starting position. Be careful not to fall over as you start to feel tired—and you will soon feel tired. Keeping your balance on one foot can be tough. Repeat with your right limb for the leg strength to carry a backpack to Nepal and back.

NOTE   Keep your back straight throughout the exercise.

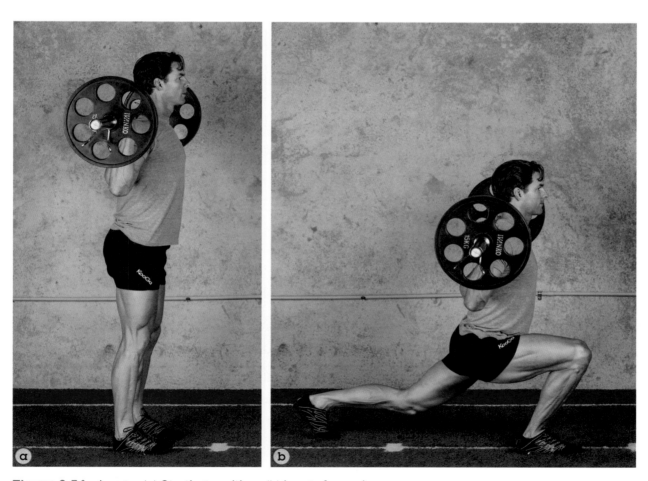

Figure 3.54   Lunge. *(a)* Starting position. *(b)* Lunge forward.

Split Squat

Overinflated arms are nothing if you don't have a set of legs to back them up.

Muscles

Quads, hamstrings, glutes, abs

Execution

1. Stand in the lunge position with your right foot forward (figure 3.55a). If you're more advanced, rest a barbell across the back of your shoulders or hold a dumbbell in each hand.
2. Bend both knees until your back knee is about three centimetres off the ground (figure 3.55b). Rise back up to the starting position.
3. Switch legs and go again. Push starting your car by yourself will no longer be a problem.

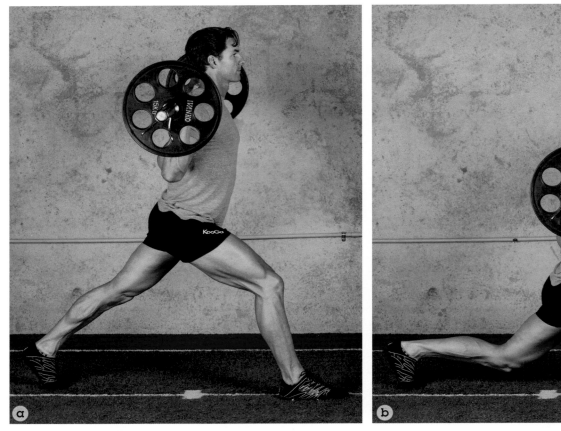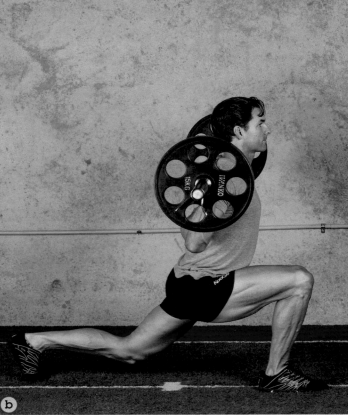

Figure 3.55 Split squat. *(a)* Starting position. *(b)* Bend your knees and lower yourself towards the ground.

Leg Press

Carve out teardrop-shaped slabs of muscle above each knee that'll kickstart another machine—your bicycle—into going faster.

Muscles

Quads, hamstrings, glutes, calves

Execution

1. Slot yourself in a leg-press machine for a mini man-versus-machine battle that'll make John Connor proud. Place your back and glutes flat against the back pad and your feet hip-width apart on the platform above you.
2. Press the weight up until your legs are straight. Do not lock your knees (figure 3.56a).
3. Release the support bar and slowly lower the weight until your legs are bent to 90 degrees (figure 3.56b). Push the weight back up until your legs are straight, keeping your knees unlocked.

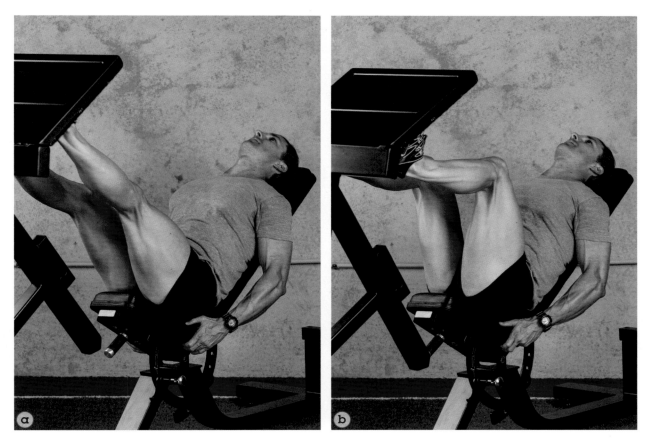

Figure 3.56 Leg press. *(a)* Straighten your legs. *(b)* Lower the weight until your legs are bent to 90 degrees.

Leg Extension

Time for a bit of man-versus-machine action. By the end of your battle against the weight stack you'll have the power to boot a soccer ball into the next post code.

Muscles

Quads

Execution

1. Sit at a leg-extension machine with your buttocks flush against the seat. Tuck your ankles under the footpads.
2. Slowly extend your legs up and forward until they are straight in front of you. Do not lock your knees (figure 3.57).
3. Pause and then slowly bend your knees until your legs are lowered back down.

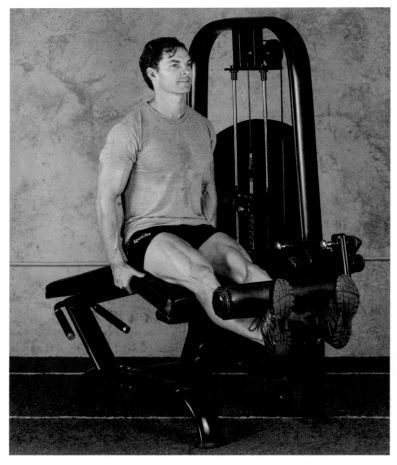

Figure 3.57　Leg extension.

Jumping Split Squat

This exercise is aptly named for its ability to rip the crotch out of unsuspecting training shorts. Beware, those who wear running shorts.

Muscles

Glutes, hamstrings, quads, calves, core

Execution

1. Stand in the lunge position with your right leg forward, your left leg behind you and your knees slightly bent (figure 3.58a). If you wish, hold a light weight plate or dumbbell in each hand and let it rest against your sides.
2. Bend your knees and jump up (figure 3.58b). Cross your legs while in the air and land with your left foot forward and your right foot behind you.
3. Bend your knees when you land to absorb the impact.

NOTE   If you have knee issues, do these with your body weight only.

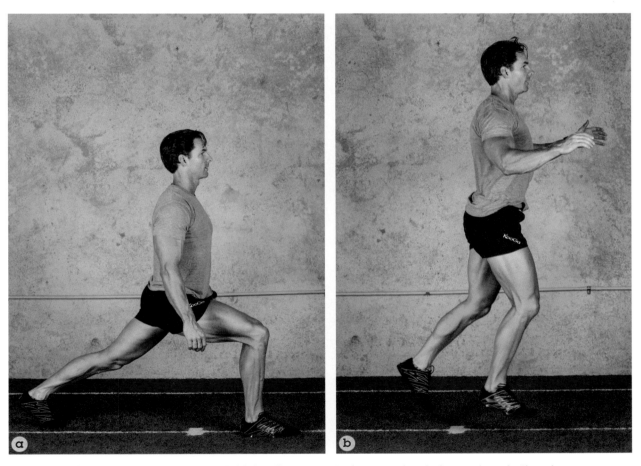

Figure 3.58 Jumping split squat. *(a)* Initial split squat. *(b)* Jump and switch your legs in the air.

Hamstring Curl

Hamstrings may not be flashy muscles you flex for your buddies, but they are responsible for the glory when you side-step an opponent on a sport pitch. And that's something you'll want to flex in public.

Muscles

Hamstrings, glutes

Execution

1. Lie on a hamstring machine with your torso pressed flat on the platform. Place your ankles under the pads.
2. Bend your legs and curl the pads up to your glutes (figure 3.59).
3. Take three to four seconds to lower the pads to the starting position. It's pretty tough to get this one wrong because there's only one way to work this machine.

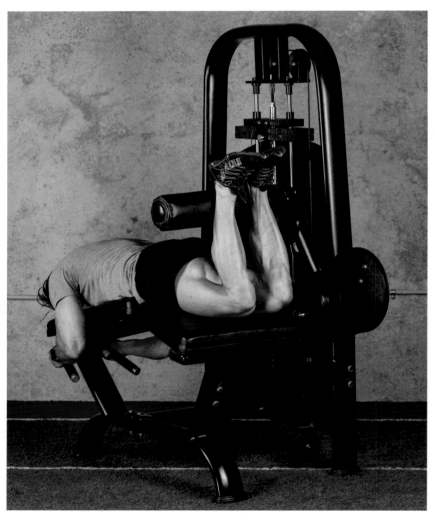

Figure 3.59   Hamstring curl.

Stiff-Legged Deadlift

This move will help your back and legs stand tall in your golden years when your mates are hobbled over their walking sticks.

Muscles

Hamstrings, lower back, abs

Execution

1. The form of this exercise is the same as that of the traditional deadlift except you keep your knees straight, though not completely locked, throughout the lift. Stick a barbell in front of you and grab it with an overhand grip (figure 3.60a).
2. Straighten your back and pick up the barbell. Keep it as close to your body as possible (figure 3.60b).
3. Take two to three seconds to lower the barbell to the starting position. This will strengthen and stretch your hammies, which is good for the sport pitch as well as for freeing up some new positions behind closed doors.

NOTE Don't sacrifice form by rounding your shoulders forward to get a bigger range of motion.

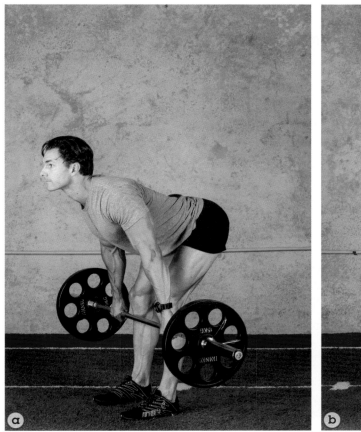
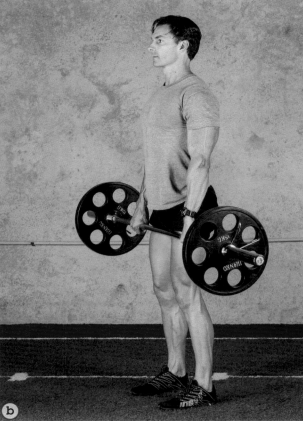

Figure 3.60 Stiff-legged deadlift. (a) Starting position. (b) Pick up the barbell.

Seated Calf Raise

This exercise will help you develop calves that can stand up to the chunkiest of sneakers.

Muscles

Calves

Execution

1. Sit on the edge of a bench and rest the balls of your feet on a step or box with your heels hanging off the edge. Place weights on your knees and hold them in place with your hands.

2. Push down on the toes of your feet and raise your heels as high as you can (figure 3.61a). Don't worry—no one will accuse you of impersonating a ballerina.

3. Pause, lower your heels towards the floor as far as you can (figure 3.61b) and then raise them again. Keep going for calves that look like cows. Alternatively, you can use the seated calf machine and save yourself the trouble of holding the weights.

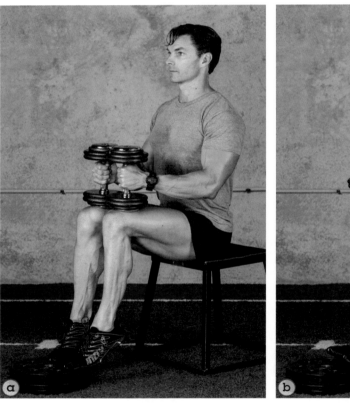
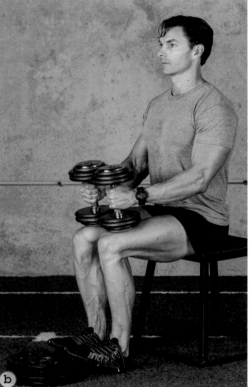

Figure 3.61 Seated calf raise. *(a)* Raise your heels. *(b)* Lower your heels.

Standing Calf Raise

Carved lower legs are what count in boardies. Start to shore up for the summer now.

Muscles

Calves, abs

Execution

1. Rest the balls of your feet on the edge of a step, raised platform, or weight plate. Two thirds of both feet should be suspended in midair. Hold onto a support for balance if you need to.

2. Lower your heels towards the ground (figure 3.62a). Just before your heels touch the ground, rise up onto your toes (figure 3.62b) and hold this position for three to five seconds. Regardless of the rep counts in the workouts, you can do as many reps as you can bear to jackhammer more size into your lower legs.

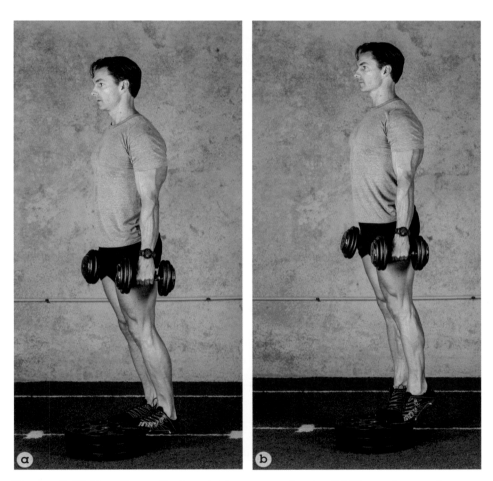

Figure 3.62 Standing calf raise. *(a)* Lower your heels. *(b)* Rise onto your toes.

Where Now?

You've now had a good look at the kind of stuff you'll be doing. Feeling a little nervous? You shouldn't. It's very much the same as starting a new job. The first day leaves you feeling as though you're in way over your head. But after a month at the grind it becomes second nature and so routine that you laugh about feeling nervous about it. Remember this moment. If this is the first time you've considered taking exercise seriously, it is the last time you'll ever feel anxious about it. You can also take solace in the fact that the next chapter is all about something you know plenty about: chilling out. You've no doubt dented a couch in your time. Keep reading to find out how doing that and other relaxing tasks will help you achieve your goals faster.

Cooling Down and Stretching

4

Stretching is like taxes. Neither are things you really want to do, but both can carry some pretty serious penalties if you ignore them. There's no question that flexibility is important. If you didn't stretch, you'd end up with a posture that required you to ring church bells. However, it is difficult to find any huge benefit in being able to do the splits.

There are different kinds of stretching—seven to be exact—but the main kinds you should concern yourself with are static and dynamic stretches. Static stretches involve keeping a muscle at the end of its range of motion, such as touching your toes and holding the position. These stretches pull your muscle fibres apart, which means they'll have a farther distance to travel when you contract them during exercise. You should save these for your cool-down after exercise.

For your warm-up, perform dynamic stretches. Slowly and rhythmically mimic the movements you'll be doing during your training session. This strategy will shoot blood into your working muscles and lube up your joints, making you more prepared for that bench press or sprint race.

That's the long and short of stretching. The following is a quick list of facts you need to know before you stretch out on the mat. Get ready to have a few myths busted.

Stretching Won't Cure Your Cowboy Swagger

The idea that stretching after a workout prevents stiffness and pain is a myth. Cochrane Researchers (Herbert, de Noronha and Kamper, 2010) analysed 10 trials on stretching and found that it did nothing to heal the post-workout hurt regardless of whether it was performed before or after a workout. That's right: Your junior-school sport coach was wrong.

Stretching Doesn't Completely Stop Injuries

Stretching before a run will not safeguard you against hobbles. In a study presented at the 2011 Annual Meeting of the American Academy of Orthopaedic Surgeons, Pereles and McDevitt (2011) analysed almost 3,000 runners and found that stretching before exercise neither prevented nor caused injury. That's your license to scoff at marathoners stretching at the starting line.

Your Heart Will Thank You

Long periods of stretching will keep your ticker in metronomic health. Research in *International Journal of Medical Engineering and Informatics* (Sunkaria, Kumar and Saxena, 2010) shows that heart rate variability, a sign of a healthy heart, is better in yoga practitioners—people who stretch regularly—than in nonpractitioners. Seems all that rhythmic breathing calms you from the inside out.

You'll Fix Your Back

Yoga is more effective for treating low-back pain than conventional exercise or getting a self-care book about the condition, according to a study in *Annals of Internal Medicine* (Sherman et al., 2005). Touch your toes regularly and you won't be pimping a walking stick anymore.

It'll Put a Smile on Your Face

Stretching for long periods of time is brilliant for improving your mood and lowering anxiety. No wonder yoga instructors always seem just a little bit smug.

Half a Minute Is All You Need

When it comes to stretching, a quick game is a good game. Research in *Physical Therapy* (Bandy, Irion and Briggler, 1997) found that holding a stretch for 30 seconds increased flexibility as much as holding the same stretch for 60 seconds. Don't waste a precious minute on a single muscle. Spread your time across all your muscles instead.

Once a Day Is Enough

Like anything else, stretching is addictive, but there's no need to overindulge. Research in *Physical Therapy* (Bandy, Irion and Briggler, 1997) found that stretching once a day yielded the same flexibility as stretching three times a day. Even if your ambitions are to be a yogi master, limit yourself to one stretch a day.

Hot and Cold Can Be Good

Treating your muscles with hot or cold packs can increase the effectiveness of the stretch, found research in *Physician and Sports Medicine* (Shrier and Gossal, 2000). For the best results, ice or heat the muscle you're stretching.

Be Quick to Be Powerful

Stretching your muscles dynamically before training will improve the power of the muscles you've stretched, found research in *Journal of Strength and Conditioning Research* (Yamaguchi and Ishii, 2005). The same can't be said for static stretching or not stretching at all.

Run to Stretch

If you're a runner or any other kind of athlete, you should stretch even though the benefits aren't always crystal clear. Research in *Clinical Journal of Sports Medicine* (Shrier, 2004) found that regular stretching improves force, jump height and speed, although no evidence suggests that it improves running economy.

You might notice that a lot of the information about the benefits seems to be contradictory, but at least you know that stretching, like your taxes, does produce some return on your exercise investment. Why should you bother stretching? You never did it when you were a youngster and you felt pretty good back then. That's actually the most important reason you should stretch. One of the whips Father Time uses in his aging arsenal is inflexibility. As you get older your muscles shrink and start to do exactly what they've been trained to do over the years: lock into bad positions. Many geriatrics adopt a hunched-over posture not because they've lost a penny but because they've subconsciously trained their bodies over the years to adapt to that position. If you sit at a desk or drive a car for long periods of time, your body adjusts by finding the easiest way to hold that arrangement. It starts to lock your fascia, tendons, muscles and ligaments into whatever position you've put them in over the years. Trouble rears its head and pain becomes a problem when you can't get out of the posture you've created. This is when stretching can be beneficial: It helps you hit the reset button on your muscles and put them back in their natural position.

Full-Body Stretch Routine

Performing the following stretching routine takes only about 10 minutes. Do it after any workout while your muscles are still warm, or do it in front of the television if you need to be distracted in order to drudge through the boredom of stretching. You can even use very light weights on some of the moves to go deeper into each stretch. This strategy will help improve your range of motion and flexibility more than the garden-variety bodyweight stretches will. Instead of trying to touch your toes, use a one- or two-kilogram dumbbell to help you hold each stretch for as long as you need to rest between sets. It's a good idea to do these stretches between sets during a workout, especially if you find stretching boring. You have to do the routine only once a week if you're already flexible or three times a week if you move like a rusty shed door. It doesn't require a great deal of time and will keep you broad chested and wide shouldered, which will instantly make you look bigger and leaner.

Inner Thighs

Sit with your feet together and your back straight. Push down on your knees with your elbows (figure 4.1). Hold for 30 seconds.

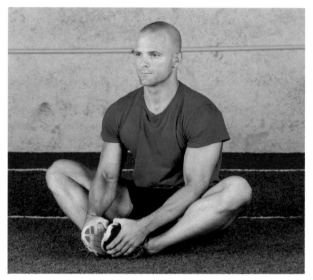

Figure 4.1   Inner-thigh stretch.

Hamstrings

Sit on the ground with your back straight, your legs out in front of you and your knees straight. Touch your feet with both hands (figure 4.2) and hold for 30 seconds.

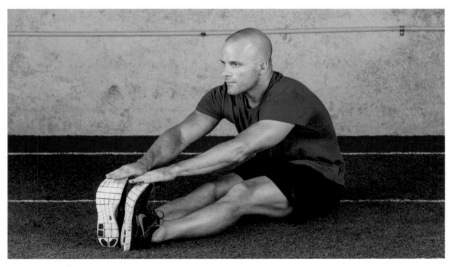

Figure 4.2   Hamstring stretch.

Spine

Begin in the hamstring-stretch position (figure 4.2). Keep your left leg stretched out in front of you and cross your right leg over the thigh of your left leg. Place your left elbow on your right knee and twist your body away from your outstretched leg (figure 4.3). Hold for 30 seconds, then switch sides.

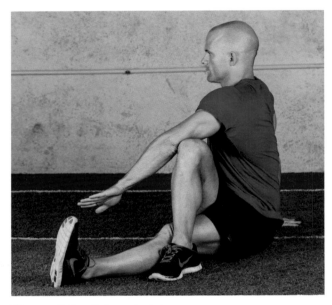

Figure 4.3   Spine stretch.

Glutes

Lie on your back. Bring your left knee to your chest and place your right foot on top of your left thigh. Hold your left leg in place with both hands and pull it towards you to go deeper into the stretch (figure 4.4). Hold for 30 seconds, then switch sides.

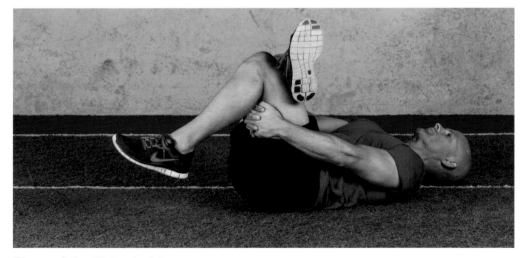

Figure 4.4   Glute stretch.

Core and Lower Back

Lie on the ground with your legs straight and arms outstretched. Bring your left knee over your right leg and hold it as close to your waist as possible with your right hand (figure 4.5). Leave your left arm outstretched. Hold for 30 seconds, then switch sides.

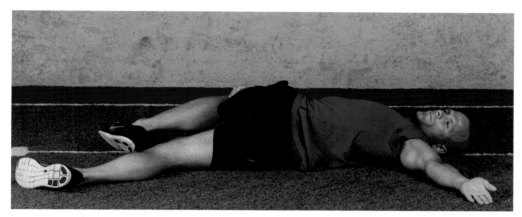

Figure 4.5   Core and lower-back stretch.

Calves

Get into a push-up position and rest the toes of your right foot on the heel of your left foot. Push back and try to touch your left heel to the ground (figure 4.6). Hold for 30 seconds, then switch sides.

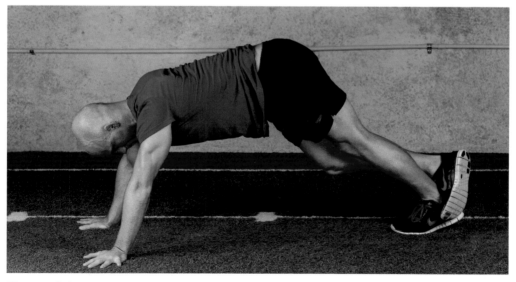

Figure 4.4   Calf stretch.

Lower Back

Assume a push-up position. Drop onto your elbows so that you're in the same position as the Egyptian Sphinx. Push your chest up (figure 4.7) and hold for 30 seconds.

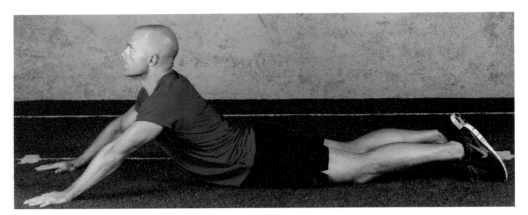

Figure 4.7   Lower-back stretch.

Lats

Assume a push-up position. Get to your knees and rest the palms of your hands on the ground. Try to sit back onto your heels (figure 4.8). Hold for 30 seconds at the deepest part of the stretch.

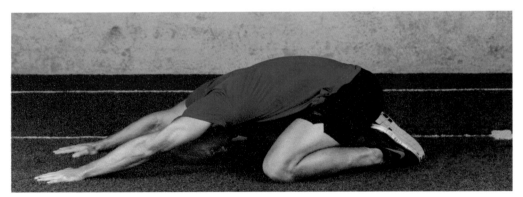

Figure 4.8   Lat stretch.

Quads

Stand on one foot (hold onto a railing if you need to) and bring the heel of your other leg towards your glutes. Hold your heel there with your hand for 30 seconds (figure 4.9), then switch legs.

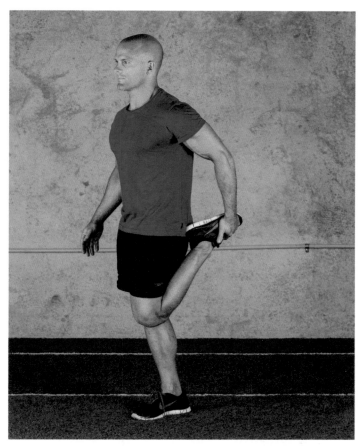

Figure 4.9 Quad stretch.

Chest

Stand with your feet shoulder-width apart and hold your hands together behind your back. Push your chest up and your shoulders back and down until your feel the stretch in your chest (figure 4.10). Hold for 30 seconds.

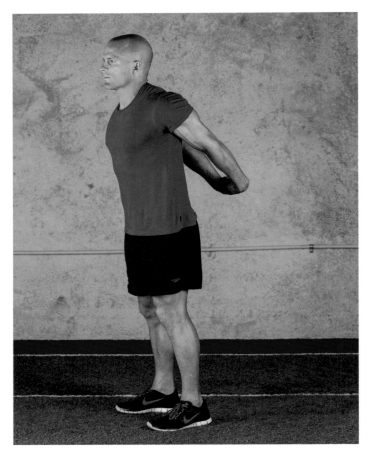

Figure 4.10 Chest stretch.

Rest and Recovery Postworkout

Many exercisers furiously pound the steel or treadmill during every free moment to make the most of their muscles. The peril of this is that the rewards often don't fit the efforts. Overtraining occurs when you exercise above and beyond your body's ability to adapt positively to working out. In short, you turn a positive into a negative. It's like galloping on a horse all day every day. For a while the horse will get stronger and faster, but without rest it will eventually tire out and muster only a lame canter. The solution to overtraining is the simplest of them all: Cut yourself some slack, do nothing and kick back. When people finally take a day off in their weekly strength programmes they often start to get stronger and bigger. That's because muscles grow during rest. So relax, put your feet up and read on to learn the secrets of doing nothing at all.

Get Out

Make your rest day active by leaving the house. To maintain fitness without burning out, a bloke needs active recovery. This means doing something other than the typical workout, such as a long walk or an activity that is recreational but not as intense as exercise. Croquet, anyone?

Think About Tomorrow

Doing a mental run-through of tomorrow's session will prepare your body better than any supplement or coach. Athletes who think about competition and success in their sport before bed often report faster running times and better performance. It's called mental prep. You're competing against yourself, so before bed challenge yourself to reach higher goals in tomorrow's session. You'll sleep your way to a better workout.

Triple Up on Fish Oil

If you feel like you can barely get out of bed or have had a particularly gruelling workout, be sure to load up on extra fish oil. You can take upwards of 12 1,000-milligram tablets a day to accelerate away from agonisingly painful muscles, especially after a hectic sport match or workout. The added fat will also give you a welcome boost in muscle growth. Just don't take fish oil before a date.

Eat Up

This is your day off, after all, so relax, treat yourself and pig out. If you want to put on muscle you have to put in the time at the table. Increase your protein intake on your rest days by approximately 25 per cent to cover your bases and make sure your muscles grow to their full potential. But eat your vice meals in moderation by taking them slowly. You don't want to undo all your hard work. You'll eat less but still feel satisfied if you take the time to enjoy your food. Try closing your eyes for 10 seconds midmeal to gauge your hunger. No longer feeling hungry? Stop eating.

Have a Lie-In

You probably need no encouragement to do this. Sleep is what helps you recover, and athletes who often sleep out (that is, sleep until they feel they have had enough) can get an advantage over their peers and perform better in competition the next day. Pump out more pillow time and you'll push more reps the next day. Tell her that if she tries to wake you up.

Stretch Away Stress

On your day off, substitute your couch-warming sessions with some time on the floor. Stretch for 10 minutes the muscle groups you last trained and the ones you are going to work the next day. This'll help you recover faster and prep you for the next day's session.

Melt Aches Away

If you don't have the luxury of a jumbo freezer to fuel a rest-day ice bath, try the polar opposite: a warm bath. It can be just as soothing for your aching muscles. How hot is hot enough to sizzle off your soreness? Our bodies are made up of 70 per cent water, so to maximise healing try get the water temperature near 36 degrees Celsius, your body's natural temperature. Use a thermometer if you have to. Much hotter and it becomes a monkey bath that'll have you going 'Oo-oo-aa-aa!' Add some Dead Sea salts to increase the recovery properties of the bath.

Keep Shaking

Just because you're not sweating doesn't mean your supplement plan should stand still. Your muscles demand nutrients to recover, so be sure to give them the fuel they need to rebuild and repair, even on your days off—this is when they need it most. Worried about the cost? If there's one thing you shouldn't play penny pincher with, it's protein. Stick with one to three protein shakes each day, spread out as evenly as possible, and your muscles will always be financed with the building blocks they need to grow.

Enjoy Your Lungs

Breathe in all the way down to your belly button. Hold for 5 to 10 seconds and exhale all the way out. Do five of these breaths three times a day and your energy level will be consistently higher throughout the day. Deep breathing disperses oxygen to all areas of your body and allows you to give 100 per cent in tomorrow's workout.

Keep Drinking

Drink 2 to 3 litres of water a day to remain hydrated and keep your energy levels high. A 500-millilitre glass of water before every meal has been proven to improve energy and help digest food, which allows you to gain its full nutritional value. Water makes up 70 per cent of your body and 85 per cent of your brain. Getting fully hydrated for a workout begins the day before.

Where Now?

You've trained, recovered and recuperated. The only thing left to do is reap the rewards: improved muscle tone and lower body fat. Now is not the time to rest on your laurels. You still have to challenge your muscles, and the best way to do this is move onto more advanced workouts. So keep reading because if you thought exercise was supposed to get easier, you're wrong. It's always supposed to be tough. That's how you force progress upon yourself.

Total Muscle Gaining for Beginners

Being new to weightlifting is one of the biggest muscle-building and fitness-inducing advantages you can have. Here's how to maximise your rewards.

Everyone has to start somewhere. Even the fittest of the fit had to walk into a gym a little wet behind the biceps. Fortunately, you've already put your best foot forward by educating yourself before you start training. When it comes to building muscle, losing weight and getting fit, it's far easier to go wrong than it is in to blindly stumble onto the right formula. When you're a total novice the best thing you can do is ease into training. If you strain so hard that the veins in your forehead read like a road map, the next day you'll feel stiffer than the Tin Man after a dip in the Pacific. Yes, it's only natural and expected to experience a little post-workout pain, but you shouldn't be bumping up the share price of your favourite ibuprofen. This is not the route you have to take.

The following is the most basic muscle-building plan for the everyman. If you have any injuries, see a professional to figure out whether you can do these moves. That said, you should expect to feel comfortable with all of these exercises. Some trainers may argue that these are advanced exercises and that novices should use machines first. However, these exercises involve essential, everyday actions (performed with a weight) that even a 5-year-old can do with a smile. If you can't perform these exercises, see a medical professional about fixing your imbalances before you start any kind of exercise programme. If you have a persistent, irresolvable injury, simply leave out the exercises you can't do and replace them with the nearest machine equivalent that your gym has to offer. See chapter 3 for detailed instructions about how to do the exercises. In less than four weeks you'll probably have to fork out some money for a few new shirts, it's a small price to pay for sleeve-splitting arms.

Getting Started

Perform the following workouts two to four times a week and perform a different workout each day (see tables 5.1 through 5.4). You don't need to do the workouts on the days of the week listed here—these are included just as an illustration—but make sure to either do them two days in a row with a rest day afterwards or alternate between rest and training days. Rest for 60 to 90 seconds between each set. Figure out during the first fortnight what weights you're capable of pushing. After this, try to increase the weights by 3 to 7 per cent each week. In a few short weeks you'll be the proud owner of a newly refurbished body made of box-fresh muscle.

BEGINNER'S PROGRAMME

WORKOUT 1 (MONDAY)

Table 5.1   Beginner's Programme Workout 1

Exercise	Sets	Reps
1. Squat (body weight)	3	15
2. Dumbbell flat chest press	3	15
3. Overhand-grip pull-up	3	15
4. Dumbbell deadlift	3	15
5. Lateral raise	3	15
6. Hammer curl	3	15
7. Triceps push-down	3	15
8. Bicycle crunch	3	15

Cardio

After the weights workout, jog, walk, elliptical train, row or cycle for 5 to 15 minutes.

WORKOUT 2 (TUESDAY)

Table 5.2   Beginner's Programme Workout 2

Exercise	Sets	Reps
1. Dumbbell incline chest press	3	12
2. Step-up (body weight or dumbbell)	3	12
3. Dumbbell bent-over row	3	12
4. Lunge (body weight or dumbbell)	3	12
5. Dumbbell seated shoulder press	3	12
6. Plank	3	60 sec.

Cardio

After the weights workout, jog, walk, elliptical train, row or cycle for 5 to 15 minutes.

WORKOUT 3 (THURSDAY)

Table 5.3   Beginner's Programme Workout 3

Exercise	Sets	Reps
1. Split squat (dumbbell)	3	15
2. Power clean	3	15
3. Parallel bar dip	3	15
4. Incline reverse fly	3	15
5. Lying leg raise	3	15
6. Seated calf raise	3	25
7. EZ-bar curl	3	15
8. Close-grip bench press	3	15

Cardio

After the weights workout, jog, walk, elliptical train, row or cycle for 5 to 15 minutes.

WORKOUT 4 (FRIDAY)

Table 5.4   Beginner's Programme Workout 4

Exercise	Sets	Reps
1. Squat (dumbbell)	3	12
2. Underhand-grip pull-up	3	12
3. Dumbbell chest fly	3	12
4. Dumbbell upright row	3	12
5. Single-arm dumbbell row	3	12
6. Good morning	3	12

Cardio

After the weights workout, jog, walk, elliptical train, row or cycle for 5 to 15 minutes.

Progressing the Programme

Phase 1 (weeks 1-8): Stick with the programme for around 2 months. However, if you have a little experience and your muscle building and fitness progression become stagnant, move onto phase 2. Try to increase the weights by 2 to 7 per cent each week. If you initially do bodyweight exercises such as squats, progress to doing weighted versions of those exercises in order to continually challenge yourself.

Phase 2 (weeks 8-12): Do 12 reps instead of 15. Increase the weights from phase 1 by 10 to 15 per cent and keep resting for a maximum of 60 seconds between sets.

Phase 3 (weeks 12-18): Do 10 reps. Do 4 sets instead of 3 and rest for 45 seconds between sets. Increase the weights from phase 2 by 10 to 15 per cent.

Finished? Well done: You're officially a weightlifter. Now try a few of the other beginner's workouts for another two to four months and you quickly progress to an intermediate lifter with the arms to match.

More Beginner Workouts

There's more than one way to get started. Don't be fooled into thinking that the grass is greener in someone else's programme. You might look at a guy who has the physique you want and see that his routine is totally different from yours. However, you don't need to do what he's doing to look like him. When you're a beginner, sticking to your guns produces the quickest gains.

You undoubtedly value your time and demand results right now, so you want the very best programme. Just don't chop and change too much. You see, no litmus test can tell you exactly how much muscle you'll add by the end of each programme. If a programme professes to build a specific amount of muscle or burn an exact amount of fat, its developers are simply guessing. Yes, workouts do differ slightly in effectiveness, but not by the pronounced effect that abs salesmen on the Internet would have you believe. In fact, the world's best programme done without focus will produce smaller results than an average programme done with determination, dedication and heart. The ugly truth is that all fitness- and muscle-building systems work. How well they work is based on your attitude and motivation.

With this in mind, all of the following well-respected beginner approaches are proven to stack on muscle quickly. Simply perform the exercises listed in the beginner's workout, keeping the exercise order the same if you like. If you become more experienced or just want a little change after two to three months, incorporate a few new exercises for the same muscle groups. But do keep off of machines. Yes, the flashy new contraptions are high tech and excellent, but no machine can compete with the mass- and fitness-building prowess of free weight. Once you have the exercises down pat, put them into action using the parameters outlined here. You can perform the exercises in the order specified in the beginner's workout or you can rearrange the order to first work your favourite muscles or the muscles you feel you need the most growth in. Stick to each muscle-building technique for six to eight weeks or until your gains start to taper off, then take a one-week break from all exercise and choose another muscle-building technique.

Injured Man's Plan

Do this super-slow programme if you need to work around an injury and if you're not training to improve at sport.

Super Slow

- Do full-body workouts and draw out each rep until even those little pink weights feel heavy.
- Do 1 or 2 sets of 6 to 8 reps of 12 exercises; do 1 exercise per muscle group. Perform 1 set of most exercises. However, you can perform 2 sets of exercises for body parts that you specifically want to grow.
- Take 5 seconds to lower the weights and 10 seconds to raise them.
- Perform 3 or 4 sessions per week.
- Take 1 minute of rest between each set and alternate resting and training days.
- Start with exercises for your legs and use a new set of exercises in each session each week. Do 10 to 12 exercises in each workout.

Equipment-Sparse Workout

Do this programme if you're working out at home and have access to only very light weights—it has a knack for making these weights feel extra heavy. In this static-training programme, you'll train your muscles without moving them. You'll hold weight in a fixed position for a set amount of time to resist gravity. The length of the muscle doesn't change and no visible movement occurs at the joint. This is called a static hold.

Static Training

- Warm up with 2 sets of 12 reps, using a full range of motion, of each exercise you're going to train statically. Do 2 or 3 sets of static holds, lasting 10 to 40 seconds, of each exercise. At the end of each static-hold set, reduce the weight by 40 per cent and do 6 full-range reps.
- In the warm-up sets, take 1 second to lower the weights and 1 second to raise them.

- Perform 2 to 4 sessions per week.
- Take 2 minutes of rest between each static-hold set. Alternate between resting and training days or take a resting day after training for 2 or 3 days.
- Perform full-body workouts and do 1 or 2 exercises for each major muscle group. Do 8 to 10 exercises in each workout.

Strength Builder

Do this programme if you want to build power and strength while devoting a good chunk of time to each session. In this pyramid-training programme, you'll start with light weights and do a high number of reps. On each successive set you'll increase the weight and decrease the number of reps. On the final one or two sets you'll reduce the weight and again do a high number of reps.

Pyramid Training

- On set 1 do 12 to 15 reps. (Remember that you'll increase the weight on each successive set.) On set 2 do 8 to 10 reps. On set 3 do 6 reps, and on set 4 do 4 reps. On set 5, decrease the weight to the initial level and do 12 reps or go until your muscles fail.
- Take 1 to 2 seconds to lower the weights and 1 to 2 seconds to raise them.
- Perform 2 to 5 sessions per week.
- Take 1 to 2 minutes of rest between sets and take a rest day after every 2 training days.
- Do full-body workouts (perform 1 or 2 moves per major muscle group) or body-part training routines (train 1 or 2 muscle groups per session).
- Pair the following muscles: chest and biceps, back and triceps, shoulders and abs. Train legs on their own. If you do body-part training, perform 3 or 4 exercises for each body part. Do 7 or 8 exercises in each workout.

Time-Poor Man's Workout

Do this quick-circuit programme if you are training during your lunch hour or can't commit a lot of time to exercise. To save time you'll do circuit-style workouts using compound, multijoint exercises such as squats, deadlifts or bench presses that target all major muscle groups. You'll rest briefly between sets to keep the intensity high and workouts short.

Quick Circuits

- To add muscle, do 4 to 6 sets of 8 to 12 reps of 4 to 12 exercises. To burn fat, do 4 to 6 sets of 15 to 20 reps of 4 to 12 exercises. To increase strength, do 4 to 6 reps of 4 to 8 exercises; do more sets and rest for longer periods.
- Take 2 to 4 seconds to lower the weights and 1 to 2 seconds to raise them.
- Perform 2 to 5 sessions per week.
- Take 20 to 60 seconds of rest between sets or do the moves as a no-rest circuit without any breaks. Take a rest day after 2 or 3 training days.
- Perform only free-weight exercises and never use machines. The best exercises are those that work the most muscle, such as squats, deadlifts, bench presses and pull-ups.

Burn Fat and Build Muscle

Do this programme if you want to get leaner while adding muscle. You'll also improve your sport performance; this is great if you've hit a muscle-building plateau. In this pulse-training programme, you'll perform 15 reps in each set. Perform the first 5 reps super fast, the next 5 reps slow and the last 5 reps at normal speed.

Pulse Training

- Use a weight you can manage 25 reps with, and never exceed 15 reps of 3 sets on each exercise.
- For the first 5 reps take 1 second to lower the weights and 1 second to raise them. For the next 5 reps take 4 seconds to lower the weights and 4 seconds to raise them. For the final 5 reps take 2 seconds to lower the weights and 2 seconds to raise them.
- Perform 2 to 5 sessions per week.

- Take 1 to 2 minutes of rest between each set and take a rest day after every 2 training days.
- For both the body-part and full-body workouts, train the biggest muscle groups first and their supporting cast afterwards. Pair the following muscles: chest and triceps, back and biceps, shoulders and abs. Train legs on their own. For body-part workouts do 3 or 4 exercises for each body part. For full-body workouts do 1 exercise for each muscle, alternating between upper- and lower-body exercises.

Where Next?

Congrats. You've now taken the first step towards transforming yourself and you can be proud of the work you've done. To continue improving, turn to the next chapter to learn ways to recover after tough sessions. When you're done, keep reading because chapter 6 presents intermediate workouts. Prepare yourself because the best (yes, that's you) is about to get better.

Total Muscle Gaining for Intermediates

You've been soldiering at it for a little while. The notches on your weight belt are mounting up and you greet the gym's receptionist by name. You've earned your spot under the squat rack, but now you want a little more. If you're not a crusty veteran just yet but no longer a baby, this is how to add to the burgeoning muscle investments you've already made. To make it to the intermediate level, you should have four to six months of training behind you.

The first thing you're going to increase is intensity, which refers to the sweat factor of your workouts. But don't dive into a 10-rep yawn-a-thon just yet because there are several ways to increase intensity; the best of these are listed in 'Refresh Your Workout'. The most well-respected and researched method is to use supersets. During a superset, you move from one exercise to the next without resting between sets. You've no doubt seen or heard of supersets or may have already given them a crack. But there's more to it than lumping any old exercises together. Recent research at Syracuse University (Kelleher et al., 2010) compared supersets with traditional straight sets—the ones you did in the beginner workouts. The researchers found that supersets burned more calories than did traditional straight sets and that the exercisers finished their sessions significantly faster. You may be thinking, 'I don't care about being ripped. I want muscle.' Well, that's exactly what you'll get. You burn more calories because your muscles have to work harder, which makes them grow bigger. You'll get both bigger and leaner in less time. You should now be starting to see the link between other super things such as heroes, sizing and Mario. What's more, you'll get results even faster if you choose your exercises wisely. Pairing antagonistic (opposing) muscle groups such as the back and chest or biceps and triceps shores you against injuries and boosts your muscle gains. Starting to get the picture? Train your body back to front and your muscles will become supersized. Keep reading to buy into this two-for-one muscle bargain.

Full-Body Intermediate Workouts

The intermediate workouts that follow stick with the full-body scheme. However, you can train two or three body parts in each session if you're tempted to try something completely different. If you choose this route, pair the following muscle groups together in the same workout.

Workout 1 (Monday): chest and back

Workout 2 (Tuesday): biceps and triceps

Workout 3 (Thursday): hamstrings, quadriceps, calves and glutes

Workout 4 (Friday): shoulders, abs and lower back

Wednesday, Saturday and Sunday are rest days.

Perform the same exercises listed in the full-body workouts that follow (see tables 6.1 through 6.4). Take a rest day after every 2 or 3 training days to make sure your body has enough recovery time. Take a 1- to 2-minute rest after each superset, but don't take a break between the two exercises in a superset. The workout should take 45 to 60 minutes. If you're consistently taking longer than an hour, then either do only 2 sets per superset or hurry the hell up, slacker.

INTERMEDIATE PROGRAMME

WORKOUT 1 (MONDAY)

Table 6.1
Intermediate Programme Workout 1

Exercise	Sets	Reps
Superset 1 (legs)		
1. Squat (barbell)	3	8
2. Dumbbell deadlift	3	8
Superset 2 (chest, back)		
3. Dumbbell flat chest press	3	8
4. Dumbbell bent-over row	3	8
Superset 3 (shoulders)		
5. Dumbbell seated shoulder press	3	8
6. Dumbbell flat pullover	3	8
Superset 4 (core)		
7. Lying leg raise	3	8
8. Back extension	3	8
Superset 5 (arms)		
9. Cable rope curl	3	8
10. Rope push-down	3	8

Cardio

After the weights workout, jog, walk, elliptical train, row or cycle for 5 to 15 minutes. During this workout, sprint for 10 seconds and then go easy for 30 seconds. Repeat until you've done as much as you can manage.

WORKOUT 2 (TUESDAY)

Table 6.2 **Intermediate Programme Workout 2**

Exercise	Sets	Reps
Superset 1 (chest, back)		
1. Dumbbell incline chest press	3	8
2. Dumbbell incline row	3	8
Superset 2 (legs)		
3. Lunge (dumbbell)	3	8
4. Good morning	3	8
Superset 3 (arms)		
5. Hammer curl	3	8
6. Standing triceps extension	3	8
Superset 4 (shoulders)		
7. Lateral raise	3	8
8. Incline reverse fly	3	8
Superset 5 (core)		
9. Hanging leg raise	3	8
10. Single-leg plank	3	60 sec.

Cardio

After the weights workout, jog, walk, elliptical train, row or cycle for 5 to 15 minutes. During this workout, sprint for 15 seconds and then go easy for 45 seconds. Repeat until you've done as much as you can manage.

WORKOUT 3 (THURSDAY)

Table 6.3 **Intermediate Programme Workout 3**

Exercise	Sets	Reps
Superset 1 (arms)		
1. Close-grip bench press	3	8
2. Barbell biceps curl	3	8
Superset 2 (shoulders)		
3. Arnold press	3	8
4. Dumbbell front raise	3	8
Superset 3 (legs)		
5. Hamstring curl	3	8
6. Split squat (dumbbell)	3	8
Superset 4 (chest)		
7. Inverted row	3	8
8. Dumbbell chest fly	3	8
Superset 5 (core)		
9. Superman	3	60 sec.
10. Barbell rollout	3	8

Cardio

After the weights workout, jog, walk, elliptical train, row or cycle for 5 to 15 minutes. During this workout, sprint for 30 seconds and then go easy for 90 seconds. Repeat until you've done as much as you can manage.

WORKOUT 4 (FRIDAY)

Table 6.4   Intermediate Programme Workout 4

Exercise	Sets	Reps
Superset 1 (chest, back)		
1. Overhand-grip pull-up	3	8
2. Parallel bar dip	3	8
Superset 2 (legs)		
3. Stiff-legged deadlift (barbell)	3	8
4. Step-up	3	8
Superset 3 (arms)		
5. EZ-bar skull crusher	3	8
6. EZ-bar curl	3	8
Superset 4 (core)		
7. Side plank	3	8
8. Lying leg raise with pike	3	8
Superset 5 (shoulders, calves)		
9. Cable face pull	3	8
10. Standing calf raise	3	8

Cardio

After the weights workout, jog, walk, elliptical train, row or cycle for 5 to 15 minutes. During this workout, sprint for 60 seconds and then go easy for 120 seconds. Repeat until you've done as much as you can manage.

Progressing the Programme

Phase 1 (weeks 1-6): Stick with the programme. However, if you feel your gains tapering off or backpedalling by week 4, then move to phase 2. Increase the weights by 2 to 5 per cent each week.

Phase 2 (weeks 6-12): Do 6 reps instead of 8. Increase the weights from phase 1 by 5 to 10 per cent and rest for a maximum of 60 seconds between sets. Again, increase the weights by at least 2 to 5 per cent each week.

Phase 3 (weeks 12-18): Do 12 reps of each exercise and rest for 45 seconds between sets.

That's it. You've no doubt fielded a few compliments about your box-fresh muscles. Now take a week off and then try the other intermediate workouts that follow.

More Intermediate Workouts

Already progressed from the first plan? The following workouts will keep you on a muscle-winning streak for years to come.

As is the case with beginner's workouts, there's always more than one way to do something. Whether you have sweated more than a sauna or less than Henry VIII, you'll benefit from mixing things up. Use the following guidelines to craft new workouts using the same exercises you've used to build your existing brawn. Feel free to use new exercises that you haven't tried. They'll add much-needed variety and help keep you interested and motivated.

The moves listed in chapter 3 are some of the very best for each muscle group. Use each of the techniques that follow for four to six weeks, but remember to do a little self-diagnosis. If you feel your gains tapering off, take a week off and switch to a new technique. Remember that progress isn't always linear or constant. Sometimes it comes in batches when you least expect it. You might train hard for weeks with no results and then all of a sudden progress slaps you in the face and your best lift jumps up by 20 kilograms or you stack on 2 kilograms of muscle. The results can seem instant and almost effortless but they are actually the work of months of consistent and persistent effort. So treat your muscles like a player, letting them bounce from one technique to the next, and you'll soon be rewarded with an avalanche of growth.

Size and Strength Builder

Do this programme if you want to build muscle size and strength at the same time. This system can be a little monotonous, so it requires focus and drive. This technique calls for 5 sets of 5 reps of each exercise using the same weight; this is called your working weight. You'll gradually increase it by 2 to 5 per cent each week.

5 × 5

- Do 5 sets of 5 repetitions of 3 or 4 exercises per muscle group. Train 2 or 3 muscle groups in each session.
- Take 2 seconds to lower the weights and 1 to 2 seconds to raise them.
- Perform 2 to 4 sessions per week.
- To build strength, rest for 3 minutes between sets. To build size, rest for 90 seconds between sets. For the middle road, take 2-minute breaks. To recover fully, take at least 1 rest day after every 2 training days.
- You can train by body part (train 1-3 muscles per session) or train in upper–lower body splits (train upper body in one workout and lower body in a separate workout). For body-part training, work your biggest muscles first and pair with noncompeting muscles, such as chest with biceps or back with triceps. Use only compound, multijoint exercises such as bench presses, squats, deadlifts, dips and barbell rows.

Tall Man's Plan

Do this programme if you have long limbs. This plan is excellent for isolating muscle groups, which can be tough if you're lanky. In this programme, you'll do a set of an isolation exercise for a muscle you're targeting and then do a compound, multijoint exercise for the same muscle. Doing the isolation move forces the targeted muscle to work harder during the compound move.

Pre-Exhaust Training

- Perform 10 to 15 reps of the isolation move and then do 6 to 10 reps of the compound exercise for the same muscle. That's a single superset. Do 2 or 3 supersets for each muscle group and train 1 or 2 muscle groups per workout.
- Take 2 seconds to lower the weights and 2 seconds to raise them during both the initial isolation move and the compound move that follows.

- Perform 1 to 4 sessions per week.
- Do the isolation and compound moves as a superset without resting between them. It's useful to set up both exercise stations before you start. Take 1 to 2 minutes of rest after each superset, and alternate training and rest days.
- Do body-part training and train 1 to 3 muscles in a workout. Work your targeted muscle and its supporting cast in the same workout. Train these muscles together: chest, triceps and shoulders; back and biceps; legs and abs. Perform 4 to 6 exercises per body part—2 or 3 isolation moves and 2 or 3 compound moves. Exercises on machines and single-joint exercises such as push-downs are best for isolation moves; free weights are best for compound exercises.

Cover Model Plan

Do this programme if you want to build muscle while losing fat but you don't fancy getting lean by running on a treadmill. To achieve the seemingly impossible—becoming large and lean at the same time—you'll alternate between weeks of low reps with heavy weights to build muscle and high reps with low weights to accelerate calorie-burning potential.

Large and Lean

- Alternate between a fat-burning phase (phase 1) and a muscle-building phase (phase 2). In phase 1, do 4 or 5 sets of 12 to 20 reps of each exercise. In phase 2, do 4 or 5 sets of 4 to 12 reps of each exercise using the most weight you can.
- In phase 1 (fat burning), take 1 second to lower the weights and 1 second to raise them; fast reps burn more calories. In phase 2 (muscle building), take 1 to 2 seconds to lower the weights and 1 to 2 seconds to forcefully raise them.
- Perform 4 sessions per week.
- In phase 1, take 15 to 30 seconds of rest between sets to keep your heart pumping. In phase 2, take 60 to 90 seconds of rest between sets. For both phases, either

train for 2 days and then take a rest day or alternate rest and training days.

- Do body-part training. In phase 1, couple the following muscles in a workout: back and biceps; legs and abs; chest and abs; shoulders and triceps. In phase 2, couple these muscles: chest and abs; quads and hamstrings; biceps and triceps; back and shoulders. Train 1 or 2 body parts per workout and do 2 to 4 compound, multijoint exercises for each. Do a new move in each phase to give your muscles a challenge. Avoid isolation exercises; they aren't good for building muscle or burning calories.

Blue-Collar Muscle

Do this programme if you work a physical job that can sap your strength.

In this high-intensity programme, you'll do short, very intense bursts of training followed by big spurts of rest to allow more recovery. The activity is brief and infrequent and you'll give 100 per cent. A high volume of exercise is unnecessary to grow. Intensity and rest work better.

High-Intensity Training

- Do just 1 set of 8 to 12 reps for each body part. Try to do more reps of each exercise than you did in your previous workout. When you can manage 12 reps with perfect form of an exercise, increase the weight by 3 to 5 per cent.

- Take 4 seconds to raise the weights and 4 seconds to lower them. Lift and lower the weights smoothly.

- Perform 1 to 4 sessions per week.

- Don't rest between sets. The time it takes you to put away the weights you've used and rack up the next set is all you need to recover. Alternate training and rest days.

- Do full-body workouts. Work your largest muscles (quads, hamstrings and glutes) first when you're fresh and then train your smaller muscles (shoulders, biceps, triceps and calves) at the end of the workout. Pick one compound, mul-

tijoint exercise that you can lift the most weight with for each muscle group and stick with it for the entire programme.

Sportsman's Muscle Builder

Do this speed-training programme if you want to improve your sport performance and overall endurance. It is also great for busting through a muscle-gaining plateau. As the name suggests, you'll perform reps as quickly as possible. Instead of just lowering a weight you'll push and pull it against gravity so that your muscles are responsible for every single inch of movement.

Speed Training

- Perform 3 to 5 sets of 15 to 30 repetitions (perform fewer, such as 4 to 6, if you want to build power) of 3 to 5 exercises for each muscle group. Use light weights; heavier weights won't allow you lift at breakneck speed.

- Lower and raise the weight as fast as you can.

- Perform 2 to 5 sessions per week.

- Take 45 to 60 seconds of rest between sets. Either take 1 or 2 rest days after every 2 training days or alternate training and rest days.

- You can do body-part training (work 2 muscle groups per session), an upper–lower body split or a full-body routine. Pair these muscles in the same workout: chest and abs; shoulders and biceps; back and triceps. Do legs on their own. Do 2 to 4 exercises for each body part. The best strategy is to exclusively perform compound, multijoint exercises. However, you can opt to do compound, multijoint moves for the first 1 to 3 exercises and then finish off with careful lifting on machine and isolation moves.

Refresh Your Workout

Hit your workout's refresh button by including these intensity-increasing tricks. On your mark. Get set. Grow.

Boredom. It affects everything, and your muscles are no exception. If you haven't been hitting your goals fast enough, you need to break the tedium. Quickly. Variety is vital because your body is the most adaptable thing you own—yes, even more than your iPhone. If you nag it with the same tedious routine, you'll look like the before picture rather than the after picture. If you're impatient about hitting your goals—and you should be—every sweat session should be tougher than a boiled pigeon. The fix? Hit the refresh button of any workout by including these intensity-increasing techniques on an ad hoc basis. Use them when you feel that a muscle group needs a little boost. Don't create an entire workout around these tips. Rather, throw them into an existing routine to make it more effective. They're pretty good at busting boredom and they'll revive your enthusiasm. Your visits to the stackhouse will start coughing up fast results that the redhead in accounts will comment on soon.

Drop Sets

When performing drop sets you do 6 to 10 reps of an exercise or as many as it takes for your muscles to fail. Then decrease the weight by 50 per cent and crank out another 6 to 10 reps with the reduced poundage. Drop sets fatigue your muscles in a short time, get your heart going and give you an impressive pump. To go one better, you can even do several drops sets of one exercise.

You can use drop sets in two ways. You can either do a drop set of each exercise in an entire workout or you can do them on the final two or three exercises of your session in order to get an extra muscle-burning kick before you hit the showers. Whichever line of attack you choose, do six reps with perfect form, then reduce the weight by half and complete another six reps. Warning: Drop sets will probably make your muscles feel like they have a curry stewing inside.

Eccentric Sets

In eccentric sets you take three to four seconds to lower a weight, or yourself, in order to force your muscles to work during the lowering por-

tion of an exercise instead of the lifting part. Dwelling on the negative will offer a positive gift to your muscles: size.

It's best to perform eccentric sets with a training partner. Getting trapped under the bar is fun only at the Keg and Whistle. Get your partner to boost as much of the weight as possible during the lifting phase, then lower all of it yourself. If you don't have a training partner, you can use machines instead of free weights in some instances. For example, if you use the biceps curl machine, you can raise the weight with both limbs and then lower it with one. Your spare limb becomes your training cohort. Unlike some partners, it's never late.

Cheat Reps

In cheat reps you use momentum from the rest of your body to overcome a sticking point as you tire at the end of a set. Most muscles fail on the lifting portion of an exercise before they fail on the lowering portion. Use momentum from the rest of your body to quickly and explosively lift a weight to the end position. Then take three times as long to lower it back to the starting position.

This technique is ideal for sport exercises that build explosive power, such as explosive push-ups or the power clean. But be careful: Cheat on only one or two exercises, do it early in your workout when you're fresh and thoroughly warm up first. Cheat reps can lead to injury, so only intermediate to advanced lifters should perform them.

Pre-Exhaust Sets

In pre-exhaust sets you pre-exhaust a muscle with an isolation exercise and then work it to failure with a compound, multijoint exercise. It's the gym-based equivalent of cleaning the bath with a toothbrush and then, as your fingers get tired, switching to a big brush. Doing the isolation move forces the targeted muscle to work harder during the compound move. Do pre-exhaust sets at the beginning of your workout while your muscles are still fresh.

Pre-exhaust sets are excellent time savers that target muscle groups very accurately and are perfect for muscles that work across multiple joints, such as the chest and shoulders. To isolate your chest, do a set of shoulder presses followed by a set of bench presses. You can better isolate your quads by doing a set of leg extensions before you do squats. You can also do postexhaust sets, which are the reverse of pre-exhaust sets. In a postexhaust set, do squats first and then a set of leg extensions. You can even set up an entire routine based on pre-exhaust sets.

Rest Pause

The rest pause method was developed by former Mr. Olympia Mike Mentzer, author of *High-Intensity Training the Mike Mentzer Way* (McGraw-Hill). In this method you take brief (5-20 seconds) rest periods during a set to give yourself extra energy to push out more reps. The extra energy will help you do 10 reps with a weight you can normally manage 5 reps with. This drives strength and size into your muscles.

Use this method on exercises that demand maximum effort, such as squats or bench presses. Use a weight you can manage three or four reps with. Finish the reps, rack the weight and rest for 15 to 20 seconds. Then try for another two or three reps. Repeat as many times as you can. In this case, resting is certainly not the pursuit of slackers.

Half Reps

When performing half reps you lift a weight through an incomplete range of motion of an exercise. Half reps are like a mini rep done with more weight than you'd usually use. If you've become stuck on the same weight for squats, you can use half reps to build the strength to blast through your sticking point (for example, standing up from the deepest part of the squat). Perform half reps through that sticking point to the midpoint of the exercise (for example, the part of the squat where you haven't stood up completely). This strengthens your muscles though that section of the lift and enables you to push more weight when you do reps through the full range of motion.

Half reps are great for starting and finishing a workout. At the start, use half reps to blast through your weak points of an exercise while you're still fresh so you can get stronger in an exercise you've stagnated on. At the finish, do them through your strongest parts of an exercise—after you've done all your reps using full range of motion—to build more strength endurance in that muscle. Yes, sometimes a half-hearted approach can pay dividends.

Static Holds

In static holds you hold a weight in a fixed position for 10 to 20 seconds to resist against gravity. Muscles grow in proportion to the tension they're placed under. Holding a weight in a stationary position creates tension and stresses your muscle fibres enough to cause growth. Some experts claim that static holds are as good as dynamic training (the traditional up-and-down, full-range-of-motion method) for building muscle and strength.

Do static holds at the end of a set for any muscle group and hold the weight at the point where the most tension is on your muscles. For example, instead of bringing a biceps curl all the way up to your shoulder, stop when your forearm and upper arm form a 90-degree angle and hold the weight there for 10 to 15 seconds—if you can fight the pain for that long.

Centurion Sets

In centurion sets you perform 100 repetitions in each set. Warning: Few people survive this gigantic task and most retreat to the safety of their old routine. But if you can push past the pain, this stimulus is so foreign to your muscles that it'll bust you out of any training rut and increase muscle development, separation and definition. When you return to a standard programme of heavier weights and lower reps, you'll shuttle on more size.

Perform 100 reps of two to four exercises and do one set per exercise. Use a weight that's 30 to 40 per cent of your 1RM. Perform the sets with a partner or use drop sets to break past the pain barrier that the 80th rep will bring. Take a 10-second break when the pain is unbearable. Centurion sets work great for calves and bodyweight moves, especially when you're on a business trip or are training in a gym that has only small weights.

Doubles

Doubles involve doing a three-exercise super-set for the same muscle group without resting between moves. With this method you do an exercise for a muscle group, then do a new exercise for the same muscle and, finally, repeat the first exercise. For example, for your chest you'd do bench presses, then flys, then bench presses again.

You can perform doubles on the first two or three exercises of a routine or you can create an entire routine based around doubles. Do 2 to 4 sets of 4 to 10 reps of both the first and second exercises. A lot of lifters say they're able to do more reps on the second set of the first exercise. Nobody knows why this works, but take strength gains where you can get them.

Cluster Sets

In cluster sets you perform 5 to 10 exercises, one after another without rest, using the same weight. Think of it as a giant superset. Cluster sets add a fluid form of resistance and have an aerobic element, which damages your muscles enough to force them to grow. They also train your body's lactate system with a mix of strength and cardio work, making your muscles release lactic acid. This forces your body to release growth hormone, the catalyst responsible for adding muscle and reducing fat.

Perform cluster sets one of two ways. Option 1: Do a 5-exercise circuit for 4 or 5 sets of 6 reps. Perform 2 circuits in a workout. Option 2: Do a 10-exercise circuit of 4 or 5 sets of 6 reps. Perform this circuit only once for a full-body workout.

Jump Sets

In jump sets you do a set of an exercise for one muscle group, rest for a few minutes and then do a set for the muscle opposite to the muscle you just worked. You then rest and do another set of the first exercise. Alternating between the exercises helps you preserve your strength and boosts recovery by providing more rest for the body parts but in the same workout time. This allows you to use more weight for each exercise.

If you plan to do 5 sets of pull-ups and 5 sets of bench presses, do 3 sets of pull-ups and 3 sets of bench presses. Then go back and do the remaining 2 sets of pull-ups and 2 sets of bench presses. The extra rest will allow you to be stronger than you normally would on the last two sets. You can base an entire routine around this concept.

Peak Contraction

With the peak concentration method you flex and squeeze a muscle when it's under the most stress during a rep. You can do this on any rep and on any exercise at any point in a set. Arnold Schwarzenegger is of fan of this intensity booster and credited it with giving his biceps a bigger peak.

To use this method, flex your biceps at the top of a curl and hold the position for one to two seconds. Squeeze the muscle as hard as you can or until the pain becomes too much. You'll soon turn your molehills into mountains.

Rep Targeting

In rep targeting you pick a target number of reps for an exercise and then pump out that number of reps in as many sets as it takes. Progress by increasing the total number of reps you do each week. It's a great strategy for bodyweight exercises, where you can't always easily reduce the resistance.

Set a goal to do 50 pull-ups. Perhaps you can do only 15 on the first set. Take a rest and then do another set. Perhaps you get just 10. Rest for another minute and then keep going until you reach your goal of 50 reps. You can also make the amount of time you rest between sets proportionate to the amount of reps you have left to get to your target. For example, if your target is 50 and you've already done 30 reps, your rest period is 20 seconds. If you get 10 more reps on the next set, this leaves you with 10 reps to go. You'll rest for 10 seconds and go again.

Challenging Combinations

Use these techniques to buff some new shine onto your existing routine. You can even combine the techniques to multiply their effectiveness. The combinations are immense: 13 to the power of 13, which is whole lot of permutations. Try a few of these examples.

- A rest pause set followed by drop sets
- An eccentric set followed by a centurion set
- A double followed by a drop set
- Half reps combined with static holds
- Superset eccentric sets combined with drop sets of full reps
- A drop set at the end of an exercise in a cluster set
- A double of two static holds and a normal move
- An eccentric set followed by a static hold
- The rest pause technique with half reps
- Drop sets combined with peak contractions

Where Now?

Congratulations: You're no longer a middle-of-the-range lifter and are probably tempted to stop reading because you think you know it all. That viewpoint is perfectly understandable given that people have no doubt complimented you on your physique. But blokes whose physiques are even better than yours look the way they do because of a thirst for knowledge and an insane amount of hard work. Even though you're now an advanced lifter you can still learn a trick or two about how to improve on your improvements. Keep reading because those extra kilograms of lean muscle are within reach.

Total Muscle Gaining for Advanced Lifters

Once you've been training for more than a year, you're an advanced lifter. At this point it becomes harder to add muscle. Here's how you can accelerate your gains.

To see fast gains and bring a lagging muscle group up to speed, advanced lifters should train at least three times a week. If each workout lasts about an hour, this adds up to 3 hours out of a 168-hour week—that's not a lot to ask. You also don't want to neglect your other muscles. After all, it took sweat and hard work to get the rest of your physique looking good and you don't want to unravel all the hard yards. This chapter describes the best ways to train the muscle groups outlined in chapter 3. Being an advanced lifter, you should already know how to do all the exercises listed and probably won't need to refer back to the exercise descriptions. There are several approaches and it's nearly impossible to tell how much better one works than the next. Your best bet? Try them all over the course of a year and by the end your experiment you will have a very obvious conclusion: size.

Arm-Building Workouts

Want big arms? Here's the information you need in order to grab them with an iron fist.

ARMS FOR THE MAN WITH PLENTY OF TIME

Do the exercises listed in table 7.1 one after another and rest for 45 to 60 seconds between sets. Each rep should take 3 to 4 seconds.

Table 7.1 Straight Sets

Exercise	Sets	Reps
1. Underhand-grip pull-up	4	10
2. Dumbbell deadlift	4	10
3. Hammer curl	3	8
4. EZ-bar curl	4	8
5. Close-grip bench press	4	8
6. EZ-bar skull crusher	4	8
7. Triceps push-down	5	12
8. Back extension	4	12

WORKOUT FOR THE BLOKE WHO WANTS ARM STRENGTH

Use as much weight as you can manage for each set (see table 7.2) so that you fail on the final rep, especially for the sets of 6 and 4 repetitions. Rest for 60 seconds between sets.

Table 7.2 Pyramid Sets

Exercise	Sets	Reps
1. Barbell biceps curl	5	12, 10, 6, 4, 4
2. Close-grip bench press	5	12, 10, 6, 4, 4
3. Hammer curl	4	10, 8, 6, 6
4. Standing triceps extension	4	10, 8, 6, 6
5. EZ-bar curl	3	10, 8, 6
6. EZ-bar skull crusher	3	10, 8, 6
7. Back extension	2	15, 12
8. Power clean	2	6, 6

WORKOUT FOR HARD-TO-GROW ARMS

In each superset (see table 7.3), complete each exercise directly after the next. Rest for 45 to 60 seconds afterwards.

Table 7.3 Supersets

Exercise	Sets	Reps
Superset 1		
1. Underhand-grip pull-up	4	10
2. Parallel bar dip	4	10
Superset 2		
3. EZ-bar curl	4	12
4. EZ-bar skull crusher	4	12
Superset 3		
5. Hammer curl	3	8
6. Standing triceps extension	3	8
Superset 4		
7. Cable rope curl	4	15
8. Rope push-down	4	15

SPORT-SPECIFIC GUNS FOR ATHLETES

The goal of this workout (see table 7.4) is to complete all 60 repetitions in 60 seconds, so do the repetitions at breakneck speed and pick a small weight. You can even use elasticized bands. Take as much rest as you need between sets so that you feel fully refreshed before each set. You can even tack this on to the end of another workout; it should take only about 15 to 20 minutes.

Table 7.4 Fast Reps

Exercise	Sets	Reps
1. Hammer curl	3-4	60
2. EZ-bar skull crusher	3-4	60
3. Rope push-down	3-4	60
4. Cable rope curl	3-4	60

WORKOUT FOR GUYS WITH A HIGH PAIN THRESHOLD

For the first two exercises (see table 7.5), complete the 50 reps in as few sets as possible but take rest when you need it. This workout is for the advanced lifter. If you can't do at least 8 to 10 reps of these two exercises, stick to a full-body strength workout rather than specialising on arms. Don't be surprised by the inclusion of other exercises, such as squats, that seemingly have nothing to do with arms. They'll increase your overall musculature, which will bolster the size of your arms. Take the leap of faith and tighter sleeves will be yours.

Table 7.5 No-Curl Arms

Exercise	Sets	Reps
1. Underhand-grip pull-up	As needed	50
2. Parallel bar dips	As needed	50
3. Squat (barbell)	5	5
4. Dumbbell flat chest press	5	5
5. Dumbbell deadlift	4	10, 8, 8, 6
6. Back extension	3	12

Shoulder Workouts

Strong shoulders help you build your back, chest and arms to their fullest potential. Keep reading for the workouts to get it all.

BUILD BIG SHOULDERS QUICKLY

Shoulders are a comparatively small muscle group. You might want to do this workout on a day when you're not really up to training because it's easier than training your legs or chest. Or you can pair it with an abs or arm workout. Do the exercises one after another (see table 7.6) and rest for 45 to 60 seconds between bouts. Use perfect form to protect your most valuable asset: your V-shape.

Table 7.6   Straight Sets

Exercise	Sets	Reps
1. Power clean	4	6
2. Dumbbell seated shoulder press	3	12
3. Lateral raise	4	12
4. Dumbbell front raise	4	15
5. Incline reverse fly	3	10

DEVELOP SIZE AND STRENGTH

This is a maximum-effort programme (see table 7.7), so load up and don't be afraid to push your limits. Be sure to rope in a spotter when you can. You should fail on the final rep, especially for the sets of 6 repetitions. Rest for 60 seconds between sets and you'll soon find your suit jackets tightening.

Table 7.7   Pyramid Sets

Exercise	Sets	Reps
1. Arnold press	5	15, 10, 6, 6, 10
2. Lateral raise	5	15, 10, 6, 6, 10
3. Dumbbell seated shoulder press	4	10, 8, 6, 6
4. Incline reverse fly	3	15, 12, 12
5. Dumbbell upright row	4	15, 12, 10, 8
6. Dumbbell front raise	3	10, 8, 8

SHOTGUN SPORT ENDURANCE INTO YOUR SHOULDERS

Shoulders can take a huge amount of punishment. This workout (see table 7.8) primes them for endurance. Don't get too cavalier: Be sure to use weights that are significantly lighter than those you'd normally use. You'll recover quickly between sets, so don't take too much rest—45 to 60 seconds should be enough to feel the sizzle in your end caps.

Table 7.8   Stamina

Exercise	Sets	Reps
1. Dumbbell deadlift	3	20
2. Lateral raise	3	20
3. Dumbbell seated shoulder press	3	20
4. Incline reverse fly	3	20
5. Dumbbell upright row	3	20
6. Dumbbell front raise	3	20

SHOULDERS FOR THE MAN SHORT ON TIME

Sometimes you're in a rush and need a quick fix for your shoulders. This is the workout for that time. Grab a modest-size set of dumbbells and do all of these exercises (table 7.9) as one large set without resting or putting the dumbbells down. To work all three heads of your shoulders and fast-track their growth, rest for 1 to 3 minutes after you're done and then go again.

Table 7.9   High Reps, Big Weights

Exercise	Sets	Reps
1. Dumbbell seated shoulder press	3-5	6
2. Lateral raise	3-5	6
3. Dumbbell upright row	3-5	6
4. Dumbbell front raise	3-5	6
5. Incline reverse fly	3-5	6

BUILD YOUR ENTIRE BODY AND SHOULDERS

This workout (table 7.10) includes a mix of several techniques. The pyramids at the beginning shift the most weight and build strength. Straight sets totally fatigue your muscles while giving other parts of your shoulder a break. Dip into a variety of heavy and super-light weights so that you fatigue on the final reps. The technical term for the after effects is *killer*.

Table 7.10 Complete Package

Exercise	Sets	Reps
1. Dumbbell deadlift	5	15, 12, 8, 8, 10
2. Lateral raise	4	10
3. Dumbbell seated shoulder press	4	12, 8, 8, 10
4. Incline reverse fly	4	10
5. Dumbbell front raise	4	20

Chest Workouts

Boost the size of your frontage with these workouts that pinpoint growth onto your pecs.

ADD MUSCLE MASS TO YOUR CHEST FAST

Do the exercises listed in table 7.11 one after another and rest for 45 seconds between sets. Feel free to substitute your favourite chest exercises, such as barbell flat chest press, for any of the dumbbell exercises listed, but always start with the pressing exercises.

Table 7.11 Straight Sets

Exercise	Sets	Reps
1. Dumbbell incline chest press	4	10
2. Dumbbell flat chest press	3	8
3. Parallel bar dip	4	12
4. Push-up	3	15
5. Dumbbell flat chest fly	8	8

WORKOUT FOR THE MAN WHO WANTS SIZE AND STRENGTH

Use as much weight as you can manage for each set (see table 7.12) so that you fail on the final rep, especially for the sets of 6 and 4 repetitions. Rest for 60 seconds between sets.

Table 7.12 Pyramid Sets

Exercise	Sets	Reps
1. Dumbbell flat chest press	5	12, 8, 6, 4, 10
2. Dumbbell incline chest press	4	10, 8, 6, 4
3. Dumbbell flat chest fly	4	10, 8, 8, 8
4. Dumbbell flat pullover	3	12, 10, 8
5. Push-up	4	15, 12, 10, 10

WORKOUT FOR THE TALL GUY WHO STRUGGLES TO ADD MASS TO HIS CHEST

Growing your chest can be difficult because it has two very apt helpers: the triceps and shoulders. These supporting muscles often steal the effort from your pecs, which explains why incline presses can leave you with smouldering shoulders but an upper chest softer than Helen Mirren. To solve this conundrum, do pre-exhaust sets consisting of an isolation chest exercise immediately followed by a compound, multijoint chest exercise (table 7.13). The initial isolation move forces your pecs to work harder during the compound move. This gives you more chest burn for your efforts. Rest for 60 seconds after each superset.

Table 7.13 Pre-Exhaust Training

Exercise	Sets	Reps
Superset 1		
1. Cable crossover	4	12
2. Dumbbell incline chest press	4	6
Superset 2		
3. Dumbbell chest fly	4	12
4. Dumbbell incline chest press	4	6
Superset 3		
5. Push-up	4	12
6. Parallel bar dip	4	6

WORKOUT FOR PURE STRENGTH AND PUSHING POWER

In this workout (table 7.14) you'll do a group of 3 sets, called a wave, of a single exercise. After each set, increase the weights by 10 to 30 per cent and decrease the number of reps. After each wave you'll do a second wave (another 3 sets) of the same exercise, but this time you'll be able to use bigger weights and push past old limits because the first wave primes your nervous system for heavy lifting. Rest for 1 to 2 minutes between each set and do a 15-rep warm-up set of each exercise. Stick to it for a month and you'll soon be rewarded with muscle worthy of any beach.

Table 7.14   Strength Wave Loading

Exercise	Sets	Reps
Exercise 1		
1. Dumbbell flat chest press (two waves)	3	6, 3, 2
2. Dumbbell flat chest press (two waves)	3	6, 3, 2
Exercise 2		
3. Dumbbell incline chest press (two waves)	3	6, 3, 2
4. Dumbbell incline chest press (two waves)	3	6, 3, 2
Straight sets		
5. Parallel bar dip	4	10
6. Dumbbell flat pullover	3	12

SPORTSMAN'S CHEST WORKOUT

In this workout (table 7.15) you'll perform a set of a heavy strength exercise, rest for 45 seconds and then do a set of a plyometric moves using a similar movement pattern for the same muscle. This builds power, size and fast-moving muscles that excel on the sport pitch. Explosive moves recruit more muscle fibres than strength moves do. Doing an explosive move before a strength move makes your body think a higher workload is coming, so it recruits more muscle fibres; this helps you lift heavier. Rest for 1 to 2 minutes between sets to minimise your fatigue and optimise your power throughout the workout. If you recover quickly, reduce the rest time. Alternate between training and rest days when possible.

Table 7.15   Power Training

Exercise	Sets	Reps
Superset 1		
1. Dumbbell flat chest press	4	8
2. Explosive push-up	4	4
Superset 2		
3. Dumbbell incline chest press	4	8
4. Medicine ball lying throw	4	4
Superset 3		
5. Parallel bar dip	4	8
6. Explosive push-up	4	4

Back Workouts

Strong back muscles help you stand tall and look lean better than any other muscles do. Carve your torso into perfect shape with these hard-hitting workouts.

SHOTGUN MUSCLE ONTO YOUR BACK FAST

You can tack a biceps or shoulder workout onto the end of this workout (table 7.16) if your schedule allows it. Do the exercises one after another and rest for 1 to 2 minutes between sets to carve out the straight lines that'll build solid upper-back strength.

Table 7.16   Straight Sets

Exercise	Sets	Reps
1. Overhand-grip pull-up	4	8-10
2. Single-arm dumbbell row	3	10
3. Power clean	4	6
4. Inverted row	4	10
5. Cable face pull	3	15

BUILD SIZE and Strength Quickly

Use as much weight as you can for each set (table 7.17). You should fail on the final rep, especially for the final sets. Rest for 1 to 2 minutes between sets and work towards a muscle scorching that'll make your chest feel jealous.

Table 7.17 Pyramid Sets

Exercise	Sets	Reps
1. Weighted overhand-grip pull-up	5	15, 10, 6, 6, 10
2. Dumbbell bent-over row	5	15, 10, 6, 6, 10
3. Single-arm dumbbell row	4	10, 8, 6, 6
4. Dumbbell flat pullover	4	15, 12, 10, 8
5. Cable face pull	3	10, 8, 8
6. Back extension	3	15

SPORTSMAN'S BACK-SPECIFIC WORKOUT

The aim? Go big, then rest big. The idea is to shift more weight than you ever imagined you could. Raise the weights as quickly as you can but take your time returning them to starting position. Rest for 1 to 2 minutes between each set (table 7.18), rope in a spotter if you can and don't wimp out—a big back demands big weights.

Table 7.18 Power Training

Exercise	Sets	Reps
1. Power clean	6	3
2. Dumbbell bent-over row	5	4
3. Weighted overhand-grip pull-up	6	5
4. Dumbbell incline row	6	3

BUILD STRENGTH AND MASS

This workout (table 7.19) may seem easy enough, especially if you've been on a high-rep scheme before, but when done correctly it's tougher than a rat sandwich. Pick a weight and stick to it for the entire exercise. It should be heavy enough that the first 2 sets feel easy but hard enough that you fail on the final 3 sets. Trial and error are the best judges, but remember to increase the weight by 2 to 5 per cent each week in order to progress. Rest for 1 to 2 minutes between sets. The next time you high-five someone—to be ironic, of course—he'll blow on his fingers.

Table 7.19 5 × 5

Exercise	Sets	Reps
1. Weighted overhand-grip pull-up	5	5
2. Dumbbell deadlift	5	5
3. Single-arm dumbbell row	5	5
4. Dumbbell incline row	5	5
5. Dumbbell flat pullover	5	5

BUILD SPORT ENDURANCE IN YOUR BACK

Your back, like your legs, often can respond to very high rep ranges. It's not something you should do all the time, but it's worth targeting your endurance fibres every few months to help break out of a muscle-building plateau. Exercise selection is crucial (see table 7.20), especially if you can't do many reps of bodyweight exercises, so stick to the cables and free weights. Rest for 45 to 60 seconds between each set and give yourself a long stretch afterwards to keep those muscles limber.

Table 7.20 High Reps

Exercise	Sets	Reps
1. Dumbbell bent-over row	3	20
2. Dumbbell deadlift	3	15
3. Dumbbell incline row	3	20
4. Cable face pull	3	15
5. Good morning	4	12

Abs Workouts

Every muscle relies on your abs, hips and lower back, collectively known as your core. Your core is your base and your centre of attraction. Here's everything you need to sculpt a rock-solid midsection.

BUILD HARD AB MUSCLES FAST

Table 7.21 shows undoubtedly the most simplistic abs programme in existence, so do it at the start of your workout if you're desperate for some progress in your gut or at the end if you're after a balanced approach to all your muscles. Do 1 to 4 sessions a week. Perform the exercises one after another and rest for 30 to 60 seconds between sets. Just make sure you don't eat a big meal beforehand or you may taste it a second time.

Table 7.21 Straight Sets

Exercise	Sets	Reps
1. Bicycle crunch	3	10
2. Plank	4	60 sec.
3. Lying leg raise	3	8
4. Hanging leg raise	4	12

BURN FAT WHILE BUILDING ABS

Use as much weight as you can manage for each set (see table 7.22) and remember not to rest between the exercises of each superset. Speed up the transition from one move to the next by setting up both stations before you start. Rest for 60 seconds after each superset. Do this workout 1 to 3 times a week for a rock-solid core that'll ward off injuries to your trunk and improve your stability and power in other exercises, giving you more muscle everywhere.

Table 7.22 Core Supersets

Exercise	Sets	Reps
Superset 1		
1. Good morning	4	10
2. Lying leg raise with pike	4	10
Superset 2		
3. Barbell rollout	3	12
4. Back extension	3	12
Superset 3		
5. Plank	4	60 sec.
6. Superman	4	60 sec.

BUILD ABS THAT'LL PERFORM ON THE SPORT PITCH

Do not use heavy loads in this workout (see table 7.23). The goal is to perform the exercises as quickly as possible with perfect form. Remember that last part: *perfect form*. If you feel your form faltering, slightly reduce the speed until you achieve perfect form again. Rest

just 30 seconds between bouts and do not use any momentum to cheat through the reps. You can even slot this workout in between bouts of cardio exercises.

Table 7.23 High Reps

Exercise	Sets	Reps
1. Bicycle crunch	3	15
2. Lying leg raise	3	12
3. Barbell rollout	4	10
4. Hanging leg raise	3	12

DEVELOP STRENGTH AND AN INJURY-PROOF BACK

Ab strength is not something you traditionally boast to mates about. That's because the results—six-packs—speak louder than words. The occasional bout with big weights will give you results, especially if you've been doing a few months of high-rep workouts. Be sure to warm up your entire body before you load up the weights; if you don't, the slow, heavy movements can cause an injury. For the first two exercises (see table 7.24) hold a dumbbell between your legs. For the weighted plank get a mate to place a weight on your back. For the crunches hold a small weight in each hand. You should strain and fail on the final rep, so don't be afraid to reach for weights that are bigger than you think you can manage. Rest for 1 to 2 minutes between sets. Do this workout 1 or 2 times a week for Hulk-strength abs.

Table 7.24 Power

Exercise	Sets	Reps
1. Hanging leg raise	5	6
2. Lying leg raise	5	6
3. Plank (weighted)	5	6
4. Bicycle crunch	5	6

BUILD YOUR ENTIRE BODY AND ABS AT THE SAME TIME

These full-body exercises (table 7.25) rope in your abs to a huge degree by making them flex to brace against the loads placed on the rest of your body. Abs are, in essence, a supporting muscle in every one of these exercises. This technique is used often by lifters who have low levels of body fat because their abs show up regardless of whether they target them. The benefit? More muscle everywhere, including your abs.

Table 7.25   Full-Body Abs Builder

Exercise	Sets	Reps
1. Squat (barbell)	5	7
2. Dumbbell deadlift	4	7
3. Overhand-grip pull-up	4	7
4. Dumbbell flat chest press	4	7
5. Power clean	3	6
6. Dumbbell front raise	4	10
7. Side plank	4	90 sec.

Leg Workouts

Work your lower body not solely to debone your chicken legs—that's just a bonus—but to get lean and more muscular everywhere.

QUICKLY ADD MUSCLE MASS TO LEGS

Table 7.26 is probably the most simplistic leg programme. Do the exercises one after another and rest for 45 to 60 seconds between sets, but go easy if it's your first time isolating your legs. The next day they'll ache like you owe the mob money.

Table 7.26   Straight Sets

Exercise	Sets	Reps
1. Step-up	4	8 each leg
2. Squat	5	10-12
3. Lunge	4	8 each leg
4. Split squat	3	8
5. Hamstring curl	3	15

BUILD SIZE AND STRENGTH

Use as much weight as you can manage for each set (see table 7.27). You should fail on the final rep, especially for the sets of 6 repetitions. Rest for 60 seconds between sets and work towards setting a fire in the belly of your muscles.

Table 7.27   Pyramid Sets

Exercise	Sets	Reps
1. Squat	5	15, 10, 6, 6, 10
2. Dumbbell deadlift	5	15, 10, 6, 6, 10
3. Lunge	4	10, 8, 6, 6
4. Good morning	4	15, 12, 10, 8
5. Step-up	3	10, 8, 8
6. Stiff-legged deadlift	3	15, 12, 12

SPORTSMAN'S LEG-BUILDING WORKOUT

This workout (table 7.28) may include only a few exercises, but your goal is to push as much weight as possible on every single set and take a heap of rest between bouts. Lower yourself or the weight slowly and then explode back to the starting position. Warm up with 12 to 15 reps of each exercise before you start, and rest for 1 to 3 minutes between sets. This workout will add a lot of strength to your legs as quick as a flash.

Table 7.28   Power Training

Exercise	Sets	Reps
1. Squat	7	3
2. Dumbbell deadlift	7	4
3. Split squat	6	4
4. Good morning	6	3

WORKOUT FOR THE MAN WITH PLENTY OF TIME TO TRAIN

The glory of this routine (table 7.29) is its simplicity. Doing 5 reps of 5 sets builds mass and strength in equal proportions. Make sure to rest 1 to 3 minutes between each set. Every week try to increase the amount of weight you use.

Table 7.29   5 × 5 Training

Exercise	Sets	Reps
1. Step-up	5	5
2. Squat	5	5
3. Lunge	5	5
4. Split squat	5	5
5. Dumbbell deadlift	5	5

WORKOUT FOR THE MAN WITH LEGS THAT REFUSE TO GROW

Drop sets (table 7.30) are excellent for legs. The first set allows you to shift heavy weights, thereby building strength and muscle, and the drop set that follows works the muscle fibres that the heavy set missed. Each set includes a drop set, so you'll do a set of 6 reps, reduce the weight by 30 per cent and then do another set of 6 reps. Throw in another drop set if you can still stand and your legs will be sweltering with size.

Table 7.30   Drop Sets

Exercise	Sets	Reps
1. Squat	5	6
2. Dumbbell deadlift	4	6
3. Split squat	4	6
4. Leg extension	4	6
5. Stiff-legged deadlift	4	6

Calf Workouts

Use these workouts to carve calves that'll stand out when you're wearing boardshorts.

BUILD LOWER-BODY ENDURANCE FOR SPORT

Do these exercises (table 7.31) one after another and rest for 45 seconds between sets. Complete this workout 2 to 4 times a week if you're desperate to quell any taunts about your chicken legs.

Table 7.31   Straight Sets

Exercise	Sets	Reps
1. Seated calf raise	4	25
2. Standing calf raise	5	15
3. Hamstring curl	3	20

BUILD STRENGTH AND SIZE

Use as much weight as you can manage for each set (table 7.32) so that you fail on the final rep, especially for the sets of 6 and 4 repetitions. Rest for 60 seconds between sets.

Table 7.32   Pyramid Sets

Exercise	Sets	Reps
1. Seated calf raise	5	25, 20, 15, 6, 4
2. Standing calf raise	4	25, 15, 12, 10
3. Hamstring curl	3	30, 20, 10

WORKOUT FOR THE MAN SHORT ON TIME

Pair this workout (table 7.33) with your upper-thigh session. After each set of an upper-thigh exercise, grab a machine or find a step and pump out 15 reps very quickly. Knock off from your amount of rest the time it takes you to complete all the reps. Alternatively, mix this in with any upper-body session.

Table 7.33   Jump Sets

Exercise	Sets	Reps
1. Standing calf raise	4	15
2. Seated calf raise	4	15

STIMULUS PACKAGE FOR STUBBORN, HARD-TO-GROW CALVES

Complete 100 reps (table 7.34) while taking as many rest periods as you need (or none if you can handle the pain). Do not rush the repetitions but keep them slow and controlled. Take 2 seconds to lift your ankles and 2 seconds to lower them, and try not to lose count. Take just 30 to 60 seconds of rest, as long as you need for the pain to subside, between each set.

Table 7.34   Centurion Sets

Exercise	Sets	Reps
1. Standing calf raise	2	100
2. Seated calf raise	2	100

WORKOUT FOR THE MAN WITH LIMITED EQUIPMENT OR A HOME GYM

You can mix this workout (table 7.35) in with another workout or just do it on its own anytime, anywhere. Pump out as many super-fast repetitions as you can muster. Feel free to bounce at the bottom of each repetition. Those who are man enough to bust through the pain barrier will be rewarded with lower legs that resemble cows, not calves.

Table 7.35 Sets to Failure

Exercise	Sets	Reps
1. Standing calf raise	4	As many as possible
2. Seated calf raise	4	As many as possible

Scheduling Workouts

You have a wealth of workouts at your fingertips. Now you should look to find out how you can piece them all together. The number of combinations and options available is staggering, which can make it a little tough to choose. Start by figuring out how many days a week your schedule allows you to exercise. Once you've created a conservative estimate it's time to piece the puzzle together. The following sections describe how to build your muscles based on the time you have in your schedule. There is no right or wrong way to create a weekly plan; simply create a plan that best suits your lifestyle. Break out your diary and get planning.

Three Workouts a Week

Training three times a week means you can still follow full-body regimens. A full-body programme may offer the best results, but it does present the option of concentrating on specific body parts. If you follow the routines in this chapter, you'll be trying to finish mammoth sessions and will end up burnt out. To get around this, adapt your programme following this simple rule: Choose your system and then make sure you never do more than 24 sets in a workout. You should always limit your workouts to an hour, so you'll have to pick and choose your favourite exercises to make this happen. You don't even have to use the same system for all your body parts. You might use pyramids for arms and do supersets for legs. It will work better if you follow a single system for every muscle group, but there really are

no rules except to keep consistent and give it all you've got.

Option 1: Push–Pull Split

Monday: Chest, back, abs
Tuesday: Upper legs, calves
Wednesday: Rest
Thursday: Biceps, triceps, shoulders
Friday, Saturday, Sunday: Rest

Option 2: Group Supporting Muscles

Monday: Chest, triceps, shoulders
Tuesday: Upper legs, calves
Wednesday: Rest
Thursday: Back, biceps, abs
Friday, Saturday, Sunday: Rest

Option 3: Build Up a Weak Body Part

This example programme focuses on growing arms, but you can focus on another body part if you wish.

Monday: Biceps, chest, triceps, shoulders
Tuesday: Rest
Wednesday: Upper legs, calves
Thursday: Rest
Friday: Back, biceps, triceps, abs
Saturday, Sunday: Rest

Four Workouts a Week

You're now committed enough to begin working one to three body parts in every session in true bodybuilder style. You can still do full-body workouts, but this approach helps you target lagging body parts that you might want to bring up. This is where the 'no pain, no gain' theory comes in. You'll load a muscle with such a high volume of work that it'll take almost a full week to recover, repair and then grow. You'll work only a few muscles in each session, so these sessions won't overfatigue your body the way four gruelling full-body workouts every week might. See which approach works for you and your schedule and continue to adapt the workouts as explained earlier so that your workouts remain short and sweaty.

Option 1: Keep the Weekend Free

Monday: Chest, biceps, abs
Tuesday: Calves, upper legs
Wednesday: Rest
Thursday: Back, triceps
Friday: Shoulders, abs
Saturday, Sunday: Rest

Option 2: All-Week Training

Monday: Chest, triceps, abs
Tuesday: Rest
Wednesday: Back, biceps
Thursday: Rest
Friday: Upper legs, calves
Saturday: Rest
Sunday: Shoulders or other problem body part

Option 3: Saturday Lifter

Monday: Back, shoulders
Tuesday: Upper legs, calves
Wednesday: Chest, abs
Thursday, Friday: Rest
Saturday: Biceps, triceps
Sunday: Rest

Five Workouts a Week

You can now give all your muscles the attention they deserve. A full-body routine will be too taxing on your body, so it's best to train one or two body parts in each workout, just like you would if you were training four days a week.

Pay attention to how your body is coping when you're training this many times a week. If you're feeling tired and yawning your way through the day, give yourself a rest. Be sure to take a full week off from all exercise after six to eight weeks of training five days a week; this stops you from hedging towards overtraining. You can even train a lagging body part twice in one week to speed up its progress and you won't have to adapt the workouts in this chapter much, if at all.

Option 1: Even Split

Monday: Chest
Tuesday: Upper legs, calves
Wednesday: Rest
Thursday: Back
Friday: Biceps, triceps
Saturday: Rest
Sunday: Shoulders, abs

Option 2: Work a Problem Area

This example programme focuses on the chest.
Monday: Chest
Tuesday: Biceps, triceps
Wednesday: Upper legs, calves
Thursday: Rest
Friday: Chest
Saturday: Shoulders, abs
Sunday: Rest

Option 3: Rest All Weekend

Monday: Chest
Tuesday: Upper legs, calves
Wednesday: Back
Thursday: Shoulders, abs
Friday: Biceps, triceps
Saturday, Sunday: Rest

Six Workouts a Week

A quick word on training this many times a week: Try not to do it. It brings you very close to burnout and unless your diet is spot on you'll be walking a tightrope with more muscle on one side and the depths of overtraining on the other. What's more, your gains may not be as pronounced as you think. One study in *European Journal of Applied Physiology* (Bell et al., 2000) in which lifters trained either three or six days a week using the same programmes found that the guys doing just three sessions gained as much muscle as the guys doing six sessions. If you must do six sessions a week, do it for one or two weeks followed by a week of three sessions and keep each session to 30 to 40 minutes so that you're not rolling out a sleeping bag in the gym. That's not to say you can't do it, so here are some example programmes, but remember: Sometimes more really is less.

Option 1: Maximum Recovery Split

Monday: Chest

Tuesday: Hamstrings, calves

Wednesday: Biceps, abs

Thursday: Shoulders, triceps

Friday: Quads

Saturday: Back

Sunday: Rest

Option 2: Growth-Maximising Split

Monday: Chest, shoulders, triceps

Tuesday: Back, biceps, abs

Wednesday: Upper legs, calves

Thursday: Rest

Friday: Chest, shoulders, triceps

Saturday: Back, biceps, abs

Sunday: Upper legs, calves

Option 3: Bring Up a Problem Part

This example programme focuses on the shoulders.

Monday: Shoulders

Tuesday: Chest

Wednesday: Biceps, triceps

Thursday: Back

Friday: Shoulders

Saturday: Upper legs, calves

Sunday: Rest

Seven Workouts a Week

Oh, now you're just being overly keen.

Where Now?

By this point you're no doubt turning a few heads when you walk down the street. You should be proud of that. You've put in the hard yards and deserve all the accolades you get. But a steadfast desire to improve is often yoked to perfectionism. That can mean that you're never really happy with how your body looks, no matter how good you actually do look. That's not a bad thing and can be a gift that brings out the best in you. But if you've got enough bulk and muscle, what's the next step? The next chapter on fat burning teaches you how to strip the fat off your physique so that it looks like it's carved from stone. Unless you're sporting a body-fat percentage so low that the veins on your muscles look like a road map, keep reading to find out how to get your abs—and every other muscle—to pop even more than they already do.

Minor Slimming

Getting memorably lean isn't a guessing game. This chapter contains the hard and fast facts that will help you successfully torch calories.

No one sets out to be overweight. Most of the time weight sneaks up on you like a credit card bill from a night out. One moment you're looking good and the next there's a little bit more to love. But there's no point in looking through the rearview mirror. It's far better to look at what's ahead. Most blokes' Pavlovian response to trouser tightening is a beeline for the cardiovascular machines at the gym, but is that really the best plan of attack? Perhaps not for everyone. Not all exercise is created equal. Just look at infomercials, gyms, exercise classes and personal trainers—they all profess to be the most effective fat burner.

Burning fat is not always a cut-and-dry affair. Locker room debates rage on about which type of exercise will put you on the fastest route to ripped. With inflight Internet, 10-second 100-metre sprints and 24-hour deadlines, the pace of life is ever hastening. Your results should follow suit.

Before you lace up your trainers you need to observe the first rule of success for long-term fat loss: Do what you love. This is the biggest hiccup with all forms of exercise. You may not enjoy getting yelled at by a beefed-up instructor or relish the chance to numb your crotch with hours on a bicycle saddle. If you don't like what you do, days when you don't feel like exercising will probably outnumber days when you do. When choosing your fat-burning ammunition, pick a form of exercise you

enjoy the most. Like squash? Go for it. The real secret to health is a sustainable exercise routine, not a two- or three-month blitzkrieg on your love handles.

If enjoyment comes second to results, you'll want to know what works and what doesn't. Here are the best fat-burning methods, ranked according to their effectiveness.

1. Weightlifting circuits. Do several sets of weightlifting without resting between sets. Rest only after completing each circuit.

2. High-intensity cardio. Alternate between 20 to 30 seconds of extremely hard cardiovascular work and 60 seconds of rest during which you keep exercising at a slow pace.

3. Interval training. Alternate between 60 to 90 seconds of hard cardiovascular work and 2 to 3 minutes of rest during which you keep exercising at a slow pace.

4. Cardioacceleration. Alternate between a set of weightlifting and 30 to 60 seconds of cardio exercise.

5. Threshold training. Alternate between 90 to 120 seconds of hard cardiovascular work and 3 to 4 minutes of rest during which you keep exercising at a slow pace.

6. Steady-state cardio. Spend 30 to 90 minutes (or even more) on one activity. This is how runners and cyclists train.

7. Everyday exercise. Toss a Frisbee or go for a light walk.

Sport and exercise classes fall somewhere in the middle. They're not ranked because each sport and class burns different quantities of calories depending on variables such as the league, your experience and how often you practise or play matches. You simply can't compare the calorie demands of a fourth-grade football game with those of a premiership final. These variables make it tough to rank the effectiveness of these modalities. However, thanks to intermittent nature of these activities they're somewhere in the top three, so do them rather than going for a long run or bike ride. Keep reading to find out how and why these ranking were formed and how you can put them into practise to lose those stubborn fat layers once and for all. The final five kilograms is yours to lose.

1. Weightlifting Circuits

The cast-iron, no-fail route to fat loss involves getting sweaty using weights.

To lose a lot of your gut quickly, don't think of lifting weights as an option. Consider it a necessity. Why? If you don't pump iron, part of the weight you lose may come from muscle. If you drop nine kilograms without lifting, about two kilograms of that will be hard-earned muscle. More muscle means you burn more calories with everything you do. That includes lifting your coffee cup to take a sip of your brew.

Dumbbells: Metabolism Kickers

Getting to grips with weights affects how your body burns energy. A study at West Virginia University (Bryner et al., 1999) compared weightlifting and cardiovascular exercise and found that pumping iron actually speeds up metabolism—the rate at which you fry calories—when you're doing nothing at all. The lifters in the study peeled off an average of 14.5 kilograms and saw their metabolism rates increase by 4 per cent. The participants who did aerobics lost more weight—an average of 18 kilograms—but that included 4 kilograms of muscle. Consequently, their metabolisms slowed down by an average of 14 per cent.

Those folks with slower metabolisms will have more trouble keeping the weight off in the future. You can easily avoid this problem if you build muscle while dropping fat.

The resistance-based circuits in the following workouts target all your larger muscles: chest, back, arms, core and legs. According to the study by Bryner and colleagues (1999), hard exercise such as circuits signals the body to burn more calories of fat in the hours after a workout. Whether you're lazing on the beach or surfing the net, you'll be zapping your love handles for free.

What's more, the harder you tackle your workouts the more growth hormone is released, which in turn stimulates muscle growth and flicks your fat burners into over-drive. Recruit the legs—your biggest muscles—for the biggest release of growth hormone and the best results. Most of the workouts in this chapter start with the legs while you're still fresh because that's where you'll put on the most muscle. It doesn't matter if you always wear trousers. Training your legs will make your upper body look better and leaner.

Muscle Burns Fat the Easy Way

The overall goal of lifting weights to burn fat is to increase your energy expenditure in the long term by adding muscle all over so that your metabolism hikes up and prevents future fat gain. Even though your shirt size will decrease, your weight might increase as you add muscle. Remember: Don't treat the scale as gospel because it doesn't take your body-fat levels into account. A kilogram of fat takes up a lot more space than a kilogram of dense muscle. Rather, take readings with a tape measure or get a personal trainer to take your body-fat percentage. These numbers are perfect points of reference to plot your improvements against. You may not always notice a difference in your physique because change happens daily in small increments, but the figures will help you keep track of your progress and will be a great source of motivation. Having the will to stick to it guarantees you a body you'll be proud of that doesn't come at the cost of a normal life. The workouts that follow can be finished in 40 to 50 minutes. These quick bursts of effort are the gold standard for all exercise. What are you waiting for? Your newer, leaner self is waiting at the end of these programmes.

What to Do

Do the exercises (see tables 8.1 through 8.3) one after the other without rest until you've ticked off every move. Then take a one- to three-minute break during which you stretch or just walk around the gym to get your breath back. The trick to this workout is to set up all the exercise stations before you kick off each circuit. Because this isn't always possible in crowded gyms, you can adapt the exercise as you're pumping out the reps. If a crew of dudes set up camp on the squat rack and you need to use it, simply do your squats with a set of dumbbells.

The key to success is not your exercise selection or the size of the weight you push but the intensity of your workout. The higher the intensity (which means the less rest), the bigger the calorie burn and the faster you'll get results. Do not spend time waiting for machines; that is never an excuse and you know it. Adapt your workouts on the fly and your physique will follow your lead.

WEIGHTLIFTING CIRCUIT WORKOUTS

Table 8.1 Weightlifting Circuit Workout 1 (Monday)

Exercise	Sets	Reps
1. Squat	3-5	12-15
2. Dumbbell flat chest press	3-5	12-15
3. Dumbbell bent-over row	3-5	12-15
4. Dumbbell deadlift	3-5	12-15
5. Arnold press	3-5	12-15
6. Barbell biceps curl	3-5	12-15

Table 8.2 Weightlifting Circuit Workout 2 (Tuesday)

Exercise	Sets	Reps
1. Step-up	3-5	12-15
2. Inverted row	3-5	12-15
3. Dumbbell incline chest press	3-5	12-15
4. Power clean	3-5	12-15
5. Close-grip bench press	3-5	12-15
6. Hanging leg raise	3-5	12-15

Table 8.3 Weightlifting Circuit Workout 3 (Thursday)

Exercise	Sets	Reps
1. Parallel bar dip	3-5	12-15
2. Overhand-grip pull-up	3-5	12-15
3. Lunge	3-5	12-15
4. Stiff-legged deadlift	3-5	12-15
5. Lateral raise	3-5	12-15
6. Barbell rollout	3-5	12-15

Challenging Change-Ups

These set and rep parameters aren't the only ways to burn fat, although they are the most commonly accepted. High reps do burn more calories, but what happens after the workout often counts the most towards your losses. Using weights so heavy you can manage only six reps increases your metabolism more than doing sets of a higher number of reps does, found a study in *Scandinavian Journal of Medicine and Science in Sports* (Mjølsnes et al., 2004). The effects of using big weights last longer than you might think, and your body uses up calories to recover after a heavy lifting session. This hikes up your metabolism, so you'll burn more calories long after you've left the gym.

This strategy is more for the advanced lifter who has already mastered perfect form on these moves and who has a very clear idea of how much weight he can push for 6 reps. If you're not failing on the final rep, you aren't using enough weight to achieve these gains. If you use weights that you can comfortably do 15 reps with, you will fail on all accounts. The take-home message? The more experienced you are, the fewer repetitions you can do.

But that doesn't mean you can give yourself more rest. Remember the secret ingredient: intensity.

2. High-Intensity Cardio

Warm up your running shoes because this system is about to burn holes in them. Warning: It's not for the faint hearted or weak willed.

Before you get started, know that one big difference exists between interval training and high-intensity training (HIT). The principles are similar in that they both alternate periods of hard work and rest, but HIT is brutal. It has a single function: to obliterate every scrap of energy you have in the shortest time possible. If you're brave enough to do it properly you shouldn't have a breath left in you to whine about how tired you are. Blokes often do it improperly by doing the working part of the intervals slowly. For HIT to work it needs to be puke-worthy and the veins on your forehead should be bulging.

Think of interval training and HIT as the moon and the sun: both are big round things you'll find above you, but they're not the same entity. Interval training is the moon—it'll give light. But the superior entity, the sun, a.k.a. HIT, is best for seeing things such as your abs.

Not every man has a built-in dungeon master he can turn on during a workout. The best way to do HIT and push past your pain barriers is to have a training partner or personal trainer tell you what to do. It works best if his or her attitude is that of a sadistic drill sergeant rather than a respectable professional.

Hit the Spot

Even though HIT is tougher than a rat sandwich, you can take solace in the knowledge that it works bloody well. You'll incinerate your fat stores by elevating your postexercise oxygen consumption, which is the extra oxygen your body uses after you've finished sweating. The more oxygen you breathe in after training, the more calories your body burns. After a strenuous bout of HIT, your body gobbles up more oxygen than normal so that it can return to its pre-exercise state. This raises your metabolism because you're burning more calories to fund the recovery process. Studies in *Sports Medicine* (Børsheim and Bahr, 2003) found that this elevated calorie expenditure can last from 15 minutes to 48 hours depending on how your body reacts. You could be burning more calories for free while you kick back on the couch.

Go Ape on Your Gut

You'd be hard pressed to find a more muscled and leaner beast than a silverback gorilla. Although it might not look like it, these gorillas are one of our closest relatives; our DNA matches 99 per cent. But, if we're so similar, why can these 275-kilogram animals effortlessly pump out single-arm pull-ups like they weigh as much as a marmoset? Understanding how these gorillas got their impressively lean musculature is the key to figuring out why HIT works.

Again, their secret can be summed up in one word: intensity. These gorillas relax for most of the day but when they do work—such as when fighting off a rival—they go at it with 100 per cent intensity. Their activity is brief, fierce and uses all of their muscles, which forces them to grow to bodybuilder-like proportions sans the potbelly.

Luckily, it's pretty easy to use their strategy to build more muscle, get fitter and carve away body fat. The key is frugality with your time. If you tried to exercise a gorilla with the workload most blokes use to get leaner and build muscle, you'd probably kill it. You don't need hours of hard slog to look like the leader of the pack. Limiting your training sessions to 55 minutes or less maximises your muscle-building hormone testosterone. When you slog away for more than an hour, levels of the stress hormone cortisol begin to increase. Cortisol in the right amounts is actually very important for growing muscles, but too much is bad because excess amounts can eat away at muscles while making you feel grumpy and listless. You're better off keeping your sweat sessions short and sweet, even if you find the time to do only one session a week.

High-Intensity Workouts

Before you do these workouts, remember that this system will not work if you're unable to smash each set with the fiercest intensity. They're not the best kind of thing to do on a treadmill; the consequences could be tragic if you suddenly lose the legs to keep going. What's more, it often takes exercise machines a while to speed up and slow down. Because these intervals are very short, this may cause you to lose track of how long you've really trained at your maximum. It's always better to train outside and see yourself going somewhere rather than mimicking a hamster in a wheel. Once you've found a patch of grass, choose workouts that include periods of hard work that you can manage. If you're a total beginner, don't assume you can sprint at full pace for 20 seconds. This is a deceptively long period of time, even for super-fit punters, and this is exactly where a lot of exercisers fail with HIT. You're better off building a base level of fitness with interval training.

Always remember to do a thorough warm-up and then give it everything you've got in your tank. Now take a deep breath and get ready to use the fat-burning power of your lungs to exhale your podgy bits.

What to Do

Do the following workouts using any kind of modality. Mixing it up—alternating between running, cycling, rowing, swimming, whatever—delivers a more balanced form of fitness and a greater calorie burn. Do 2 to 4 workouts a week. Repeat the same workout if you like, alternate among the ones that follow or feel free to make up your workouts as you go along.

HIGH-INTENSITY CARDIO WORKOUTS

WORKOUT 1: BEGINNER

1. Warm up for 5 to 10 minutes with the activity you plan to train.
2. Sprint for 5 seconds and then exercise at a low intensity (for example, walk) for 30 seconds or until you've got your breath back. Repeat 10 times.
3. Cool down with a slow effort for 10 to 12 minutes.

WORKOUT 2: INTERMEDIATE

1. Warm up for 5 to 10 minutes with the activity you plan to train.
2. Sprint for 10 seconds and then exercise at a low intensity (for example, walk) for 40 seconds or until you've got your breath back. Repeat 10 times.
3. Cool down with a slow effort for 10 to 12 minutes.

WORKOUT 3: ADVANCED

1. Warm up for 5 minutes with the activity you plan to train.
2. Sprint for 15 seconds and then exercise at a low intensity (for example, walk) for 50 seconds or until you've got your breath back. Repeat 10 to 15 times.
3. Cool down with a slow effort for 5 minutes.

WORKOUT 4: SPORTSMAN

1. Warm up for 5 to 10 minutes with the activity you plan to train.
2. Sprint for 12 seconds and then exercise at a low intensity (for example, walk) for 40 seconds or until you've got your breath back. Repeat 4 times and then choose a different activity. For example, if you've just cycled, switch to rowing.
3. Sprint for 12 seconds and then exercise at a low intensity (for example, walk) for 40 seconds or until you've got your breath back. Repeat 4 times and then choose a different activity.
4. Sprint for 12 seconds and then exercise at a low intensity (for example, walk) for 40 seconds or until you've got your breath back. Repeat 4 times.
5. Cool down with a slow effort for 4 minutes.

Break the Pain Barrier

HIT demands a high threshold for pain and exhaustion. Use these mental tricks to keep going when you have nothing left to give.

- Dedicate an interval to a person you admire. You're less likely to give up or give a shoddy effort on his or her mile.
- If you play sport, mentally replay some of your greatest moments. It will give you the confidence to carry on and distract you from the pain.
- Blast your favourite music. This improves stamina, strength and power and will help you tackle the working parts of the intervals with vigour.
- Count backward instead of forward. This brings you mentally closer to your end goal of finishing the workout.
- Close your eyes and visualise finishing the next interval faster than the previous one. Now stand up and do it.
- Repeat a single motivational mantra in your mind or say it aloud. Say a phrase such as *don't think, just do* or a word as simple as *energy*.
- Break the intervals into steps and then count the steps to distract yourself.

3. Interval Training

Interval training—HIT's little brother—will help you get fit faster. And leaner to boot.

Imagine you've just heard that your favourite band is giving away a limited number of free tickets to their final gig. Problem is, you're on the other side of a congested city centre and you have a big distance to cover. You need to get to that ticket office—fast! Instead of taking a cab or a train, you run. What would your strategy be? If you run at the fastest pace you could manage, you'll likely get out the blocks quickly but slow down as you get to the finish line—the exact spot where other punters are racing for the final tickets. A better option would be to run as fast as you can for one to two minutes and then jog at a moderate pace to catch your breath. When you get to the final leg you'll still have something in the tank for the final dash and will arrive faster than you would if you'd jogged at a steady pace. The result? Tickets are yours and you look a little leaner and feel a little fitter because you used the third most effective training tool on the planet: interval training.

How it Works

Interval training was once a buzzword that meant 'do less, gain more' or 'twice the burn in half the time'. You've probably heard all the headlines. The bottom line is that it works because you get fitter and leaner when your body adapts to a workload that's higher than it's used to. Interval training works on the same principles as HIT in that it alternates between work and rest. That's exactly why it's so effective.

It would be impossible to work hard for a long period of time such as running a marathon. To force your muscles to work beyond their limits you need to insert a little break. These rest periods, during which you're still moving at a slow pace, help your energy stores recover. When your battery is recharged you can go at it again at breakneck intensity until your battery is empty again. If you remember what the salesman said when you got your iPhone, running the battery all the way down is best for its longevity.

The same is true for your longevity, body fat and overall fitness. The breaks help you work at an intensity that's far higher than you're used to, which fast tracks your gains. A Laval University study (Tremblay, Simoneau and Bouchard, 1994) found that this kind of training burns up to three times as much fat as plodding along at a continuous pace does. If you're interested in performing better, interval training is your best option. Research in *European Journal of Applied Physiology* (Weston et al., 1997) showed that cyclists who did just six interval-training sessions improved their time trials in a 40-kilometre race. If more free time, quicker results and a better performance are on your agenda, keep your sweat sessions short and sweet.

Difference Between HIT and Interval Training

HIT and interval training may seem like the same animal, but the difference lies in the toughness. HIT spikes your heart rate up to 90 to 95 per cent of your maximum whereas interval training gets your heart rate up to about 80 to 85 per cent of your maximum. Because you work at a slightly lower intensity, interval training lets you train longer during the working part of the interval. Interval training is ideal for sports such as football in which you run flat out for around 60 seconds on attack and then ease back during defence. Interval training also encourages you to vary the length of your intervals in order to produce a broader form of fitness. Interval training also favours gym-based exercise equipment such as treadmills, stationary bikes and elliptical cross-trainers. It often takes these machines a while to speed up and slow down, which gives you the flexibility to do longer intervals that might better suit your sport or schedule. HIT, on the other hand, is more like a U.S. customs officer: It's super strict, allows no room for variation and demands all-out effort on every single interval. Make sure you have the stomach for whichever approach you choose or your lack of self-knowledge will make your results fall flat.

INTERVAL-TRAINING WORKOUTS

Do the following workouts using any kind of modality. Mixing it up—alternating between running, cycling, rowing, swimming, whatever—delivers a more balanced form of fitness and a greater calorie burn. Do 2 to 4 workouts a week. Repeat the same workout if you like, alternate between the ones that follow or feel free to make up your workouts as you go along.

WORKOUT 1: BEGINNER

1. Warm up for 5 to 10 minutes with the activity you plan to train.
2. Sprint or move quickly for 30 seconds and then exercise at a low intensity (for example, walk) for 60 seconds or until you've got your breath back. Repeat 5 to 10 times.
3. Cool down with a slow effort for 10 to 12 minutes.

WORKOUT 2: INTERMEDIATE

1. Warm up for 5 to 10 minutes with the activity you plan to train.
2. Sprint or move quickly for 60 seconds and then exercise at a low intensity (for example, walk) for 120 seconds or until you've got your breath back. Repeat 5 to 10 times.
3. Cool down with a slow effort for 10 to 12 minutes.

WORKOUT 3: ADVANCED

1. Warm up for 5 minutes with the activity you plan to train.
2. Sprint or move quickly for 90 seconds and then exercise at a low intensity (for example, walk) for 90 seconds or until you've got your breath back. Repeat 10 to 15 times.
3. Cool down with a slow effort for 5 minutes.

WORKOUT 4: SPORTSMAN

1. Warm up for 5 to 10 minutes with the activity you plan to train.
2. Sprint or move quickly for 30 seconds and then exercise at a low intensity (for example, walk) for 60 seconds or until you've got your breath back. Repeat 3 times, increasing your sprint and rest times by 10 seconds after each bout. (You should sprint for 60 seconds on the final bout.) Then choose a different activity. For example, if you've just cycled, switch to rowing.
3. Sprint for 40 seconds and then exercise at a low intensity (for example, walk) for 60 seconds or until you've got your breath back. Repeat 3 times, increasing your sprint and rest time by 20 seconds after each bout. Choose a different activity.
4. Sprint for 60 seconds and then exercise at a low intensity (for example, walk) for

60 seconds or until you've got your breath back. Repeat 4 times.

5. Cool down with a slow effort for 4 minutes.

4. Cardioacceleration

This abomination of fat burning and muscle building will quell postworkout stiffness and give you the most well-rounded form of fitness.

Boxing. Spin. Body pump. Membership to even the most vanilla gym offers a lot of fat-burning choices. If you're like most blokes these choices can be overwhelming, and it's tough to know whether some varieties work better than others.

Most exercise classes follow a pretty set formula in which you alternate between bouts of strength moves and cardio. You do a few push-ups and then hit the bag or skip. Fortunately, the boffins at the University of California (Davis et al., 2008) were also tired of these ambiguous choices and decided to test the effectiveness of several kinds of training. In this study one group did cardio, another group did resistance training and a final group ran for 30 to 60 seconds after each weightlifting set. This last option is similar to what you do in most boot camp-style exercise classes. Even though each group did the same amount of work, the combination group experienced

- 35 per cent greater improvement in lower-body strength,
- 53 per cent greater improvement in lower-body endurance,
- 28 per cent greater improvement in lower-body flexibility,
- 144 per cent greater improvement in upper-body flexibility,
- 82 per cent greater improvement in muscle gains and
- 991 per cent greater loss of fat mass.

The hybrid approach got rid of more wobbles and built more muscle. This approach is like a polar bear breeding with a grizzly bear to make a super bear. The researchers didn't mention how intense each session was, which is why this training method comes in at number four in terms of effectiveness. It's tough to tell whether a cardioacceleration session would be better than a high-intensity weightlifting or cardio session because the size of the weights used and speed of the intervals performed in the study weren't mentioned. Furthermore, this is a one-off study, so there's no reason to brush aside well-established training modalities such as interval training. That's not to say cardioacceleration doesn't work. The study results are staggering to say the least, and the method is well worth a try. In fact, what more could you ask for? Building muscle and power while burning fat is the holy grail of exercise. Fortunately, the labcoats proved that the two are not mutually exclusive.

World's Most Brutal Fitness Fad

The hybrid concept is deceptively simple, and another form of this kind of training spawned a fitness fad of epic proportions called Cross-Fit. A trainer named Greg Glassman thought that doing cardio at one time and then lifting weights separately was bloody annoying. He was certainly onto something; if you're time poor, this split is not a good use of your time. Luckily, Glassman thought outside the box and merged cardio and weightlifting to create CrossFit. It is probably more effective than weight circuits and is arguably the most ferocious calorie burner there is, provided it's done at the right intensity. This subjectivity about how intense workouts should be is why it's further down the rankings. This fat burner will slap on muscle and kick you into shape for every activity life can throw at you. It includes a mix of gymnastics moves, weight-lifting exercises and brief, intense cardio training. Olympians, soldiers, police officers, fire fighters and even housewives use it to get fit enough to be ready for anything. The best bit: Everyone uses the same programme. You see, the needs of Igor the 140-kilogram Bulgarian weightlifter and your granddad differ by degree, not by kind. We're all the same. Everyone has to stand up, sit down, lift boxes off the floor and push things overhead. All that changes for each programme is the size of the weights. If a workout calls for eight reps using your heaviest weight, the powerlifter might crank out reps using a 250-kilogram weight whereas gramps might use his shopping bags. You use weights you feel comfortable with and in the end you're fit enough to shovel dirt, haul rocks, cut down trees, lift weights, pump out pull-ups, sprint faster and do everything better while looking your very leanest. Be warned: This is some of the most gut-wrenching exercise you'll ever do, so have a puke bucket handy.

Workouts

The regimens that follow can be divided into two types: cardioacceleration as outlined by the University of California study (Davis et al., 2008) and CrossFit. If you're a beginner, start with the cardioacceleration regimens because they will help you build a base of fitness. (That's not to say they won't work for fitter athletes. You can always ramp up the intensity of the weights you push and the speed at which you do the cardio.) The best thing about cardioacceleration is that the people who did it reported next to no stiffness the day after training. This is particularly appealing for beginners, who can feel like they've been to the panel beaters after a tough exercise session. This pain can deter a lot of beginners because it restricts daily life to the point that even a flight of stairs can elicit feelings of dread. This system also works fantastically well for people who have a home gym setup with a treadmill or rowing machine; they can even leave the mill whizzing away while doing their weights exercises. If you don't have a cardio machine you can do a 60-second run around the block between sets for exactly the same effect. If you do your workout in a gym, try to set up your weightlifting stations close to the cardio machines to minimise the transition time. The more intense your workout, the better the results you'll get.

The CrossFit-variety workouts are usually undertaken only by people who are already fit. A thriving web community in which people post their own workouts and try to outperform one another surrounds this training animal. It gets so extreme that CrossFit has been labelled a cult. (However, the only thing they're likely to burn is fat, so it's a good cult as far as cults go.) You can do CrossFit-type training in three basic ways. You can aim to do as many circuits as you can in a set time frame, you can simply aim to finish the circuit or you can race against a clock. Remember to use weights that you are comfortable with because if you go too big you won't finish each circuit. Oh, and bring a buddy. This form of training is a lot more fun when you have competition, and you'll need someone to spur you on.

CARDIOACCELERATION WORKOUTS

Do all of the exercises one after another as a giant circuit and then rest for one to three minutes after each circuit. Alternate between workouts 1 and 2 (tables 8.4 and 8.5) and leave a day of rest between each workout. Use different cardio equipment as much as possible to ensure that you don't stick to just one form of exercise.

Table 8.4 Cardioacceleration Workout 1

Exercise	Sets	Reps
Warm up with a 5-minute jog		
1. Squat	3-4	12
Run, cycle or row for 60 seconds		
2. Dumbbell flat chest press	3-4	12
Run, cycle or row for 60 seconds		
3. Dumbbell bent-over row	3-4	12
Run, cycle or row for 60 seconds		
4. Dumbbell deadlift	3-4	12
Run, cycle or row for 60 seconds		
5. Dumbbell seated shoulder press	3-4	12
Run, cycle or row for 60 seconds		
6. Barbell rollout	3-4	12
Run, cycle or row for 60 seconds		

Table 8.5 Cardioacceleration Workout 2

Exercise	Sets	Reps
Warm up with a 5-minute jog		
1. Lunge	3-4	15
Run, cycle or row for 60 seconds		
2. Inverted row	3-4	15
Run, cycle or row for 60 seconds		
3. Parallel bar dip	3-4	15
Run, cycle or row for 60 seconds		
4. Power clean	3-4	15
Run, cycle or row for 60 seconds		
5. Hammer curl	3-4	15
Run, cycle or row for 60 seconds		
6. Close-grip bench press	3-4	15
Run, cycle or row for 60 seconds		

CROSSFIT WORKOUTS

Do one of these CrossFit workouts 2 to 4 times a week. Alternate between all of them for more rounded fitness and a bigger fat-burning effect. Remember to take a day of rest between each bout or you'll burn out. Try to enjoy because you'll soon be enjoying your newly lean physique.

BEAT YOUR OWN TIME OUTDOORS

Do 3 or 4 rounds as quickly as you can without resting between the exercises. Record how long it takes you and try to beat your time next week.

1. Run 1,000 metres as fast as you can.
2. Do 50 reps of bodyweight squats.
3. Perform 50 reps of push-ups.
4. Hold the plank position for 60 seconds.

RACE AGAINST THE CLOCK

Do this circuit as fast as you can. Jot down your time and try to beat it next week to get fitter and stronger and increase your stamina.

1. Run or cycle at your own pace for 2 kilometres.
2. Perform 20 reps of inverted rows.
3. Perform 100 reps of bicycle crunches.
4. Perform 50 step-ups with each leg.
5. Run 2 kilometres.

TRY TO FINISH THIS CIRCUIT

Do the circuit just once and take as little rest as possible. Don't bother recording your time—the goal is simply to finish.

1. Perform 60 pull-ups.
2. Run 800 metres.
3. Do 60 parallel bar dips.
4. Run 800 metres.
5. Do 60 lying leg raises.
6. Run 800 metres.
7. Do 60 inverted rows.
8. Run 400 metres.

DO AS MANY ROUNDS AS YOU CAN

Big on determination but short on time? This is the answer. Do as many rounds as you can in 15 minutes or however much time you can spare. Don't rest unless you absolutely have to, and use the same weight for all sets. Write down the number of rounds you complete and then beat that number next week.

1. Do 10 dumbbell flat chest presses.
2. Do 10 squats.
3. Do 10 cable face pulls.
4. Run, row or cycle for 1 minute.

5. Threshold Training

Increase the length of your intervals to boost your sport performance, fat-burning prowess and stamina.

Imagine how you'd feel if you ran 400 or 800 metres. If you're brave enough, find a track and give it a try. Or just kick back and try to picture the exhaustion you'd feel when you rounded that final turn. Your legs would feel like they had a curry stewing inside. That feeling is what most people describe as lactic acid. They're wrong. Lactic acid is not that burn and it is not behind the soreness you feel in the days after a tough training session. Why should you care? Manipulating lactic acid is the backbone of threshold training because lactic acid is in fact a fuel. It is more friend than foe.

Lactic acid is a byproduct—not a waste product—created when your body uses glucose (energy created when you eat carbs or fat) for fuel. Not all of the glucose is used when it is fed into your muscles. What's left over seeps out of your muscle cells and into your blood. When this happens, hydrogen ions are released. The resulting salt is called lactic acid or lactate. Your liver then sets to work converting these leftovers into more fuel so you can keep exercising.

You actually produce lactate all the time, even when you walk to the corner shop for a bag of crisps. But if you train at a high intensity—such as sprinting to the corner shop for more beer—your efforts eventually outstrip your liver's ability to convert this lactic acid into fuel and it starts to build up rather than get used. This point is called your lactate threshold. You need to decrease the intensity of your training if you want to keep moving. The goal of threshold training is to improve your lactate threshold so you can train at higher intensities for longer. This type of training is fantastic for burning fat because the higher the intensity, the bigger the calorie burn.

The Scoop

Several tests can help you figure out how long and at what pace you need to exercise in order to reach this threshold. These tests differ from sport to sport and are not entirely necessary unless you're a seriously competitive sportsman, in which case you probably have a coach to guide you. But if you're looking to burn fat and get fitter, you need to know just two things. First, these intense bouts of exercise need to last 90 to 180 seconds. Second, you need to train at 85 to 90 per cent of your maximum heart rate for about 20 to 25 minutes. This session isn't continuous—you couldn't do that if you wanted to—but rather is broken up by periods of rest. More complex and accurate tests are available, but this equation gives you a near-exact figure to work towards.

In terms of intensity, threshold training is slightly harder than interval training because the working part of the intervals are longer. Most endurance-style sportsmen, such as cyclists or runners, train just below their lactate threshold so that they can increase these intervals to four to six minutes, take a two- to four-minute break and then go again. Threshold training will improve your overall pace

Calculate Your Maximum Heart Rate

Your maximum heart rate (HRmax) is the highest heart rate you can safely achieve when you exercise. You've probably heard that you can figure out your HRmax using this formula: 220 − your age. These numbers, coined by Dr. William Haskell in the 1970s, weren't actually based on a doddle of research. Haskell has since called the formula laughable and said that it was never supposed to be an absolute guide for athletes' training. Somebody should have told Polar that before they included it in their heart rate monitors. Fortunately, a study in *Journal of Exercise Physiology* (Robergs and Landwehr, 2002) examined 43 HRmax formulas and found this one to be the most accurate:

$$\text{HRmax (beats per minute)} = 205.8 - (0.685 \times \text{age}).$$

So you would calculate the HRmax of a 30-year-old man as follows:

$$205.8 - (0.685 \times 30) = 185.25 \text{ beats per minute.}$$

Don't fret if your heart rate exceeds the maximum. Research at the University of North Carolina (Kolata, 2001) found that some athletes can hold their HRmax for several minutes, and not a textbook in the world says that this is possible. So if you can get your freak on, put it to good use to beat the next bloke.

and get you leaner no matter what sport you participate in.

Threshold-Training Workouts

These workouts might look like interval training. They are, but they can be longer and tougher depending on your ability to recover and your base level of fitness. They're a good way to work up to or down from interval training, depending on how hard you're training. They consist almost exclusively of cardiovascular exercise such as running, cycling or rowing. If you're a bit of an extremist you can try to keep your heart rate up into these parameters with weights, but it'll be vomit-worthy. Most of the following workouts are focused around running because running is the most easily accessible form of training, but you can easily adapt them to any kind of exercise with a little common sense. If a workout includes hill sprints, do the sprints on a bike or crank up the resistance on the machine. The goal is to get your lungs puffing and panting. They should even feel a little pain after these intervals—that's good. This desired effect means that you're taking the rushed approach to losing your love handles.

THRESHOLD-TRAINING WORKOUTS

TRAINING FOR A SET DISTANCE

1. Warm up with a slow jog for 5 to 10 minutes.
2. Run 800 metres as quickly as you can and then jog for 2 minutes or until your breathing returns to normal.
3. Run 1,000 metres as quickly as you can and then jog for 2 minutes or until your breathing returns to normal.
4. Run 1,200 metres as quickly as you can and then jog for 2 minutes or until your breathing returns to normal.
5. Run 1,600 metres as quickly as you can and then jog for 2 minutes or until your breathing returns to normal.
6. Run 1,000 metres as quickly as you can and then jog for 2 minutes or until your breathing returns to normal.
7. Run 800 metres as quickly as you can and then jog for 2 minutes or until your breathing returns to normal.
8. Cool down with a slow jog or walk for 5 minutes.

TRAINING FOR TIME

1. Jog 2 kilometres at a slow pace to warm up.
2. Run (or cycle, swim, row, whatever) for 20 minutes at a pace or heart rate that's just below your lactic threshold.
3. Jog 1 to 2 kilometres at a slow pace to cool down. Try to increase the distance you run or your speed each week.

CARDIO MACHINES IN THE GYM

1. Jog, cycle, row or swim at a slow pace for 5 to 10 minutes to warm up.
2. Set the incline or resistance to 1 and then jog at a pace you can sustain for only 2 minutes. Reduce the speed and jog until you catch your breath but for no longer than 1 minute.
3. Increase the incline or resistance by 1 for at least another 5 bouts so that at the end of the 6 bouts the resistance is set to 6. After each bout, jog until you catch your breath but for no longer than 1 minute.
4. Exercise slowly for 5 minutes to cool down.

WORKING OUT ON A TRACK

1. Run or cycle around the track a few times to warm up.
2. Jog at a moderate pace on the straight of the track. When you get to the turn, accelerate and go as fast as you can go.
3. Once you hit the straight again, reduce your speed and jog until you hit the next curve. When you get to the turn, accelerate again and go as fast as you can. Do this at least 10 times or for as long as you can manage.

4. Slowly walk around the track for 5 minutes to cool down.

HILL SPRINTING

1. Run slowly for 5 minutes, travelling towards a hill if you can, to warm up.

2. Once you've found a hill that's at least 400 metres long, stand at the bottom. Sprint up the hill as fast as you can and then slowly run back to the bottom of the hill. Repeat this 8 to 12 times if you can.

3. Jog slowly for 5 minutes to cool down.

6. Steady-State Cardio

Set off on a fat-burning journey that'll take your body and mind places.

Ever looked in the mirror, grabbed your gut, given it a shake and realised that you've added a few extra kilos? That reflection is usually followed by the question 'Where the hell are my running shoes?' This is pretty much every bloke's knee-jerk reaction to a little unwanted expansion.

Countless articles and studies in fitness magazines or online slam same-paced cardio in favour of interval training or weight training. Let's assume you already know that going for a run around your local park is not the best way to get leaner. Then why do it? In a word: *enjoyment*. Getting out of the rat race without your phone badgering you is pretty fun once you get fit enough that you're not gasping for air every few minutes. Training in the outdoors is a 100 per cent natural form of Prozac. Research in *Environmental Science and Technology* (Thompson Coon et al., 2011) found that just 5 minutes of outdoor exercise was enough to boost mood and feelings of happiness.

If you're feeling a little stressed or miffed, going for a run on the beach or in the local park is an excellent way to decompress after a tough day. Obviously, you might reap the same benefits that you would after the same run on a treadmill thanks to all the stresses—blaring techno music, news flashes on the telly and feeling self-conscious next to the spray-tanned tank-top meathead—that a gym can bring. You should actually try to avoid running on a treadmill. When running on terra firma you propel yourself forward, whereas on the treadmill you just lift your feet, which is much easier. You're not a hamster on a wheel. If you want to go for a long run, make damn sure you get outside and soak up the physical and mental benefits of the great outdoors.

It's Addictive

Endurance athletes can be a pretty a solitary bunch, but they've definitely got a club feel about them. If you meet a fellow endurance aficionado, you know you're both getting high off the same supply. This is the euphoria you feel after a run, cycle or anything that gets your blood pumping for an extended period of time. It's the cheapest and healthiest high you can get and is most certainly addictive. But this high isn't caused by pain-killing endorphins like most people think. It's actually more akin to the buzz that a stoner gets after he puffs a bong.

When you exercise you produce a chemical called anandamide, which attaches to a cannabinoid (seeing the link?) receptor in your brain. This is the same receptor that the active ingredient in marijuana (tetrahydrocannabinol) attaches to give you feelings of relaxation, elation and a buzz similar to what Bill Clinton felt when he didn't inhale. But anandamide does more than just make you see stars and stripes. It dilates your blood vessels and the bronchial tubes in your lungs so that more oxygen gets to your muscles, helping you to run better and longer. It's produced only when your body is under enough stress. But why don't you feel chirpy enough to chat with the blonde sitting next to you after sprinting for the bus? You're likely to experience the runner's high only when running a little slower and for a decent period of time. Work towards achieving the runner's high because it'll spur you on while you train and is certain to give you a body you'll feel euphoric about.

How to Use It

Steady-state cardio is the ideal way to try a sport or even cross-train for a sport. If you want to give running, cycling, swimming, rowing or whatever a go, you'll probably plod along at the same steady pace the first time you have a crack at it. That's fine. It will help you eventually build stamina and most certainly will burn calories. It clocks into the biggest motivational plus point: enjoyment. If you like it you'll come back to it, and if you don't you can just move on. What's more, you can use steady-state cardio training to build a base level of fitness and then start to tackle the fat-burning techniques that are higher up the food chain.

In terms of guidelines, there aren't any. Simply set out and go as long or as far as you can and then return home. (Just make sure you leave enough gas in the tank to make it back.) If you're married with kids or work in a stressful job, you'll probably enjoy the peace. You can even combine several disciplines in one training session the way triathletes do. But be warned that they spend an immense amount of time exercising. This is the biggest caveat of steady-state cardio: the time. If you're willing to dedicate hours on end to getting better at a particular sport, this is the route to follow. But if you have a diary full of commitments, taking endurance exercise seriously will be like taking a second job and may become too much to handle. This type of training can be a problem if you're a bit of a social creature and don't like solitude, but it's easy enough to rope in a training partner or join a club. Once you've put all the pros and cons on the table, look at tables 8.6 and 8.7 to see which forms of exercise fry the most calories. The number of calories burned per hour is based on an 80-kilogram man (Ainsworth et al., 2000). Pick one and then jump on your bike, son.

Putting It All Together

You don't have to handcuff your fat-burning pursuits to a single technique. Here's how to combine and conquer your stored calories.

You've probably heard that avocados are good for you. But just because they're universally accepted as a health food doesn't mean you eat them on their own all the time. You probably spread some on a little bit of toast, make one into guacamole or throw a few slices of another into a salad. This way you get all

STEADY-STATE CARDIO WORKOUTS

Table 8.6 Gym Burn

Gym exercise	Calories burned in 1 hr
Stationary bike (moderate)	571
Rowing (moderate)	572
Elliptical trainer	589
Rowing (fast)	695
Step machine	735
Stationary bike (fast)	859

Table 8.7 Sport Burn

Sport	Calories burned in 1 hr
Bowling	254
Walking (moderate)	279
Golf (walking)	351
Cricket	409
Kayaking	409
Boxing (punch bag)	490
Wrestling	490
Basketball	654
Tennis	654
Walking (fast)	654
Road cycling (moderate)	654
BMX or mountain biking	695
Boxing (sparring)	736
Martial arts	818
Soccer	818
Swimming	818
Running (moderate)	900
Boxing (in the ring)	981
Squash	981
Road cycling (fast)	1301
Running (fast)	1309

the benefits of their healthy fats and vitamins without becoming sick to death of their taste. You probably could live on avocados, but you'd be far healthier if you ate a balanced diet.

When it comes to losing weight you should treat your sweat sessions like you treat avocados. Mix them up, try a new recipe and

When Exercise is a Chore

When you work with your hands and do things around the house you create impressive real-world strength that builds muscles and keeps you lean enough to earn a few beers. When household chores—such as the ones in the following list—were compared with an equivalent calorie-burning gym activity, people perceived the chores as easier even though the chores burned as many calories as the gym activity, found research in *Current Psychology* (Slotterback, Leeman and Oakes, 2006). If something seems easier you're more likely to stick to it. Your body doesn't know that you're not slogging it out in the gym, so it reacts as if you were: by building muscle and burning fat. Your muscles respond well to the tension, speed and cardiovascular demands of using tools. Jump up and chisel your body and home the old-fashioned way, just like gramps did. You may even earn a quid or two with a better-looking home and a better-looking body to fill it with.

The number of calories burned is based on an 80-kilogram man (Ainsworth et al., 2000).

Chore	Calories burned in 1 hr
Wiring and plumbing	245
Heavy cleaning (car, windows)	245
General carpentry	245
Hanging a wallboard	245
Trimming hedges or branches	286
Raking leaves	352
Planting a tree	368
Operating a floor sander	409
Cleaning gutters	409
Painting	491
Chopping and splitting wood	491
Mowing grass	491

experiment as much as possible. That way you won't get sick of relentlessly trying to burn calories. The following sections explain how to apply a perfectly balanced approach to your calorie-culling pursuits and reap the long-term benefits of having abs that show, even in winter.

Variety

There are two big players in the weight-loss game: enjoyment, which has already been mentioned, and planning. If you make a cast-iron commitment to drop fat and then set about doing it in the fastest and most efficient way possible, you'll probably choose the two top-ranked methods: weightlifting circuits and HIT. You might think that you'll tick the

enjoyment box when you see your shiny new six-pack. That's a fair assumption, but the top-ranked fat-loss methods, although very effective, are bloody tough. They're like a bitter medicine: You pinch your nose and happily take it because you know it will make you better. After two months on one of these programmes you will definitely be a few kilos lighter and happy with the results. You'll also have learned something important: Your workouts are gut-wrenchingly tough. So each time you consider exercising your brain automatically switches to hard-work mode. This can be a real problem because some days you'll be a little more tired than usual (even Usain Bolt has these days) and the thought of exercising—especially training until you feel like puking—won't elicit enjoyment. The result?

You skip the session rather than do a slightly milder form of training that you'd enjoy and that would probably rejuvenate rather than obliterate you. This is how you risk brainwashing yourself into thinking that you must do the very best type of exercise or nothing at all. Do not fall into this trap. If you're really keen to begin with, you should drip-feed yourself workouts to keep your motivation high. This strategy is far more effective in the long term than racing out of the blocks at full speed and going so hard that you eventually burn out and end up back at square one. This is why planning is so important. It helps you ration your motivation over the long haul and be lean forever rather than just over the summer.

Plan to Succeed

Make a list of all the cool activities and fitness-based stuff you'd like to do. Yes, we'd all like to go surfing in Hawaii a few times a week, but not all of us live near Maui. Limit your list to the stuff that's local, realistic and accessible. This could be running in the local park, cycling to the beach for a swim, taking up wall climbing at a rock-climbing centre, trying a boxing class, digging in the garden, whatever. Choose only stuff you actually want to do because you think you'll genuinely have fun doing it. Feel free to list things you've never done but have always wanted to try. Experiencing a new activity burns more calories than doing the stuff you're an old hand at because using new muscles burns extra calories. Once you have a minimum of 10 entries on your list, research the hell out of each one to find ways you can do them near your home or work. You'll soon have all the information you need to get started and will have no doubt whetted your appetite and stoked your motivation. Stick that list of 10 activities on your fridge so that it stares at you first thing in the morning.

Now set a goal for how much weight you aim to shift. The more weight you have to lose, the longer it will take and the more varied your training plan should be to keep you interested. If you want to shift only a few kilos, you probably need to follow a more reg-imented programme for quick results. The big thing is to pick a number and work towards it.

Click open your diary and shift, juggle or cancel things so that you can schedule the time for yourself that your body desperately craves. Mark off a 45- to 60-minute time slot in your diary for every day or at least every second day. This slot might be before you go to work, during your lunch hour, after work or even the weekends. When you look at your diary you won't see just business lunches; you'll see a commitment to your health and a promise to yourself to look precisely the way you want.

Once you know how much you want to weigh or what you want your body fat percentage to be, ask yourself another question: How good are you at following plans? Do you enjoy writing lists and crossing things off or are you more of a take-it-as-it-comes bloke who thrives on spontaneity? You can probably answer that question quickly just by looking at your clothes cupboard. If it's a jumbled mess of T-shirts and socks placed on the same shelf, chances are you're a spontaneous guy. If your shirts are folded into neat piles and placed far away from any sock, you might be better suited to preplanning your training. Both ways work but only if you're honest with yourself from the start. If you have a change of heart, it's dead easy to switch approaches.

If you're a guy who folds his T-shirts, follow the plans in this section. They outline exactly what to do based on how much weight you want to lose. The plans are quite rigid but you can always go over to the dark side with the guy with the scrunched-up T-shirts. If you're willing to embrace the randomness of the universe, a rigid training routine will not work for you in the long term. You may have tried with little success to follow a plan you got out of a magazine. That's cool. You just like being in charge of your own destiny when it suits you. Follow the rule of haphazardness and hit the shuffle button on your fat-burning sessions. Stick on your fridge your list of 10 activities you really enjoy doing. (Watching *Mad Men* shouldn't be one of them.) Each day, wake up and pick an item of fun without thinking about it or, to make it really random, have your significant other or flatmate do it for you. Do at least four items a week, which isn't so bad considering that they're fun. If you find that an activity is not fun, choose a new one. But make sure you follow this no-plan plan.

Now that you have your list you don't have to slog through the boredom of gym work or spend hours running on a treadmill. You have a firm excuse to get out there and enjoy life. Should you wish to kick up the pace of your fat burning, simply find a fat-burning workout in this book that suits your level of experience. If you get involved in a sport or activity you like doing, you'll probably benefit from a little extra training and will find yourself getting bigger thrills from the stuff you love. Fitness is life, so put aside time every day to go out, live life and have fun. Can't find the time? Then you need to change your work–life balance. There's no point in spending your health making your wealth and then spending that wealth to get back your health.

Lose the Last 5 to 10 Kilograms of Body Fat

Getting rid of that final wobble can be just as tough as getting rid of a bigger load. Here's the swiftest course of action to getting high-definition abs.

One of Mother Nature's nasty little jokes is that the first place you put on weight—above your belt—is the last place you lose it. If you've been through a bulking stage during which you stacked on muscle and a little fat, a fair bit of that mass may have settled on your stomach. Unfortunately, the world looks at that very area for signs of overall leanness. If you have abs that show, people assume that the rest of you must be lean. This is probably why abs top the most-wanted lists in trashy women's magazines. But don't feel hard done by. The fairer sex has the same conundrum except the rear end is the litmus test of fitness.

This need to reduce fat from specific areas spawned an entire generation of infomercials claiming to carve muscle from fatty areas. The fitness community desperately wanted this idea of spot reduction to work, but unfortu-

nately it doesn't. Research in *American Journal of Physiology, Endocrinology and Metabolism* (Stallknecht, Dela and Helge, 2007) even found that guys lost the tiniest amount of fat on the legs when they did a ridiculous number of leg extensions. The results proved that spot reduction has such miniscule effect that you're much better off trying something else.

The first rule of war is to know your enemy. In this case, the enemy is that stubborn bit of podge covering your abs. You can probably even poke your fingers in there and feel your six-pack under the covering layer. When your abs are no more than a fingertip away, you may be tempted to try anything and everything. Starvation, kooky fads and supplements that leave you more jittery than the cast of *Trainspotting* are all aimed at people looking to get rid of that final layer. To make matters worse, a study in *American Journal of Physiology—Regulatory, Integrative and Comparative Physiology* (Sullivan and Cameron, 2010) found that reducing your calorie intake is simply not enough to promote significant weight loss. They found that a natural body mechanism conserves energy in response to a reduction in calories. The irony is that the scientists suggest that the best way to get lean is to cut calories and step up your training, but if you're eating less you don't much feel like training. To make matters worse, you could go through all the pain and hassle of supplements and fad diets only to find that not much has changed. That's because the body is designed to hold fat. It's actually for your own good, although you may not agree. Back in the old days—long before spray tans and clothes with *Prada* sewn into the label—people who were more likely to store calories (the bigger blokes) were at an advantage because they'd be carrying a fuel reserve with them if a food shortage ever occurred. That final bit covering your abs is your camel hump that you can use in case you get trapped inside an elevator without food for a few days. Your body will use it, along with some muscle mass, as fuel if you stop eating. But don't use that as an excuse to starve yourself to get abs. Your body often hangs onto that fat when you've lost a lot of weight because it gets scared that you're eating away at your savings. This makes it hang onto the final bit of fat at all costs, which can cause some hormonal changes such as excessive cortisol and not enough testosterone. A study in *International Journal of Sports Medicine* (Karila et al., 2008) found that rapid weight loss decreases the chief hormone that builds and preserves muscle: testosterone. Hormones such as these are what can make or break your quest for a six-pack.

Don't Stress

Cortisol is a hormone that is released during times of stress. It doesn't matter whether you're stressed because your coffee is too hot or because you're not losing enough weight. The brain reacts the same way regardless of whether the stress is physical, mental or emotional and sends signals to produce more cortisol in response to the stress. This reaction can be caused by extremely low calorie diets, intense training, high volumes of training, lack of quality sleep or common daily stresses such as trouble at work or getting into a ruck with your missus. But don't get the wrong idea: Cortisol is a friend, not a foe. It's what makes your body the most adaptable thing on the planet. It cues your heart to thump faster, gives you more energy and mobilises more adrenaline—just about everything you want to happen before a hard training session. However, too much of it can make you fatigued, affect concentration, cause you to recover slower from injuries or illness and cause you to collect fat around your stomach.

A link exists between abdominal fat and cortisol in that cortisol causes you to store fat around the organs. This puts you at risk of heart disease and diabetes. Cortisol itself does not make you fat; otherwise every stockbroker on the planet would be on the next *Biggest Loser*. The trick is to maintain healthy levels. Too much can make you lose muscle tissue and reduce your levels of growth hormone, both of which in turn make you burn fewer calories. How do you keep cortisol in check? The answer is simple: balance. To keep yourself in check you need to stress yourself enough with training and balance that stress with enough

recovery time. Follow these basic rules for looking after yourself to keep your hormones working towards fat loss.

- Hit the snooze button. Sleep helps your muscles recover, increases growth hormone (a powerful fat burner) and lowers cortisol. The old adage of eight hours hold true, but nine hours will do you better.

- Get outside. Getting some sun on your back helps you absorb more minerals so you recover faster from training, found a study in *Journal of Bone and Mineral Research* (Bell et al., 1988). Other studies found that being deficient in vitamin D makes you less likely to burn fat.

- Eat to relax. Proper nutrition is easy to master. Go for natural foods and you'll have all the nutrients you need for your body to be healthy and in balance. Many cruciferous vegetables decrease your levels of oestrogen and fresh meat increases your testosterone.

- Do high-intensity workouts. The shorter and harder the better. Your cortisol levels increase after 55 to 60 minutes of training.

- Drink plenty of water. Research in *International Journal of Sports Medicine* (Maresh et al., 2006) found that being dehydrated when you train can increase cortisol and decrease testosterone. That's a double bogey against your weight-loss goals.

- Adopt a positive mindset. Worry is stress. If you rack your brain with negative thoughts you'll never get positive outcomes from your training. Do whatever it takes to see the world sunny-side up.

- Don't binge. Despite what Westerns depict, alcohol and tobacco drum your testosterone down and your cortisol up. There's no reason to be a cowboy about your health.

The Next Step

If you're really struggling to lose weight, go to a hormone clinic to get tested for imbalances.

This will help you know for certain whether you need to adopt some serious lifestyle changes or balance your hormones with medication. Once your insides are ticking along at the correct pace you can fine-tune your sweat sessions. Warning: It's not going to be an easy ride, but you'll be willing to grit through it because the results will come quickly. Unlike shifting a lot of weight, which might take a fair bit of time, the strategy for losing the final layer of fat is short and sharp. That means that it might not be overly enjoyable and will be chock full of gut-wrenching training sessions.

Rules for Losing the Final Layer

For your workouts to be effective follow these principles.

- Use the top-ranked fat-burning systems. Workouts that are more taxing build more muscle, fry more calories and deliver results quicker.

- Keep your body guessing. You get fitter because you adapt to activity. The more of a novice you are at a particular style of exercise the more calories you'll burn, so change it up often.

- Push yourself. Improve each week. Push more weight, run farther or go faster. Whatever you're doing, aim to better yourself every week. And do it in less than 60 minutes.

- Keep your motivation high. Set an end goal to hit within a fixed period of time. This will put a spark in your keenness and make it easier to reach your end point.

- Rest is as good as work. You'll go harder in your next workout if you give yourself enough time to recover. Burnout can come quickly to guys trying to shed pounds because they usually restrict calories. This creates hormone imbalances, which will backpedal your progress.

Steady-State Cardio Workouts

This short-term plan is more regimented than the six-month plan in chapter 9. Do it over four to six weeks and repeat it if you can stand it. You need to properly schedule rest due to the blitzkrieg nature of this plan, so do workout 1 on Monday, workout 2 on Tuesday and then rest on Wednesday. Do workout 3 on Thursday and workout 4 on Friday. Workout 5 is an active recovery day, so do it any time over the weekend.

In this regimen you progress every week and each workout gets a little bit tougher. By week 3 the structure and exercises used in the workouts will change dramatically. However, the techniques will be more or less the same, so you can use the base level of fitness you've built up to go harder in the new workouts. Once you hit your body-fat goal you won't have to work as hard. You can taper off the workout and watch your eating habits. The trick is to modify your training and eating so that you stay at the level of leanness that suits your lifestyle. Trying to maintain the body-fat levels of a bodybuilder is nearly impossible and massively restrictive in the long run. But you can still have a swoon-worthy six-pack and a reasonably low body-fat level that lets you have your favourite food and miss the odd workout. Tone down these workouts by doing fewer sets and taking more rest and you should be able to reap the benefits of these hard yards for years to come.

LOSE THOSE LAST POUNDS WORKOUT

WEEK 1

Workout 1: High-Intensity Weights and Cardio

This workout is full of supersets (table 8.8). Do the first exercise as heavy as you can so that you fail on the sixth rep. Do the second move straight away and then rest for 30 to 45 seconds. Once you finish, move on to the cardio session.

HIT: Go outside and sprint (or do an exercise of your choice) for 8 seconds and then jog for 30 seconds. Do this until you've trained for a total of 60 minutes.

Table 8.8   Week 1, Workout 1

Exercise	Sets	Reps
Superset 1		
1. Squat	4	6
2. Push-up	4	10
Superset 2		
3. Squat press	4	6
4. Dumbbell standing shoulder press	4	10
Superset 3		
5. Overhand-grip pull-up	4	6
6. Lunge (body weight)	4	10
Superset 4		
7. Dumbbell deadlift	4	6
8. Close-grip bench press	4	10

Workout 2: Outdoor Crossfit Session

Do the reps in the workout (table 8.9) in as many sets as you need. If you have to stop after every 10 reps, then do. Just remember that every second of slouch costs you on the body-fat scale. Do this circuit as many times as you can in 50 minutes. You're doing well if you can do it more than twice.

Table 8.9   Week 1, Workout 2

Exercise	Sets	Reps
1. Run 400 metres		
2. Squat (body weight)	1	80
3. Push-up	1	80
4. Run 1 kilometre		
5. Lying leg raise	1	80
6. Sprint 800 metres		

Workout 3: Complex Sets

In this workout (table 8.10) you'll minimise the rest period by executing all of the exercises for 1 set without putting down the barbell. This places your muscles under constant tension. You'll then rest and repeat the circuit a total of 4 times. Once you've done all of the exercises in the complex set take a 2- to 3-minute breather.

HIT: Go outside and sprint (or do an exercise of your choice) for 6 seconds and then jog for 20 seconds. Do this until you've trained for a total of 60 minutes or are too tired to walk.

Table 8.10   Week 1, Workout 3

Exercise	Sets	Reps
1. Barbell biceps curl	4	10
2. Squat press	4	8
3. Squat	4	8
4. Good morning	4	8
5. Barbell deadlift	4	8
6. Dumbbell bent-over row	4	8
7. Push-up (hands on barbell)	4	8
8. Barbell rollout	4	8

Workout 4: Interval Training

Interval training is the hard and fast way to burn fat while giving your ticker and lungs a thorough workout. In the midst of this workout you can expect to feel a burning sensation deep in your chest—that's fine. It's not a heart attack. It's merely your body working at full capacity. When it's all over and you're showering you'll feel like you've gained a brand spanking new set of lungs. Your legs, on the other hand, may not feel quite so chipper.

1. Warm up for 10 minutes with your activity of choice.
2. Sprint for 1 minute and then slow down for 2 minutes. Do this 5 times.
3. Sprint for 2 minutes and then slow down for 2 minutes. Do this 4 times.
4. Cool down for 10 minutes at a slow pace.

Workout 5: Active Recovery

Go for a walk, even if it's around a shopping centre. Just keep active so that your muscles are working.

WEEK 2

Workout 1: High-Intensity Weights and Cardio

This workout is full of supersets (table 8.11). Do the first exercise as heavy as you can so that you fail on the sixth rep. Do the second move straight away and then rest for 30 to 45 seconds. For all the sets of 6 reps, increase the weight you used in week 1 by 3 per cent. Once you finish, move on to the cardio session.

Table 8.11   Week 2, Workout 1

Exercise	Sets	Reps
Superset 1		
1. Squat	4	6
2. Push-up	4	12
Superset 2		
3. Squat press	4	6
4. Dumbbell standing shoulder press	4	12
Superset 3		
5. Overhand-grip pull-up	4	6
6. Lunge (body weight)	4	12
Superset 4		
7. Dumbbell deadlift	4	6
8. Close-grip bench press	4	12

HIT: Go outside and sprint (or do an exercise of your choice) for 8 seconds and then jog for 30 seconds. Do this until you've trained for a total of 60 minutes.

Workout 2: Outdoor Crossfit Session

Do the reps in the workout (table 8.12) in as many sets as you need. If you have to stop after every 10 reps, then do. Just remember that every second of slouch costs you on the body-fat scale. Try to do to this circuit once in less than an hour.

Table 8.12   Week 2, Workout 2

Exercise	Sets	Reps
1. Run 1 kilometre		
2. Squat (body weight)	1	90
3. Run 1 kilometre		
4. Push-up	1	90
5. Run 1 kilometre		
6. Lying leg raise	1	90
7. Run 1 kilometre		

Workout 3: Complex Sets

In this workout (table 8.13) you'll minimise the rest period by executing all of the exercises for 1 set without putting down the barbell. This places your muscles under constant tension. Once you've done all the exercises in the complex set take a 2- to 3-minute breather, repeat the circuit a total of 4 times and then crack on with the HIT that follows. Phew. It's a tough task but you'll get through it.

Table 8.13   Week 2, Workout 3

Exercise	Sets	Reps
1. Barbell biceps curl	4	10
2. Squat press	4	10
3. Squat	4	10
4. Good morning	4	10
5. Barbell deadlift	4	10
6. Dumbbell bent-over row	4	10
7. Push-up (hands on barbell)	4	10
8. Barbell rollout	4	10

HIT: Go outside and sprint (or do an exercise of your choice) for 8 seconds and then jog for 20 seconds. Do this until you've trained for a total of 60 minutes or are too tired to walk.

Workout 4: Interval Training

This workout involves slightly longer intervals. You won't be sprinting at your Usain Bolt pace, but you will learn to hit them at about 70 per cent of your maximum pace. This pace differs from person to person, so make sure you're going at the same speed for the duration of the interval. In other words, take your foot off the gas a little but not too much.

1. Warm up for 10 minutes with your activity of choice.
2. Sprint for 90 seconds and then slow down for 2 minutes. Do this 4 times.
3. Sprint for 2 minutes and then slow down for 1 minute. Do this 3 times.
4. Cool down for 10 minutes at a slow pace.

Workout 5: Active Recovery

Go for a walk (even if it's around a shopping centre), ride, swim, whatever. Just keep active so that your muscles are working—but not too hard. You should not get out of breath during this workout.

WEEK 3

Workout 1: High-Intensity Weights and Cardio

This workout is full of supersets (table 8.14). Do the first exercise as heavy as you can so that you fail on the sixth rep. Do the second move straight away and then rest for 30 to 45 seconds. For all the sets of 6 reps, increase the weights you used in week 2 by 3 per cent. Once you finish, move on to the cardio session.

Table 8.14 Week 3, Workout 1

Exercise	Sets	Reps
Superset 1		
1. Squat	4	6
2. Push-up	4	14
Superset 2		
3. Squat press	4	6
4. Dumbbell standing shoulder press	4	14
Superset 3		
5. Overhand-grip pull-up	4	6
6. Lunge (body weight)	4	14
Superset 4		
7. Dumbbell deadlift	4	6
8. Close-grip bench press	4	14

HIT: Go outside and sprint (or do an exercise of your choice) for 8 seconds and then jog for 30 seconds. Do this until you've trained for a total of 60 minutes.

Workout 2: Outdoor Crossfit Session

Do the reps in the workout (table 8.15) in as many sets as you need. If you have to stop after every 10 reps, then do. Just remember every second of slouch costs you on the body-fat scale. Try to do to this circuit once in less than an hour.

Table 8.15 Week 3, Workout 2

Exercise	Sets	Reps
1. Run 1 kilometre		
2. Squat (body weight)	1	100
3. Run 1 kilometre		
4. Push-up	1	100
5. Run 1 kilometre		
6. Lying leg raise	1	100
7. Run 1 kilometre		

Workout 3: Complex Sets

In this workout (table 8.16) you'll minimise the rest period by executing all of the exercises for 1 set without putting down the barbell This places your muscles under constant tension. Once you've done all the exercises in the complex set take a 2- to 3-minute breather, repeat the circuit 4 times and then do the HIT that follows.

Table 8.16 Week 3, Workout 3

Exercise	Sets	Reps
1. Barbell biceps curl	4	12
2. Squat press	4	12
3. Squat	4	12
4. Good morning	4	12
5. Barbell deadlift	4	12
6. Dumbbell bent-over row	4	12
7. Push-up (hands on barbell)	4	12
8. Barbell rollout	4	12

HIT: Go outside and sprint (or do an exercise of your choice) for 10 seconds and then jog for 20 seconds. Do this until you've trained for a total of 60 minutes or are too tired to walk.

Workout 4: Interval Training

The intervals are getting even longer. Although you're getting stronger and fitter, you'll need to learn how to productively manage your built-in accelerator.

1. Warm up for 10 minutes with your activity of choice.
2. Sprint for 2 minutes and then slow down for 2 minutes. Do this 3 times.
3. Sprint for 3 minutes and then slow down for 1 minute. Do this 2 times.
4. Cool down for 10 minutes at a slow pace.

Workout 5: Active Recovery

Go for a walk (even if it's around a shopping centre), ride, swim, whatever. Just keep active so that your muscles are working—but not too hard. You should not get out of breath during this workout.

WEEK 4

Workout 1: High-Intensity Weights and Cardio

This workout consists of trisets (table 8.17). Do the first exercise as heavy as you can so that you fail on the sixth rep. Do the second and third moves straight away and then rest for 30 to 45 seconds. For all the sets of 6 reps, increase the weights you used in week 3 by 3 per cent. Once you finish, move on to the cardio session.

Table 8.17   Week 4, Workout 1

Exercise	Sets	Reps
Triset 1		
1. Squat	3	6
2. Push-up	3	14
3. Standing calf raise	3	10
Triset 2		
4. Squat press	3	6
5. Dumbbell standing shoulder press	3	14
6. Hanging leg raise	3	10
Triset 3		
7. Overhand-grip pull-up	3	6
8. Lunge (body weight)	3	14
9. Hammer curl	3	10
Triset 4		
10. Dumbbell deadlift	3	6
11. Close-grip bench press	3	14
12. Bicycle crunch	3	10

HIT: Go outside and sprint (or do an exercise of your choice) for 8 seconds and then jog for 25 seconds. Do this until you've trained for a total of 60 minutes.

Workout 2: Weights Crossfit Session

Try to do this circuit (table 8.18) at least twice in 60 minutes. If you can do it a third time, go for it.

Table 8.18   Week 4, Workout 2

Exercise	Sets	Reps
1. Squat press	1	50
2. Cycle 1 kilometre		
3. Dumbbell flat chest press	1	50
4. Row 1 kilometre		
5. Power clean	1	50
6. Run 1 kilometre		
7. Squat	1	50
8. Elliptical cross-train 1 kilometre		

Workout 3: Complex Sets

In this workout (table 8.19) you'll minimise the rest period by executing all of the exercises for 1 set without putting down the dumbbells. This places your muscles under constant tension. Once you've done all the exercises in the complex set take a 2- to 3-minute breather, repeat the circuit 4 times and then do the high-intensity intervals that follow.

Table 8.19   Week 4, Workout 3

Exercise	Sets	Reps
1. Hammer curl	4	8
2. Triceps extension	4	8
3. Split squat (dumbbells)	4	8
4. Lateral raise	4	8
5. Arnold press	4	8
6. Dumbbell incline row	4	8
7. Push-up (hands on dumbbells)	4	8
8. Side plank	4	30 sec.

HIT: Go outside and sprint (or do an exercise of your choice) for 10 seconds and then jog for 20 seconds. Do this until you've trained for a total of 60 minutes.

Workout 4: Outdoor Cardioacceleration

Do this workout (table 8.20) 2 to 4 times depending on how much rest you take. The ideal method is to go for a run and then drop and do the next bodyweight exercise.

Table 8.20   Week 4, Workout 4

Exercise	Reps
1. Run for 5 minutes to warm up	
2. Push-up	15
3. Run for 1 minute	
4. Squat (body weight)	15
5. Run for 1 minute	
6. Bicycle crunch	15
7. Run for 1 minute	
8. Split squat	15
9. Run for 1 minute	
10. Single-leg dumbbell deadlift	15

Workout 5: Active Recovery

Go for a walk (even if it's around a shopping centre), ride, swim, whatever. Just keep active so that your muscles are working—but not too hard. You should not get out of breath during this workout.

WEEK 5

Workout 1: High-Intensity Weights and Cardio

This workout is full of trisets (table 8.21). Do the first exercise as heavy as you can so that you fail on the sixth rep. Do the second and third moves straight away and then rest for 30 to 45 seconds. For all the sets of 6 reps, increase the weights you used in week 4 by 3 per cent. Once you finish, move on to the cardio session.

HIT: Go outside and sprint (or do an exercise of your choice) for 10 seconds and then jog for 25 seconds. Do this until you've trained for a total of 60 minutes.

Table 8.21   Week 5, Workout 1

Exercise	Sets	Reps
Triset 1		
1. Squat	3	6
2. Push-up	3	14
3. Standing calf raise	3	12
Triset 2		
4. Squat press	3	6
5. Dumbbell standing shoulder press	3	14
6. Hanging leg raise	3	12
Triset 3		
7. Overhand-grip pull-up	3	6
8. Lunge (body weight)	3	14
9. Hammer curl	3	12
Triset 4		
10. Dumbbell deadlift	3	6
11. Close-grip bench press	3	14
12. Bicycle crunch	3	12

Workout 2: Weights Crossfit Session

Try to repeat this circuit (table 8.22) at least twice in 60 minutes. If you can do it a third time, go for it.

Table 8.22   Week 5, Workout 2

Exercise	Sets	Reps
1. Squat press	1	60
2. Cycle 1 kilometre		
3. Dumbbell flat chest press	1	60
4. Row 1 kilometre		
5. Power clean	1	60
6. Run 1 kilometre		
7. Squat	1	60
8. Elliptical cross-train 1 kilometre		

Workout 3: Complex Sets

In this workout (table 8.23) you'll minimise the rest period by executing all of the exercises for 1 set without putting down the dumbbells. This places your muscles under constant tension. Once you've done all the exercises in the complex set take a 2- to 3-minute breather, repeat the circuit 4 times and then do the high-intensity intervals that follow.

Table 8.23   Week 5, Workout 3

Exercise	Sets	Reps
1. Hammer curl	4	10
2. Triceps extension	4	10
3. Split squat (dumbbells)	4	10
4. Lateral raise	4	10
5. Arnold press	4	10
6. Dumbbell incline row	4	10
7. Push-up (hands on dumbbells)	4	10
8. Side plank	4	40 sec.

HIT: Go outside and sprint (or do an exercise of your choice) for 12 seconds and then jog for 20 seconds. Do this until you've trained for a total of 60 minutes.

Workout 4: Outdoor Cardioacceleration

Do this workout (table 8.24) 2 to 4 times depending on how much rest you take. The ideal method is to go for a run and then drop and do the next bodyweight exercise. Take a breather between the reps if you need to.

Table 8.24   Week 5, Workout 4

Exercise	Reps
1. Run for 5 minutes to warm up	
2. Push-up	20
3. Run for 1 minute	
4. Squat (body weight)	20
5. Run for 1 minute	
6. Bicycle crunch	20
7. Run for 1 minute	
8. Split squat	20
9. Run for 1 minute	
10. Single-leg dumbbell deadlift	20

Workout 5: Active Recovery

Go for a walk (even if it's around a shopping centre), ride, swim, whatever. Just keep active so that your muscles are working—but not too hard. You should not get out of breath during this workout.

WEEK 6

Workout 1: High-Intensity Weights and Cardio

This workout is full of trisets (table 8.25). Do the first exercise as heavy as you can so that you fail on the sixth rep. Do the second and third moves straight away using the most weight you can manage for 14 and 10 reps, respectively, and then rest for 30 to 45 seconds. For all the sets of 6 reps, increase the weights you used in week 5 by 3 per cent. Once you finish, move on to the cardio session.

Table 8.25   Week 6, Workout 1

Exercise	Sets	Reps
Triset 1		
1. Squat	3	8
2. Push-up	3	14
3. Standing calf raise	3	10
Triset 2		
4. Squat press	3	8
5. Dumbbell standing shoulder press	3	14
6. Hanging leg raise	3	10
Triset 3		
7. Overhand-grip pull-up	3	8
8. Lunge (body weight)	3	14
9. Hammer curl	3	10
Triset 4		
10. Dumbbell deadlift	3	8
11. Close-grip bench press	3	14
12. Bicycle crunch	3	10

HIT: Go outside and sprint (or do an exercise of your choice) for 8 seconds and then jog for 25 seconds. Do this until you've trained for a total of 60 minutes.

Workout 2: Weights Crossfit Session

Try to repeat this circuit (table 8.26) at least twice in 60 minutes. If you can do it a third time, go for it.

Table 8.26   Week 6, Workout 2

Exercise	Reps
1. Squat press	70
2. Cycle 1 kilometre	
3. Dumbbell flat chest press	70
4. Row 1 kilometre	
5. Power clean	70
6. Run 1 kilometre	
7. Squat	70
8. Elliptical cross-train 1 kilometre	

Workout 3: Complex Sets

In this workout (table 8.27) you'll minimise the rest period by executing all of the exercises for 1 set without putting down the dumbbells. This places your muscles under constant tension. Once you've done all the exercises in the complex set take a 2- to 3-minute breather, repeat the circuit 4 times and then do the high-intensity intervals that follow.

Table 8.27   Week 6, Workout 3

Exercise	Sets	Reps
1. Hammer curl	4	12
2. Triceps extension	4	12
3. Split squat (dumbbells)	4	12
4. Lateral raise	4	12
5. Arnold press	4	12
6. Dumbbell incline row	4	12
7. Push-up (hands on dumbbells)	4	12
8. Side plank	4	50 sec.

HIT: Go outside and sprint (or do an exercise of your choice) for 15 seconds and then jog for 30 seconds. Do this until you've trained for a total of 60 minutes.

Workout 4: Outdoor Cardioacceleration

Do this workout (table 8.28) 2 to 4 times depending on how much rest you take. The ideal method is to go for a run and then drop and do the next bodyweight exercise.

Table 8.28   Week 6, Workout 4

Exercise	Reps
1. Run for 5 minutes to warm up	
2. Push-up	20
3. Run for 1 minute	
4. Squat (body weight)	20
5. Run for 1 minute	
6. Bicycle crunch	20
7. Run for 1 minute	
8. Split squat	20
9. Run for 1 minute	
10. Single-leg dumbbell deadlift	20

Workout 5: Active Recovery

Go for a walk (even if it's around a shopping centre), ride, swim, whatever. Just keep active so that your muscles are working—but not too hard. You should not get out of breath during this workout.

That's it. Congratulations: You've now flushed a significant amount of body fat and should be able to rock your abs swagger the next time the sun rears its head.

Where Next?

If you have more than 10 kilograms to get rid of, go to chapter 9 for a complete long-term plan that'll create lasting weight loss. If you're already happy with what you've got, move on to the time-poor man's training plans in chapter 10 so you'll know what to do when you have less free time than you'd like. You can also move on to the workouts that offer double results (chapter 11) and finish off with sport-specific workouts (chapter 12) that will help you put your newly lean body to the test against your fellow man.

9

Major Trimming

Got a way to go? Need to lose more than 10 kilograms of body fat? Here's the plan that'll get you leaner in the long term.

If you have a long road ahead of you, you've probably considered a diet. You may have even tried some sort of brand-name eating plan: Atkins, South Beach, Lemon Detox. If you have, chances are you've experienced what the labcoats are slowly getting their overefficient brains around. Research in *Psychology of Health and Medicine* (Amigo and Fernandez, 2007) found that people who dieted regularly—especially blokes who yo-yo dieted—did get very noticeable results in the short term. But in the long term they returned to their normal weight and continued to strain the scale as they always had. Does this hard-and-fast approach work? Yes, and it works very well. But the rapid results also lead to a rapid loss of motivation and you often end up slipping into your old training and eating habits with frankenfood such as hotdogs.

If you revert to your old habits with food—your biggest player in the success or failure of any weight-loss goal—it doesn't take a Nostradamus to predict that the same thing is likely to happen in the exercise arena. Amigo and Fernandez (2007) did state that the best way to lose weight in the long term is to make lifestyle changes. That advice may be vague, but that doesn't mean you can't take something from it. Small daily changes make it easier to change your everyday life for good. Rather than setting a time limit—say,

dieting and exercising for 2 months so you can lose 10 kilograms—aim to make permanent changes that you want to make and that are easy. It's like deciding to add an extra serving of veggies on your dinner plate rather than going on a diet where you eat nothing but flatulence-worthy cabbage.

Consider the lifestyle approach because training is far tougher than eating. It demands time, money and effort, so it's best not to dive into it while forgoing all the things you enjoy. A better bet is to strike a balance so that you earn your cheat activities such as devouring an entire bucket of KFC. Imagine if you saw the bottom of that bucket every day. It wouldn't taste as good as it would if you ate it once a month. The exercise plans that follow start off easy so you can still lead a normal life without experiencing a drastic change. You won't have to take anything away; you'll just do a little movement to counterbalance your lack of movement. Someone with absolutely no form of fitness at all can do these workouts. Yes, even if you get out of breath going up the stairs in your house. The programmes start off light and include a few spots for you to celebrate your uniqueness and do the activities you enjoy. Equally, they afford you the flexibility to cut out the things you detest. Don't like running? No problem. No rule says you have to buy a gym membership and use a treadmill if you want to be fit and lean. The goal is to slowly make a lifestyle change rather than a one-off blitz.

One thing you should strive for is consistency. That's where the lifestyle aspect comes into play. You'll slowly build up your fitness, willpower and enjoyment of using your body the way it is supposed to be used without yo-yoing back to the starting point. Be warned that these programmes may not be what you'd get if you were employing a personal trainer every day. A trainer would likely have you hitting the weights and treadmill with excitable vigour, and that would get you fast results. Unfortunately, having a trainer can be a bit like going on a crash-course diet. You'll get results very fast because someone pushes you through the tough bits when you feel like giving up. But do you plan on employing a personal trainer forever? Unlikely. When your motivation or money run out you'll be left with noticeable results that you're very happy with, but you'll be in danger of slipping back into your old habits without someone reminding you about sessions or asking what you've eaten. What follows is not the strategy that the world's best trainer would give you because that programme would work only if he was working for free and measuring, coaxing and evaluating your every movement. What follows is the best programme you can use to slowly develop your own motivation, find a love for working your muscles and create a sustainable lifestyle pattern that has you shedding fat every month—well, until you're satisfied that you're exactly as lean as you've always planned to be.

Your muscles get bored easily. If you haven't been hitting your goals fast enough you need to break the tedium—quickly. To refresh your workout you'll need to include new challenges as much as possible, and to do that you need to plan. Plan for the chaos and plan to bring in unpredictability. You don't have to get out your yearly calendar; you can get away with planning your fitness pursuits a month in advance. Planning on an ad hoc basis is probably the most effective because it lets you adjust your workouts on the fly. One month you might have a girlfriend who likes to run. The next month the same girl (or a different one) likes to stay home and watch telly or cycle. You can and must adjust your workout according to your changing life, seasons and work or family demands. This keeps things flexible and helps you slot things into their rightful place. More important, it helps you build on your previous successes or failures. If you suddenly find that you can easily whiz up hills on your bicycle you might want to use this fitness to go on a hike up a mountain or hill. But if you struggle with hill riding you know not to accept an invitation for a hiking trip until you get better at it. In life, those who adapt the best create the biggest success.

The Workouts

Although adaptability is vital for success, for practical purposes the workout plans that follow are quite rigid and include a few open spots for you to add your own flair. For the first three months you won't need a gym membership. If you stick to this programme, shell out at your local health club in month 4 because your muscles will have become strong enough to warrant training with weights. When you do go to a gym you'll already be pretty strong and will feel confident about the size of the weights you're pushing.

The plans that follow are rough guides that will help you gradually increase your fitness and ability to burn calories. You can chop and change them as much as you like; you're probably more likely to stick to a programme of your own design. They all involve training three or four days a week to give you a balance of work and recovery. You can, of course, add a few extra sessions, but try to build those sessions around the stuff that you really like doing so that you have fun more than anything else. Like going for a ride around the local park or down to the beach? Do that on the rest days because even though it burns calories it's more of a stress reliever than a conscious effort to get fitter. Give your brain and body enough of a break from your goals and training and your drive for a healthy lifestyle and a lean body will stay high for a long time.

MONTH 1: Starting Out

The workouts aren't allocated to specific days, so fit them into your schedule where you can. If you can only do them three days in a row, that's cool. However, the best strategy is to alternate between rest and training days. It's not essential, but it gives you the recovery you need to progress quickly. Be aware that even though the bodyweight workout calls for slightly fewer reps than outlined in chapter 8 you're not meant to do low reps with heavy weights. The idea is to get used to stressing your muscles gradually rather than thrash the hell out of them on the first outing. Take it easy and grab a break whenever you need it.

WEEK 1

Workout 1: Light Intervals

Run, cycle, swim, row or whatever for 1 minute and then slow down for 90 seconds. Repeat 8 times.

Workout 2: Your Choice

Do anything active that you enjoy for 30 to 40 minutes. Wii Fit doesn't count because it burns only a fraction of the calories that real-world sport does.

Workout 3: Bodyweight Circuit

Do the exercises as a circuit (table 9.1) but rest for 45 seconds between each move so that you can recover. If you find you don't need the rest you can skip it.

Table 9.1   Week 1 Bodyweight Circuit

Exercise	Sets	Reps	Rest
1. Push-up	4	6	45 sec.
2. Squat (body weight)	4	6	45 sec.
3. Lunge	4	6	45 sec.
4. Superman	4	30 sec.	45 sec.
5. Bicycle crunch	4	6	45 sec.

Run, cycle, row, swim, walk or whatever for 15 minutes at a pace you can manage.

WEEK 2

Workout 1: Light Intervals

Run, cycle, swim, row or whatever for 2 minutes and then slow down for 1 minute. Repeat 7 times.

Workout 2: Your Choice

Do anything active that you enjoy for 30 to 40 minutes.

Workout 3: Bodyweight Circuit

Do the exercises as a circuit (table 9.2) but rest for 45 seconds between each move so that you can recover. If you find you don't need the rest you can skip it.

Table 9.2   Week 2, Workout 3

Exercise	Sets	Reps	Rest
1. Split squat	4	8	45 sec.
2. Inverted row	4	8	45 sec.
3. Lunge	4	8	45 sec.
4. Incline push-up	4	8	45 sec.
5. Plank	4	8	45 sec.

Run, cycle, row, swim, walk or whatever for 15 minutes at a pace you can manage.

WEEK 3

Workout 1: Light Intervals

Run, cycle, swim, row or whatever for 3 minutes and then slow down for 1 minute. Repeat 6 times.

Workout 2: Your Choice

Do anything active that you enjoy for 30 to 40 minutes.

Workout 3: Bodyweight Circuit

Do the exercises as a circuit (table 9.3) but rest for 30 seconds between each move so that you can recover.

Table 9.3   Week 3, Workout 3

Exercise	Sets	Reps	Rest
1. Squat (body weight)	3	8	30 sec.
2. Inverted row	3	8	30 sec.
3. Incline push-up	3	8	30 sec.
4. Split squat	3	8	30 sec.
5. Lunge	3	8	30 sec.
6. Plank	3	8	30 sec.
7. Superman	3	30 sec.	30 sec.
8. Bicycle crunch	3	6	30 sec.

Run, cycle, row, swim, walk or whatever for 10 minutes at a pace you can manage.

Workout 4 (Optional): Your Choice

Do anything active you that enjoy for 30 to 40 minutes.

WEEK 4

Workout 1: Light Intervals

Run, cycle, swim, row or whatever for 4 minutes and then slow down for 2 minutes. Repeat 6 times.

Workout 2: Your Choice

Do anything active that you enjoy for 30 to 40 minutes.

Workout 3: Bodyweight Circuit

Do the exercises as a circuit (table 9.4) but rest for 30 seconds between each move so that you can recover.

Table 9.4 Week 4, Workout 3

Exercise	Sets	Reps	Rest
1. Squat (body weight)	4	8	30 sec.
2. Inverted row	4	8	30 sec.
3. Incline push-up	4	8	30 sec.
4. Split squat	4	8	30 sec.
5. Lunge	4	8	30 sec.
6. Plank	4	8	30 sec.
7. Superman	4	30 sec.	30 sec.
8. Bicycle crunch	4	6	30 sec.

Run, cycle, row, swim, walk or whatever for 10 minutes at a pace you can manage.

Workout 4 (Optional): Your Choice

Do anything active that you enjoy for 30 to 40 minutes.

MONTH 2: Seeing the Improvements

By now you should start to feel your clothes becoming looser and you should have more energy and feel fitter. That doesn't mean that exercise should be any easier. Exercise should almost always feel tough no matter how fit you are. If it does feel easy you need to shift more weight or train harder. The intensity of the workouts gradually gets tougher, but make an effort to stick to it. Once training becomes a full-fledged habit it'll seem as natural as burping after drinking a fizzy drink.

WEEK 5

Workout 1: Light Intervals

Run, cycle, swim, row or whatever for 5 minutes and then slow down for 2 minutes. Repeat 4 times.

Workout 2: Your Choice

Do anything active that you enjoy for 30 to 40 minutes.

Workout 3: Bodyweight Circuit

Do the exercises as a circuit (table 9.5) but rest for 30 seconds between each move so that you can recover.

Table 9.5 Week 5, Workout 3

Exercise	Sets	Reps	Rest
1. Squat (body weight)	4	10	30 sec.
2. Inverted row	4	10	30 sec.
3. Incline push-up	4	10	30 sec.
4. Split squat	4	10	30 sec.
5. Lunge	4	10	30 sec.
6. Plank	4	10	30 sec.
7. Superman	4	30 sec.	30 sec.
8. Bicycle crunch	4	10	30 sec.

Run, cycle, row, swim, walk or whatever for 10 minutes at a pace you can manage.

Workout 4 (Optional): Your Choice

Do anything active that you enjoy, such as a sport or a run, for 30 to 40 minutes.

WEEK 6

Workout 1: Light Intervals

Run, cycle, swim, row or whatever for 8 minutes and then slow down for 2 minutes. Repeat 3 times.

Workout 2: Your Choice

Do anything active that you enjoy for 30 to 40 minutes.

Workout 3: Bodyweight Circuit

Do the exercises as a circuit (table 9.6) but rest for 30 seconds between each move so that you can recover.

Table 9.6   Week 6, Workout 3

Exercise	Sets	Reps	Rest
1. Squat (body weight)	4	12	30 sec.
2. Inverted row	4	12	30 sec.
3. Push-up	4	12	30 sec.
4. Split squat	4	12	30 sec.
5. Lunge	4	12	30 sec.
6. Plank	4	12	30 sec.
7. Superman	4	30 sec.	30 sec.
8. Bicycle crunch	4	12	30 sec.

Run, cycle, row, swim, walk or whatever for 10 minutes at a pace you can manage.

Workout 4: Your Choice

Do anything active that you enjoy, such as a sport or even a very light walk, for 30 to 40 minutes.

WEEK 7

Workout 1: Light Intervals

Run, cycle, swim, row or whatever for 12 minutes and then slow down for 1 minute. Repeat 3 times.

Workout 2: Your Choice

Do anything active that you enjoy for 30 to 40 minutes.

Workout 3: Bodyweight Circuit

Do the exercises as a circuit (table 9.7) but rest for 30 seconds between each move so that you can recover.

Table 9.7   Week 7, Workout 3

Exercise	Sets	Reps	Rest
1. Squat (body weight)	4	15	30 sec.
2. Inverted row	4	15	30 sec.
3. Push-up	4	15	30 sec.
4. Split squat	4	15	30 sec.
5. Lunge	4	15	30 sec.
6. Plank	4	15	30 sec.
7. Superman	4	30 sec.	30 sec.
8. Bicycle crunch	4	15	30 sec.

Run, cycle, row, swim, walk or whatever for 10 minutes at a pace you can manage.

Workout 4: Your Choice

Do anything active you that enjoy, such as a sport or even a very light walk, for 30 to 40 minutes.

WEEK 8

Workout 1: Light Intervals

Run, cycle, swim, row or whatever for 15 minutes, slow down for 1 minute and then go again for another 15 minutes.

Workout 2: Your Choice

Do anything active that you enjoy for 30 to 40 minutes.

Workout 3: Bodyweight Circuit

Do the exercises as a circuit (table 9.8) and do not rest between moves. Take a 2- to 3-minute breather after you've done each move once.

Table 9.8   Week 8, Workout 3

Exercise	Sets	Reps
1. Squat (body weight)	4	15
2. Inverted row	4	15
3. Push-up	4	15
4. Split squat	4	15
5. Lunge	4	15
6. Plank	4	15
7. Superman	4	30 sec.
8. Bicycle crunch	4	15

Run, cycle, row, swim, walk or whatever for 10 minutes at a pace you can manage.

Workout 4: Your Choice

Do anything active that you enjoy, such as a sport or even a very light walk, for 30 to 40 minutes.

MONTH 3: Going Flat Out to Get Flat

You've now got a serious amount of physical exercise under your belt. If you've also adjusted your eating plan (see chapter 2) you're undoubtedly leaner and feeling better about yourself. Be warned: Most people fall off the wagon at this stage, which is actually when you can make your most pronounced gains. Simply increasing the intensity of your workouts can markedly improve your baseline level of fitness.

If you're struggling to stay motivated, turn back to chapter 1 to ensure that you stay firmly on the wagon and never return to your former self. Enjoy your workouts and start scouting for a health club or dumbbells—this is the final month of gym-free training.

WEEK 9

Workout 1: Steady-State Cardio

Run, cycle, swim, row or whatever for 30 minutes without taking a break.

Workout 2: Your Choice

Do anything active that you enjoy for 30 to 40 minutes.

Workout 3: Bodyweight Circuit

Do the exercises as a circuit (table 9.9) and do not rest between moves. Take a 2- to 3-minute breather after you've done each move once.

Table 9.9   Week 9, Workout 3

Exercise	Sets	Reps
1. Lunge (body weight)	4	15
2. Push-up	4	15
3. Squat	4	15
4. Inverted row	4	15
5. Lunge	4	15
6. Push-up plank	4	15
7. Pendulum	4	30 sec.
8. V-knee tuck	4	15

Run, cycle, row, swim, walk or whatever for 10 minutes at a pace you can manage.

Workout 4: Interval Training

1. Warm up with your activity of choice for 5 minutes.
2. Sprint (or do your activity of choice) for 20 seconds and then slow down for 40 seconds. Repeat 15 times.
3. Cool down for 5 to 10 minutes.

WEEK 10

Workout 1: Bodyweight Circuit 1

Do the exercises as a circuit (table 9.10) and do not rest between moves. Take a 2- to 3-minute breather after you've done each move once.

Table 9.10   Week 10, Workout 1

Exercise	Sets	Reps
1. Squat (body weight)	4	12
2. Inverted row	4	12
3. Push-up	4	12
4. Split squat	4	12
5. Lunge	4	12
6. Plank	4	12
7. Superman	4	30 sec.
8. Bicycle crunch	4	12

Run, cycle, row, swim, walk or whatever for 10 minutes at a pace you can manage.

Workout 2: Your Choice

Do anything active that you enjoy for 30 to 40 minutes.

Workout 3: Bodyweight Circuit 2

Do the exercises as a circuit (table 9.11) and do not rest between moves. Take a 2- to 3-minute breather after you've done each move once.

Table 9.11   Week 10, Workout 3

Exercise	Sets	Reps
1. Lunge (body weight)	4	15
2. Push-up	4	15
3. Squat	4	15
4. Inverted row	4	15
5. Lunge	4	15
6. Push-up plank	4	15
7. Pendulum	4	30 sec.
8. V-knee tuck	4	15

Run, cycle, row, swim, walk or whatever for 10 minutes at a pace you can manage.

Workout 4: Interval Training

1. Warm up with your activity of choice for 5 minutes.
2. Sprint (or do your activity of choice) for 10 seconds and then slow down for 20 seconds. Repeat 3 times. After each bout, increase the amount of time you sprint by 10 seconds until you sprint for 40 seconds and have increased your rest time to 60 seconds.

3. Reverse the process and reduce the sprint and recovery times by 10 seconds until you do a final sprint of 10 seconds.

4. Cool down at a slow pace for 5 to 10 minutes.

WEEK 11

Workout 1: Bodyweight Circuit 1

Do the exercises as a circuit (table 9.12) and do not rest between moves. Take a 2- to 3-minute breather after you've done each move once.

Table 9.12   Week 11, Workout 1

Exercise	Sets	Reps
1. Squat (body weight)	4	15
2. Inverted row	4	15
3. Push-up	4	15
4. Split squat	4	15
5. Lunge	4	15
6. Plank	4	15
7. Superman	4	60 sec.
8. Bicycle crunch	4	15

Run, cycle, row, swim, walk or whatever for 10 minutes at a pace you can manage.

Workout 2: Your Choice

Do anything active that you enjoy for 30 to 40 minutes.

Workout 3: Bodyweight Circuit 2

Do the exercises as a circuit (table 9.13) and do not rest between moves. Take a 2- to 3-minute breather after you've done each move once.

Table 9.13   Week 11, Workout 3

Exercise	Sets	Reps
1. Lunge (body weight)	4	20
2. Push-up	4	20
3. Squat	4	20
4. Inverted row	4	20
5. Lunge	4	20
6. Push-up plank	4	20
7. Pendulum	4	60 sec.
8. V-knee tuck	4	20

Run, cycle, row, swim, walk or whatever for 10 minutes at a pace you can manage.

Workout 4: Interval Training

1. Warm up with your activity of choice for 5 minutes.

2. Mark out a piece of track that's about 50 to 60 metres long. Set a stopwatch and sprint back and forth over that distance as many times as you can in 1 minute. Walk for 1 minute and then go again. Repeat 10 times and you're done for the day.

WEEK 12

Workout 1: Bodyweight Circuit 1

Do the exercises as a circuit (table 9.14) and do not rest between moves. Take a 2- to 3-minute breather after you've done each move once.

Table 9.14   Week 12, Workout 1

Exercise	Sets	Reps
1. Squat (body weight)	5	15
2. Inverted row	5	15
3. Push-up	5	15
4. Split squat	5	15
5. Lunge	5	15
6. Plank	5	15
7. Superman	5	60 sec.
8. Bicycle crunch	5	15

Run, cycle, row, swim, walk or whatever for 10 minutes at a pace you can manage.

Workout 2: Your Choice

Do anything active that you enjoy for 30 to 40 minutes.

Workout 3: Bodyweight Circuit 2

Do the exercises as a circuit (table 9.15) and do not rest between moves. Take a 2- to 3-minute breather after you've done each move once.

Table 9.15   Week 12, Workout 3

Exercise	Sets	Reps
1. Lunge (body weight)	5	20
2. Push-up	5	20
3. Squat	5	20
4. Inverted row	5	20
5. Lunge	5	20
6. Push-up plank	5	20
7. Pendulum	5	60 sec.
8. V-knee tuck	5	20

Run, cycle, row, swim, walk or whatever for 10 minutes at a pace you can manage.

Workout 4: Interval Training

1. Warm up with your activity of choice for 5 minutes.
2. Sprint (or do your activity of choice) for 10 seconds and then slow down for 20 seconds. Repeat 10 times.
3. Sprint (or do your activity of choice) for 20 seconds and then slow down for 40 seconds. Repeat 10 times.
4. Cool down for 5 to 10 minutes at a slow pace.

MONTH 4: Congratulations

If you've stuck to it, give yourself a pat on the back—you'll be able to reach it now. The third month is like a Wednesday: Once you're past it it's all smooth sailing to the weekend. Exercise should now feel like a habit. Research in *European Journal of Social Psychology* (Lally et al., 2010) found that it took on average about 66 days for something to become a routine. At about month 3 it's safe to say that you have formed a very healthy habit. The researchers also found that missing the odd day didn't reduce the chance of forming a habit, so don't feel guilty if that thing called life occasionally has you doing something else. Now that exercise is a habit you can buy a gym membership with the confidence that you'll use it. Some of the workouts this month include weightlifting exercises. You can still stick with the body-weight stuff but you'll need to find ways to make those moves harder, such as wearing a weighted vest or a backpack with a few issues of the phone book in it. Seeing a pattern? Over the next three months you'll start to include a few more of the high-intensity exercise methods that are further up the rankings. This lets you constantly challenge your body and force it to burn more calories and build extra muscle. Take a deep breath. You might need it.

WEEK 13

Workout 1: Free-Weights Circuit 1

Do the exercises as a circuit (table 9.16) and do not rest between moves. Take a 2- to 3-minute breather after you've done each move once.

Table 9.16 Week 13, Workout 1

Exercise	Sets	Reps
1. Squat (barbell)	3	10
2. Dumbbell flat chest press	3	10
3. Dumbbell bent-over row	3	10
4. Dumbbell deadlift	3	10
5. Hanging leg raise	3	10

Run, cycle, row, swim or whatever for 30 seconds and then go slow for 30 seconds. Repeat 5 times.

Workout 2: Your Choice

Do anything active that you enjoy for 30 to 40 minutes. Now is the time to increase the intensity and variety of whatever you're doing. If you've joined a gym, try a boxing, spinning or Pilates class. Habits are good, but not if they stop you from exploring the different ways your body can work.

Workout 3: Free-Weights Circuit 2

Do the exercises as a circuit (table 9.17) and do not rest between moves. Take a 2- to 3-minute breather after you've done each move once.

Table 9.17 Week 13, Workout 3

Exercise	Sets	Reps
1. Power clean	4	8
2. Leg press	4	8
3. Parallel bar dip	4	8
4. Cable face pull	4	8
5. Barbell rollout	4	8

Run, cycle, row, swim or whatever for 15 seconds and then slow down for 15 seconds. Keep alternating for a total of 10 minutes.

Workout 4: Interval Training

1. Warm up with your activity of choice for 5 minutes.
2. Sprint (or do your activity of choice) for 15 seconds and then slow down for 30 seconds. Repeat 20 times.
3. Cool down for 5 to 10 minutes.

WEEK 14

Workout 1: Free-Weights Circuit 1

Do the exercises as a circuit (table 9.18) and do not rest between moves. Take a 2- to 3-minute breather after you've done each move once.

Table 9.18 Week 14, Workout 1

Exercise	Sets	Reps
1. Squat (barbell)	3	12
2. Dumbbell flat chest press	3	12
3. Dumbbell bent-over row	3	12
4. Dumbbell deadlift	3	12
5. Hanging leg raise	3	12

Run, cycle, row, swim or whatever for 30 seconds and then go slow for 30 seconds. Repeat 5 times.

Workout 2: Your Choice

Do anything active that you enjoy for 30 to 40 minutes or take part in an exercise class at your gym.

Workout 3: Free-Weights Circuit 2

Do the exercises as a circuit (table 9.19) and do not rest between moves. Take a 2- to 3-minute breather after you've done each move once.

Table 9.19 Week 14, Workout 3

Exercise	Sets	Reps
1. Power clean	4	10
2. Leg press	4	10
3. Parallel bar dip	4	10
4. Cable face pull	4	10
5. Barbell rollout	4	10

Run, cycle, row, swim or whatever for 15 seconds and then slow down for 15 seconds. Keep alternating for a total of 10 minutes.

Workout 4: Interval Training

1. Warm up with your activity of choice for 5 minutes.

2. Find a hill that's about 50 to 60 metres long if you're running or 100 to 200 metres long if you're cycling. If you're on a machine such as a rower or elliptical trainer, crank the resistance up as high as it will go. If you're in a pool, swim with water dumb-bells. Start at the bottom of the hill and run to the top. Walk down to the bottom at a very slow pace. Do this 7 or 8 times.

3. Cool down with a slow walk for 5 to 10 minutes.

WEEK 15

Workout 1: Free-Weights Circuit 1

Do the exercises as a circuit (table 9.20) and do not rest between moves. Take a 2- to 3-minute breather after you've done each move once.

Table 9.20 Week 15, Workout 1

Exercise	Sets	Reps
1. Squat (barbell)	4	15
2. Dumbbell flat chest press	4	15
3. Dumbbell bent-over row	4	15
4. Dumbbell deadlift	4	15
5. Hanging leg raise	4	15

Run, cycle, row, swim or whatever for 10 seconds and then go slow for 10 seconds. Repeat 10 to 15 times.

Workout 2: Your Choice

Do anything active that you enjoy for 30 to 40 minutes or take part in an exercise class at your gym.

Workout 3: Free-Weights Circuit 2

Do the exercises as a circuit (table 9.21) and do not rest between moves. Take a 2- to 3-minute breather after you've done each move once.

Table 9.21 Week 15, Workout 3

Exercise	Sets	Reps
1. Power clean	4	15
2. Leg press	4	15
3. Parallel bar dip	4	15
4. Cable face pull	4	15
5. Barbell rollout	4	15

Run, cycle, row, swim or whatever for 7 seconds and then slow down for 20 seconds. Keep alternating for a total of 12 minutes.

Workout 4: Interval Training

1. Warm up with your activity of choice for 5 minutes.

2. Go at a fast pace for 2 minutes and then take it slow for 2 minutes. Repeat 7 times with whatever activity you choose.

3. Cool down with a slow walk for 5 to 10 minutes.

WEEK 16

Workout 1: Free-Weights Circuit 1

Do the exercises as a circuit (table 9.22) and do not rest between moves. Take a 2- to 3-minute breather after you've done each move once.

Table 9.22   Week 16, Workout 1

Exercise	Sets	Reps
1. Squat (barbell)	4	15
2. Dumbbell flat chest press	4	15
3. Dumbbell bent-over row	4	15
4. Dumbbell deadlift	4	15
5. Hanging leg raise	4	15

Run, cycle, row, swim or whatever for 30 seconds and then go slow for 30 seconds. Repeat 5 times.

Workout 2: Your Choice

Do anything active that you enjoy for 30 to 40 minutes or take part in an exercise class at your gym.

Workout 3: Free-Weights Circuit 2

Do the exercises as a circuit (table 9.23) and do not rest between moves. Take a 2- to 3-minute breather after you've done each move once.

Table 9.23   Week 16, Workout 3

Exercise	Sets	Reps
1. Power clean	4	15
2. Leg press	4	15
3. Parallel bar dip	4	15
4. Cable face pull	4	15
5. Barbell rollout	4	15

Run, cycle, row, swim or whatever for 15 seconds and then slow down for 15 seconds. Keep alternating for a total of 10 minutes.

Workout 4: Interval Training

1. Warm up with your activity of choice for 5 minutes.

2. Sprint (or do your activity of choice) for 15 seconds and then slow down for 30 seconds. Repeat 20 times.

3. Cool down for 5 to 10 minutes.

MONTH 5: Getting Serious

If you've stuck at it this long you've probably altered the workouts, rest periods and days off based on personal experience you've picked up along the way. That's totally expected. When you speak to like-minded people they're always happy to share their tips and tricks with you so that you can improve. By this stage one thing is certain: You look different and are sure to be fielding compliments, hopefully from the opposite sex. Now that you're getting to grips with your new self you can categorically say that you're no longer a beginner. You have strength, you're getting leaner and you are supremely fitter and healthier inside and out.

In the next step you'll follow a slightly more regimented programme. You may have noticed that your weight loss has slowed down. The weight just streams off during the first two to three months but thereafter each kilo that you lose can seem like a little victory. To give yourself something to celebrate, start to get serious about gaining muscle and losing fat by doing three gym sessions a week. It's not a lot, and the sessions shouldn't take more than 40 to 60 minutes each. The perfect schedule is to do them is on Monday, Wednesday and Friday—that gives you a day of rest between each one. But if your schedule doesn't allow for that, do them whenever you can. You'll use the same exercises for the entire month because they work a huge number of muscle fibres; this will prime you muscles for trying new moves next month. If you can commit to three gym sessions a week you'll quickly accelerate the fat off your frame. Get ready for your toughest and most successful month yet.

WEEK 17

Workout 1: Free-Weights Circuit 1

Do the exercises in each triset (table 9.24) one after another without rest. Take a 1- to 2-minute breather after you've finished each one. Always use as much weight as you can manage.

Table 9.24 Week 17, Workout 1

Exercise	Sets	Reps
Triset 1		
1. Power clean	3	5
2. Dumbbell incline chest press	3	5
3. Standing calf raise	3	5
Triset 2		
4. Overhand-grip pull-up	3	5
5. Squat (barbell)	3	5
6. Rope push-down	3	5
Triset 3		
7. Back extension	3	5
8. Hammer curl	3	5
9. Lying leg raise	3	5

Run, cycle, row, swim or whatever for 10 seconds and then slow down for 20 seconds. Keep alternating for a total of 10 to 15 minutes.

Workout 2: Free-Weights Circuit 2

Do the exercises in each triset (table 9.25) one after another without rest. This session is meant to help you recover, so tone down the weights. It's better to go easy and finish all the reps than to go heavy and fall short. Take a 1- to 2-minute breather after you've finished each triset.

Table 9.25 Week 17, Workout 2

Exercise	Sets	Reps
Triset 1		
1. Power clean	3	15
2. Dumbbell incline chest press	3	15
3. Standing calf raise	3	15
Triset 2		
4. Overhand-grip pull-up	3	15
5. Squat (barbell)	3	15
6. Rope push-down	3	15
Triset 3		
7. Back extension	3	15
8. Hammer curl	3	15
9. Lying leg raise	3	15

Run, cycle, row, swim or whatever for 20 seconds and then slow down for 40 seconds. Keep alternating for a total of 10 to 15 minutes.

Workout 3: Free-Weights Circuit 3

Do the exercises in each triset (table 9.26) one after another without rest. Don't use weights that make you fail on the 10th rep. Rather, keep them light so that you can do the sets quickly and get out of the gym within an hour. Take a 1- to 2-minute breather after you've finished each triset.

Table 9.26 Week 17, Workout 3

Exercise	Sets	Reps
Triset 1		
1. Power clean	4	10
2. Dumbbell incline chest press	4	10
3. Standing calf raise	4	10
Triset 2		
4. Overhand-grip pull-up	4	10
5. Squat (barbell)	4	10
6. Rope push-down	4	10
Triset 3		
7. Back extension	4	10
8. Hammer curl	4	10
9. Lying leg raise	4	10

Run, cycle, row, swim or whatever for 30 seconds and then slow down for 60 seconds. Keep alternating for a total of 10 to 15 minutes.

Workout 4: Your Choice

Do anything active that you enjoy for 30 to 40 minutes or take part in an exercise class at your gym.

Workout 5: Steady-State Cardio

Run, cycle or swim for 20 minutes.

WEEK 18

Workout 1: Free-Weights Circuit 1

Do the exercises in each triset (table 9.27) one after another without rest. Take a 1- to 2-minute breather after you've finished each one.

Table 9.27 Week 18, Workout 1

Exercise	Sets	Reps
Triset 1		
1. Power clean	3	5
2. Dumbbell incline chest press	3	5
3. Standing calf raise	3	5
Triset 2		
4. Overhand-grip pull-up	3	5
5. Squat (barbell)	3	5
6. Rope push-down	3	5
Triset 3		
7. Back extension	3	5
8. Hammer curl	3	5
9. Lying leg raise	3	5

Run, cycle, row, swim or whatever for 10 seconds and then slow down for 20 seconds. Keep alternating for a total of 10 to 15 minutes.

Workout 2: Free-Weights Circuit 2

Do the exercises in each triset (table 9.28) one after another without rest. This session is meant to help you recover, so tone down the weights. It's better to go easy and finish all the reps than to go heavy and fall short. Take a 1- to 2-minute breather after you've finished each triset.

Table 9.28 Week 18, Workout 2

Exercise	Sets	Reps
Triset 1		
1. Power clean	3	15
2. Dumbbell incline chest press	3	15
3. Standing calf raise	3	15
Triset 2		
4. Overhand-grip pull-up	3	15
5. Squat (barbell)	3	15
6. Rope push-down	3	15
Triset 3		
7. Back extension	3	15
8. Hammer curl	3	15
9. Lying leg raise	3	15

Run, cycle, row, swim or whatever for 20 seconds and then slow down for 40 seconds. Keep alternating for a total of 10 to 15 minutes.

Workout 3: Free-Weights Circuit 3

Do the exercises in each triset (table 9.29) one after another without rest. Don't use weights that make you fail on the 10th rep. Rather, keep them light so that you can do the sets quickly and get out of the gym within an hour. Take a 1- to 2-minute breather after you've finished each triset.

Table 9.29 Week 18, Workout 3

Exercise	Sets	Reps
Triset 1		
1. Power clean	4	10
2. Dumbbell incline chest press	4	10
3. Standing calf raise	4	10
Triset 2		
4. Overhand-grip pull-up	4	10
5. Squat (barbell)	4	10
6. Rope push-down	4	10
Triset 3		
7. Back extension	4	10
8. Hammer curl	4	10
9. Lying leg raise	4	10

Run, cycle, row, swim or whatever for 30 seconds and then slow down for 60 seconds. Keep alternating for a total of 10 to 15 minutes.

Workout 4: Your Choice

Do anything active that you enjoy for 30 to 40 minutes or take part in an exercise class at your gym.

Workout 5: Low-Intensity Class

Take part in a fairly relaxed class such as yoga at your gym or thoroughly stretch for 10 to 15 minutes.

WEEK 19

Workout 1: Free-Weights Circuit 1

Do the exercises in each triset (table 9.30) one after another without rest. Take a 1- to 2-minute breather after you've finished each one.

Table 9.30 Week 19, Workout 1

Exercise	Sets	Reps
Triset 1		
1. Power clean	3	5
2. Dumbbell incline chest press	3	5
3. Standing calf raise	3	5
Triset 2		
4. Overhand-grip pull-up	3	5
5. Squat (barbell)	3	5
6. Rope push-down	3	5
Triset 3		
7. Back extension	3	5
8. Hammer curl	3	5
9. Lying leg raise	3	5

Run, cycle, row, swim or whatever for 10 seconds and then slow down for 20 seconds. Keep alternating for a total of 10 to 15 minutes.

Workout 2: Free-Weights Circuit 2

Do the exercises in each triset (table 9.31) one after another without rest. This session is meant to help you recover, so tone down the weights. It's better to go easy and finish all the reps than to go heavy and fall short. Take a 1- to 2-minute breather after you've finished each triset.

Table 9.31 Week 19, Workout 2

Exercise	Sets	Reps
Triset 1		
1. Power clean	3	15
2. Dumbbell incline chest press	3	15
3. Standing calf raise	3	15
Triset 2		
4. Overhand-grip pull-up	3	15
5. Squat (barbell)	3	15
6. Rope push-down	3	15
Triset 3		
7. Back extension	3	15
8. Hammer curl	3	15
9. Lying leg raise	3	15

Run, cycle, row, swim or whatever for 20 seconds and then slow down for 40 seconds. Keep alternating for a total of 10 to 15 minutes.

Workout 3: Free-Weights Circuit 3

Do the exercises in each triset (table 9.32) one after another without rest. Don't use weights that make you fail on the 10th rep. Rather, keep them light so that you can do the sets quickly and get out of the gym within an hour. Take a 1- to 2-minute breather after you've finished each triset.

Table 9.32 Week 19, Workout 3

Exercise	Sets	Reps
Triset 1		
1. Power clean	4	10
2. Dumbbell incline chest press	4	10
3. Standing calf raise	4	10
Triset 2		
4. Overhand-grip pull-up	4	10
5. Squat (barbell)	4	10
6. Rope push-down	4	10
Triset 3		
7. Back extension	4	10
8. Hammer curl	4	10
9. Lying leg raise	4	10

Run, cycle, row, swim or whatever for 30 seconds and then slow down for 60 seconds. Keep alternating for a total of 10 to 15 minutes.

Workout 4: Your Choice

Do anything active that you enjoy for 30 to 40 minutes or take part in an exercise class at your gym.

Workout 5: Long Walk

Take a walk for at least 30 minutes.

WEEK 20

Workout 1: Free-Weights Circuit 1

Do the exercises in each triset (table 9.33) one after another without rest. Take a 1- to 2-minute breather after you've finished each one.

Table 9.33 Week 20, Workout 1

Exercise	Sets	Reps
Triset 1		
1. Power clean	3	5
2. Dumbbell incline chest press	3	5
3. Standing calf raise	3	5
Triset 2		
4. Overhand-grip pull-up	3	5
5. Squat (barbell)	3	5
6. Rope push-down	3	5
Triset 3		
7. Back extension	3	5
8. Hammer curl	3	5
9. Lying leg raise	3	5

Run, cycle, row, swim or whatever for 10 seconds and then slow down for 20 seconds. Keep alternating for a total of 10 to 15 minutes.

Workout 2: Free-Weights Circuit 2

Do the exercises in each triset (table 9.34) one after another without rest. This session is meant to help you recover, so tone down the weights. It's better to go easy and finish all the reps than to go heavy and fall short. Take a 1- to 2-minute breather after you've finished each triset.

Table 9.34 Week 20, Workout 2

Exercise	Sets	Reps
Triset 1		
1. Power clean	3	15
2. Dumbbell incline chest press	3	15
3. Standing calf raise	3	15
Triset 2		
4. Overhand-grip pull-up	3	15
5. Squat (barbell)	3	15
6. Rope push-down	3	15
Triset 3		
7. Back extension	3	15
8. Hammer curl	3	15
9. Lying leg raise	3	15

Run, cycle, row, swim or whatever for 20 seconds and then slow down for 40 seconds. Keep alternating for a total of 10 to 15 minutes.

Workout 3: Free-Weights Circuit 3

Do the exercises in each triset (table 9.35) one after another without rest. Don't use weights that make you fail on the 10th rep. Rather, keep them light so that you can do the sets quickly and get out of the gym within an hour. Take a 1- to 2-minute breather after you've finished each triset.

Table 9.35 Week 20, Workout 3

Exercise	Sets	Reps
Triset 1		
1. Power clean	4	10
2. Dumbbell incline chest press	4	10
3. Standing calf raise	4	10
Triset 2		
4. Overhand-grip pull-up	4	10
5. Squat (barbell)	4	10
6. Rope push-down	4	10
Triset 3		
7. Back extension	4	10
8. Hammer curl	4	10
9. Lying leg raise	4	10

Run, cycle, row, swim or whatever for 30 seconds and then slow down for 60 seconds. Keep alternating for a total of 10 to 15 minutes.

Workout 4: Your Choice

Do anything active that you enjoy for 30 to 40 minutes or take part in an exercise class at your gym.

Workout 5: Steady-State Cardio

Run, cycle or swim for 20 minutes.

MONTH 6: You're Nearly There

Your muscle and mind are now ready to use a mix of the more effective techniques. If you find this schedule too hectic and if it takes away from your normal enjoyment of exercise, change it up. Just because you can do something doesn't mean that you have to. You can always switch back to bodyweight circuits and doing activities you thoroughly enjoy, such as a sport or just walking your dog. But if you want to kick your results up a notch, hit this final month with as much passion as you can. Then move onto the plan outlined here that specialises in shifting the final kilos of fat covering your abs.

WEEK 21

Workout 1: Weightlifting Circuit

Do the exercises (table 9.36) one after another without rest and then rest for 1 to 2 minutes after you've finished the circuit. Set up the stations before you begin to minimise lag time between sets.

Table 9.36   Week 21, Workout 1

Exercise	Sets	Reps
1. Squat	4	12
2. Parallel bar dip	4	12
3. Overhand-grip pull-up	4	12
4. Good morning	4	12
5. Dumbbell seated shoulder press	4	12
6. Close-grip bench press	4	12
7. Side plank	4	60 sec.

Workout 2: High-Intensity Training

High-intensity training is different from interval training in that you have to go all out and train so hard you can taste it.

1. Warm up for 5 minutes. Find a track of open grass that you can run up and down.
2. Sprint as hard and fast as you can for 10 seconds and then walk or jog for 50 seconds. Repeat 10 to 15 times.
3. Cool down with a 10-minute jog.

Workout 3: Cardioacceleration

Do the cardio portion of this workout (table 9.37) with whatever equipment you have. Repeat the moves one after another as a circuit and then go again once you've done a set of all of them. You can even do it while going for a run or a cycle if you want to do it outdoors.

Table 9.37   Week 21, Workout 3

Exercise	Sets	Reps
1. Squat (body weight)	4	10
Run or cycle at a slow pace for 60 seconds		
2. Push-up	4	10
Run or cycle at a slow pace for 60 seconds		
3. Lunge (body weight)	4	10
Run or cycle at a slow pace for 60 seconds		
4. Parallel bar dip	4	10
Run or cycle at a slow pace for 60 seconds		
5. Chair dip	4	10
Run or cycle at a slow pace for 60 seconds		
6. Pendulum	4	10
Run or cycle at a slow pace for 60 seconds		
7. Lying leg raise	4	10
Run or cycle at a slow pace for 60 seconds		

Workout 4: Endurance Training

Run, cycle, swim, row, or whatever for at least 35 minutes. You can even do 5 to 10 minutes of each discipline to get a varied form of fitness and challenge all of your muscles.

Workout 5: Your Choice

Do anything active that you enjoy for 30 to 40 minutes or take part in an exercise class at your gym.

WEEK 22

Workout 1: Weightlifting Circuit

Do the exercises one after another without rest and then rest for 1 to 2 minutes after you've finished the circuit (table 9.38). Set up the stations before you begin to minimise the lag time between sets.

Table 9.38   Week 22, Workout 1

Exercise	Sets	Reps
1. Squat	4	12
2. Parallel bar dip	4	12
3. Overhand-grip pull-up	4	12
4. Good morning	4	12
5. Dumbbell seated shoulder press	4	12
6. Close-grip bench press	4	12
7. Side plank	4	60 sec.

Workout 2: High-Intensity Training

High-intensity training is different from interval training in that you have to go all out and train so hard you can taste it.

1. Warm up on the rowing machine for 5 minutes.
2. Set the resistance to the highest setting. Sprint as hard and fast as you can for 10 seconds and then row slowly for 50 seconds. Repeat 10 to 15 times.
3. Cool down with a 10-minute cycle on the stationary bike.

Workout 3: Cardioacceleration

Do the cardio portion of this workout (table 9.39) with whatever equipment you have. Repeat the moves one after another as a circuit and then go again once you've done a set of all of them. You can even do it while going for a run or a cycle if you want to do it outdoors.

Table 9.39   Week 22, Workout 3

Exercise	Sets	Reps
1. Squat (body weight)	4	10
Run or cycle at a slow pace for 60 seconds		
2. Push-up	4	10
Run or cycle at a slow pace for 60 seconds		
3. Lunge (body weight)	4	10
Run or cycle at a slow pace for 60 seconds		
4. Parallel bar dip	4	10
Run or cycle at a slow pace for 60 seconds		

Table 9.39, *continued*

Exercise	Sets	Reps
5. Chair dip	4	10
Run or cycle at a slow pace for 60 seconds		
6. Pendulum	4	10
Run or cycle at a slow pace for 60 seconds		
7. Lying leg raise	4	10
Run or cycle at a slow pace for 60 seconds		

Workout 4: Endurance Training

Run, cycle, swim, row or whatever for at least 35 minutes. You can even do 5 to 10 minutes of each discipline to get a varied form of fitness. Make sure you do something different than what you did in week 21.

Workout 5: Your Choice

Do anything active that you enjoy for 30 to 40 minutes or take part in an exercise class at your gym.

WEEK 23

Workout 1: Weightlifting Circuit

Do the exercises (table 9.40) one after another without rest and then rest for 1 to 2 minutes after you've finished the circuit. Set up the stations before you begin to minimise the lag time between sets.

Table 9.40   Week 23, Workout 1

Exercise	Sets	Reps
1. Squat	4	12
2. Parallel bar dip	4	12
3. Overhand-grip pull-up	4	12
4. Good morning	4	12
5. Dumbbell seated shoulder press	4	12
6. Close-grip bench press	4	12
7. Side plank	4	60 sec.

> continued

Workout 2: High-Intensity Training

High-intensity training is different from interval training in that you have to go all out and train so hard you can taste it.

1. Warm up for 5 minutes on the stationary bike or on a normal bike.
2. Set the resistance to near maximum. Sprint as hard and fast as you can for 15 seconds until your leg muscles burn and you're standing in your seat. Then cycle slowly for 50 seconds until the muscle burn disappears. Repeat 10 to 15 times.
3. Cool down with a 10-minute jog on the treadmill.

Workout 3: Cardioacceleration

Do the cardio portion of this workout (table 9.41) with whatever equipment you have. Repeat the moves one after another as a circuit and then go again once you've done a set of all of them. You can even do it while going for a run or a cycle if you want to do it outdoors.

Table 9.41   Week 23, Workout 3

Exercise	Sets	Reps
1. Squat (body weight)	4	12
Run or cycle at a slow pace for 60 seconds		
2. Push-up	4	12
Run or cycle at a slow pace for 60 seconds		
3. Lunge (body weight)	4	12
Run or cycle at a slow pace for 60 seconds		
4. Parallel bar dip	4	12
Run or cycle at a slow pace for 60 seconds		
5. Chair dip	4	12
Run or cycle at a slow pace for 60 seconds		
6. Pendulum	4	12
Run or cycle at a slow pace for 60 seconds		
7. Lying leg raise	4	12
Run or cycle at a slow pace for 60 seconds		

Workout 4: Endurance Training

Run, cycle, swim, row or whatever for at least 35 minutes. You can even do 5 to 10 minutes of each discipline to get a varied form of fitness. Make sure you do something different than what you did in week 22.

Workout 5: Your Choice

Do anything active that you enjoy for 30 to 40 minutes or take part in an exercise class at your gym.

WEEK 24

Workout 1: Weightlifting Circuit

Do the exercises (table 9.42) one after another without rest and then rest for 1 to 2 minutes after you've finished the circuit. Set up the stations before you begin to minimise the lag time between sets.

Table 9.42   Week 24, Workout 1

Exercise	Sets	Reps
1. Squat	4	12
2. Parallel bar dip	4	12
3. Overhand-grip pull-up	4	12
4. Good morning	4	12
5. Dumbbell seated shoulder press	4	12
6. Close-grip bench press	4	12
7. Side plank	4	60 sec.

Workout 2: High-Intensity Training

High-intensity training is different from interval training in that you have to go all out and train so hard you can taste it.

1. Warm up for 5 minutes either on a running track or in a swimming pool.
2. Sprint (or swim) as hard and fast as you can for 15 seconds and then walk or jog for 60 seconds. Repeat 10 to 15 times.
3. Cool down with a 10-minute jog.

Workout 3: Cardioacceleration

Do the cardio portion of this workout (table 9.43) with whatever equipment you have. Repeat the moves one after another as a circuit and then go again once you've done a set of all of them. You can even do it while going for a run or a cycle if you want to do it outdoors.

Table 9.43   Week 24, Workout 3

Exercise	Sets	Reps
1. Squat (body weight)	4	15
Run or cycle at a slow pace for 60 seconds		
2. Push-up	4	15
Run or cycle at a slow pace for 60 seconds		
3. Lunge (body weight)	4	15
Run or cycle at a slow pace for 60 seconds		
4. Parallel bar dip	4	15
Run or cycle at a slow pace for 60 seconds		
5. Chair dip	4	15
Run or cycle at a slow pace for 60 seconds		
6. Pendulum	4	15
Run or cycle at a slow pace for 60 seconds		
7. Lying leg raise	4	15
Run or cycle at a slow pace for 60 seconds		

Workout 4: Endurance Training

Run, cycle, swim, row or whatever for at least 35 minutes. You can even do 5 to 10 minutes of each discipline to get a varied form of fitness. Make sure you do something different than what you did in week 23.

Workout 5: Your Choice

Do anything active that you enjoy for 30 to 40 minutes or take part in an exercise class at your gym.

What's Next?

Now that you've clocked in for a solid six months you have no reason to slow down. You can start all over or try some workouts from other chapters. It's time to plan your own goals based on the things you enjoy the most. If you took to building muscle, go ahead and tack a few extra fat-burning sessions onto the end of your workouts. The choices are limitless. As long as you're sweating a few times a week thanks to a bit of iron mongering or kicking a ball around, you'll always be taking the steps needed to get leaner. Now take your shirt off and start to enjoy yourself.

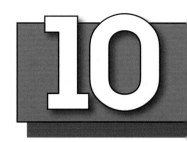

The Time-Poor Man's Workout

If you don't have time to drudge through hours in the gym in order to get muscled and fit, follow this approach to get more in less time.

Having a life is a pretty time-consuming hobby. There's work time. Family time. Travel time. Time with your significant other. Time with your buddies. You time. It makes you wonder how you can ever find time for exercise. Fortunately, you can make some steady progress by exercising for less time than it takes to wait for a meal in a restaurant.

A meagre 15 to 20 minutes is all you need to build muscle, burn fat and boost your sport performance. The only snag is that because your training sessions are so short and quick, you'll need to do them more frequently than you would if you dedicated an entire hour to each workout. For the best results do 3 to 6 sessions a week. If each session takes a measly 20 minutes, you'll dedicate a grand total of 1 to 2 hours to exercise out of a 168-hour week. You can bet the average guy spends more time unwillingly watching advertisements every week. It's the very least you can do for your body. After all, if you have a dog you'd feel guilty if you walked it any less than 2 hours a week. Here's how to make sure you get the bare minimum of exercise so that your muscles don't go lame.

Working Man's Strategy

Because you have only a small amount of time in which to train, you'll appreciate that these workouts are all short, sharp and to the point. They're geared to be as intense as possible so that you'll still get a solid exercise high, and when you hit the showers you'll know you've trained hard. These workouts are done in half the time of normal workouts. If you get an hour for lunch you can walk to the gym, train for 20 minutes, shower, walk back to work and still have time to eat your sandwich. Rather than trying to drudge through an exercise session after work, you can go straight home and relax or even hit the Rat and Parrot for a couple of guilt-free brews. What's more, you'll feel energised for the rest of your afternoon and have improved concentration and decision-making powers because your brain has taken a well-deserved break. If you're angling for a promotion, giving your memory and brain cells a boost in the middle of the day is more than a clever idea.

The following workouts can be done in a gym, in a park or at home using limited equipment. You don't have to handcuff your muscles to a particular way of training. Simply adjust your workout to your lifestyle. Going out for dinner and have only an hour at home before you have to leave? Do a home workout using a pair of dumbbells. If you're away on business and have only a small gap in which to train, do a quick bodyweight workout. If you can acclimatise your exercise approach to your current situation, your muscles will reward you by getting larger and leaner and will deceptively look like they took several hours to create.

Getting Fit in a Hurry

Follow these plans to build muscle and get fitter in the shortest time possible.

Like red and blue Star Wars lasers, only two schools of thought exist when it comes to quick workouts. The first suggests doing as many different exercises as possible in each session so that your body gets a taste for every kind of move and that no muscle—big or small—is ever overlooked. The second suggests sticking to two to four compound, multijoint exercises (such as squats and the power clean) per session because they work all your muscles and will help you become proficient at the best muscle- and strength-building exercises. Which approach is the most effectual? The truth is that they both have disadvantages and that the muscle-building and fat-burning prowess of each is equally effective. Try both approaches, each for six to eight weeks, and keep alternating to make sure you get week-on-week gains and are not stagnating. Simply follow the variety approach for a few weeks to get your muscles used to being exercised. When your gains start to taper off, switch to the multijoint-exercise approach and do very few exercises in each session. After doing both approaches for a few months you'll find the exercises that best gel with your physique and will be able to build your workouts around them. This will help you always enjoy your workouts and the gains that they bring. May the force be with you.

WORKOUTS FOR THE GUY WHO GETS BORED EASILY

Lifting weights can be boring and monotonous. Here's the plan to keep your brain and body active.

WORKOUT 1:
TOTAL-BODY MUSCLE BUILDER

Do each exercise (table 10.1) for 45 seconds, rest for 15 seconds and then go again. Once you've done a set of all of the exercises, rest for 60 seconds and repeat once.

Table 10.1   Variety Workout 1

Exercise	Sets	Reps	Rest
1. Squat	2	45 sec.	15 sec.
2. Lunge	2	45 sec.	15 sec.
3. Dumbbell flat chest press	2	45 sec.	15 sec.
4. Dumbbell bent-over row	2	45 sec.	15 sec.
5. Dumbbell deadlift	2	45 sec.	15 sec.
6. Dumbbell seated shoulder press	2	45 sec.	15 sec.
7. Hammer curl	2	45 sec.	15 sec.
8. Triceps push-down	2	45 sec.	15 sec.
9. Bicycle crunch	2	45 sec.	15 sec.

WORKOUT 2:
FAT BURNER THAT BUILDS MUSCLE

Repeat the following exercises (table 10.2) as a giant superset and perform each move one after another without rest. Once you've done a set of each exercise take a 1- to 2-minute rest. If you're after more muscle, stick to doing 10 reps using heavy weights. If you want to burn fat, do 15 reps with slightly lighter weights.

Table 10.2   Variety Workout 2

Exercise	Sets	Reps
1. Step-up	2	10-15
2. Stiff-legged deadlift	2	10-15
3. Dumbbell incline row	2	10-15
4. Dumbbell incline chest press	2	10-15
5. Good morning	2	10-15
6. EZ-bar curl	2	10-15
7. Rope push-down	2	10-15
8. Lateral raise	2	10-15
9. Barbell rollout	2	10-15

WORKOUT 3:
TOTAL-BODY ENDURANCE BUILDER

Do each exercise (table 10.3) for 40 seconds, rest for 20 seconds and then go again. Once you've done a set of all of the exercises, rest for 60 seconds and repeat once.

Table 10.3 Variety Workout 3

Exercise	Sets	Reps	Rest
1. Step-up	2	40 sec.	20 sec.
2. Stiff-legged deadlift	2	40 sec.	20 sec.
3. Dumbbell incline row	2	40 sec.	20 sec.
4. Dumbbell incline chest press	2	40 sec.	20 sec.
5. Good morning	2	40 sec.	20 sec.
6. EZ-bar curl	2	40 sec.	20 sec.
7. Rope push-down	2	40 sec.	20 sec.
8. Lateral raise	2	40 sec.	20 sec.
9. Barbell rollout	2	40 sec.	20 sec.

WORKOUT 4: SPORTSMAN'S PLAN

Repeat the following exercises (table 10.4) as a giant superset and perform each move one after another without rest. Once you've done a set of each exercise take a 1- to 2-minute rest. If you're after more muscle, stick to doing 10 reps using heavy weights. If you want to burn fat, do 15 reps with slightly lighter weights.

Table 10.4 Variety Workout 4

Exercise	Sets	Reps
1. Squat	2	10-15
2. Lunge	2	10-15
3. Dumbbell flat chest press	2	10-15
4. Dumbbell bent-over row	2	10-15
5. Dumbbell deadlift	2	10-15
6. Dumbbell seated shoulder press	2	10-15
7. Hammer curl	2	10-15
8. Triceps push-down	2	10-15
9. Bicycle crunch	2	10-15

WORKOUT 5: FAT-BURNING EXTREME

Do as many 5-rep supersets as you can in 5 to 7 minutes for each of the following superset combinations (table 10.5). Rest as long or as short as you want between each superset. Jot down the number you do and try to outperform yourself in your next workout.

Table 10.5 Variety Workout 5

Exercise	Sets	Reps
Superset 1		
1. Leg press	As many as possible	5
2. Dumbbell dead-lift	As many as possible	5
Superset 2		
3. Parallel bar dip	As many as possible	5
4. Inverted row	As many as possible	5
Superset 3		
5. Superman	As many as possible	5
6. Plank	As many as possible	5

WORKOUTS FOR THE GUY WHO LOVES CONSISTENCY

If you like to keep it straight and steady, use this plan to reinforce your intentions day after day.

WORKOUT 1: LEGS, CHEST AND BACK BUILDER

This three-lift dumbbell interval programme (table 10.6) is high intensity—so it's good for your heart—and you'll build strength if you increase the number of repetitions each time you do it. In the first 8 minutes do as many 5-repetition sets of the squat as you can. Jot your number down and try to better it next week. Move immediately to the second and third exercises, performing them as a back-to-back superset. Do as many 10-rep supersets as you can in the final 7 minutes of your 15-minute workout. If you feel sick afterward, you're working at the perfect intensity.

Table 10.6 Consistency Workout 1

Exercise	Sets	Reps
1. Squat	As many as possible	5
Superset		
2. Overhand-grip pull-up	As many as possible	10
3. Dumbbell flat chest press	As many as possible	10

WORKOUT 2:
CHEST, BACK AND ARMS BUILDER

Do the following exercises as supersets (table 10.7). Perform the moves one after another and then take a 30-second break before repeating the superset. In the second superset, take a 20-second break between the moves and do the reps as fast as you can.

Table 10.7   Consistency Workout 2

Exercise	Sets	Reps
Superset 1		
1. Dumbbell incline chest press	4	8
2. Dumbbell deadlift	4	8
Superset 2		
3. Cable rope curl	3	12
4. Rope push-down	3	12

WORKOUT 3:
FULL-BODY POWER BUILDER

Do as many 6-rep giant sets of the following exercises (table 10.8) as you can in 15 to 20 minutes. Don't rest between the exercises. Rather, take 1 minute of rest after you've done a set of every move. Jot down how many times you complete the giant set and beat that figure next week.

Table 10.8   Consistency Workout 3

Exercise	Sets	Reps
1. Power clean	As many as possible	6
2. Parallel bar dip	As many as possible	6
3. Underhand-grip pull-up	As many as possible	6

WORKOUT 4: ABS AND ARMS

Do all the reps in the first superset, rest for 1 minute and then do the exercises in the second superset (table 10.9). Keep alternating until you've done 3 or 4 sets of each exercise, depending on how much time you have.

Table 10.9   Consistency Workout 4

Exercise	Sets	Reps
Superset 1		
1. Barbell biceps curl	3-4	12
2. Plank	3-4	60 sec.
Superset 2		
3. Close-grip bench press	3-4	12
4. Barbell rollout	3-4	12

Gearing the Workouts to Burn Fat

If life has handed you a bit more around your middle that you'd like to get rid of in record time, look no further than the plans that follow.

- Do more reps. The higher your rep count, the more your body is working, provided the weights you're using are heavy enough. Doing upwards of 15 to 20 reps in each set is a terrific way to burn calories.

- Add an interval section. Simply tack a quick interval-training session to the end of your weights workout. It doesn't have to be long—5 to 10 minutes will do. You can pick an interval method from the fat-burning workouts in chapter 8.

- Do cardio between sets. You don't have to flat-out sprint, but you can alternate between riding a bike and pushing out heavy reps.

- Do 6 reps with heavy weights. Using weights so heavy you can manage only 6 reps hikes up your metabolism more than doing 12 reps does, found a study at the Norwegian University of Sport and Physical Education (Mjølsnes et al., 2004). Your body has to plumb calories into repairing the damaged muscles, and that's a surefire way to increase your metabolism.

- Eliminate rest completely. You're training for only 15 to 20 minutes—you can rest when you get home or sit at your desk. Rather, use this time to go at it 100 per cent and completely thrash yourself. You can take a well-deserved rest afterwards.

WORKOUT 5: POWER AND ENDURANCE

Complete a set of the power clean, rest for 40 seconds and then do exercises 2 to 4 as a no-rest superset (table 10.10). Rest for 40 seconds and then do the power clean again.

Table 10.10   Consistency Workout 5

Exercise	Sets	Reps
1. Power clean	3-4	8
Superset		
2. Superman	3-4	60 sec.
3. Push-up	3-4	15
4. Plank	3-4	60 sec.

The Leading Questions

Here are the answers to the questions most commonly asked about training with your nose firmly to the grind.

Q: **If I have only a few minutes to hit the rows of cardio machines, which one should I choose?**

A: The pulling power of the rower will make you hit your fitness goals faster than will any other machine. A treadmill canter is nothing more than glorified run on the spot, so it does little to build your fitness. An 80-kilogram bloke burns only about 765 calories per hour on the treadmill. Use the bike only to warm up your legs because it burns a measly 535 calories an hour. The rower ropes in the muscles of your legs, core and upper body, which are the biggest muscles in your body, and tops the charts by burning up to 802 calories an hour. It's also impact free, so you can give your muscles a good thrashing even if your joints are tired. If there's a spare seat on the rower, then jump on to get your fitness on the pull.

Q: **I want to build muscles at home to save time. I can afford a machine that costs about £250, but is it worth it?**

A: For that price you can probably get an Olympic barbell set and a used weight bench, if you hunt around. Don't worry about the equipment being secondhand because it's nearly impossible to damage steel. If you buy a used bench and weights, you might be able to find some adjustable dumbbells as well. No gimmicky machine is going to significantly help you. You need iron. Fortunately for you, it's plentiful and cheap.

Q: **During the week I do short workouts but on Saturdays I sometimes do a 2-hour workout. Afterwards I feel almost hungover. Why?**

A: That's your body telling you to chill out. You're probably dehydrated and have accumulated too much lactic acid in your system. You should hydrate and have food in your stomach before strenuous workouts. Working out too hard for too long can deplete your electrolyte stores and lead to cramping and nausea. If you insist on doing a long workout, prepping with fluids and food should help you avoid feeling like you sunk a bottle of Jack.

Q: **I have a high-profile job and a big family. How do I find the time and energy to get in shape?**

A: Time's easy: Just pick an hour when you focus on something less important than your health. That's pretty much any hour, right? Use that time for exercise and reorganise your life around it. Energy takes care of itself once you start eating five or six small meals a day, cut out junk food and alcohol and structure your life around that hour of exercise. You'll sleep better, feel better, shed fat, build muscle and have more energy. As for motivation, do you really need to be told to turn off the television for an hour and eat better? Don't spend your health getting your wealth or you'll spend your wealth getting back your health.

Q: I only have time to run in the morning before work but during winter my body just doesn't work properly when it's cold. What can I do?

A: The cold weather blows in and suddenly you're 20 years older, feeling every minor injury in every joint and muscle you've ever used, from the time you fell off your bike when you were five to last season's pulled hamstring. To prevent injury in cold weather, warm up your muscles indoors before venturing outside. When a muscle is cold it's less pliable and you're more susceptible to injury and more likely to cause a muscle pull. To feel like yourself again, do 3 sets of 12 reps of squats, push-ups and lunges in your hallway before you head outside.

Q: If I work out at lunch I'm wiped out and sore for the rest of the day. How can I recover faster?

A: You're probably rushing things and your muscles don't have enough time to recover. Give yourself at least 60 seconds rest between exercises. Also, try reducing the weight you're lifting by 10 per cent. Drink a protein shake before and after each training session and eat a solid lunch. These surplus nutrients will energise you for the rest of the afternoon and help you build muscle. Don't worry about the effect of lunch on calorie burning. Your body is the most forgiving postworkout, so your meal won't make you ache with fat.

Q: I cycle after work in the cold of the early evenings and my nose runs like a faucet. How can I stop it?

A: Get a pair running gloves with terry-cloth on the thumb and use it to wipe your nose. Alternatively, you can wear a bandana, which will act as a buffer by warming the air before it reaches your nose. Just remember to take it off before you go in the shops or the tellers might start giving you money.

Q: Is it better to lose weight first and then add muscle or vice versa?

A: The upside is that you can both lose weight and add muscle at the same time. The downside is that it takes a lot of work and dedication. Start a sound nutrition and supplement plan and train three to six days a week. You'll increase your lean body mass, which will give you more muscle. More muscle is the long-term solution to staying lean and healthy because it causes you to burn more calories when you exercise and when you laze on the couch watching television. And there's just no downside to more muscle.

Q: How can I stay focused enough to keep exercising when I really don't like the gym?

A: Your plan to get fit by visiting the gym is doomed because, well, you don't like the gym. A beginner who chooses a workout that matches his personality is more likely to improve his fitness. The seven major characteristics to consider when selecting a programme are sociability, spontaneity, self-motivation, aggressiveness, competitiveness, mental focus and risk taking. So, if you're a social, spontaneous type, consider team sports. Risk takers may like skiing or mixed martial arts. Aggressive and focused? You should love rugby. The key to winning with fitness is simply to find your perfect match.

Q: I work out in the morning before work. How long should I wait after eating to hit the gym?

A: The larger the meal (and the more fat or protein in it), the longer the wait. If you eat a typical breakfast of oats and orange juice, you should wait 30 to 45 minutes before exercising. This should be enough time to get ready and drive to your gym. You'll have to test your tolerance through trial and error. Don't exercise on an empty stomach. Raising your blood sugar with a banana or a few eggs will help you hang on to your hard-won muscle.

What's Next?

Now that your lunch-hour schedule is taken care of and you're maximizing every minute of your day, you can take your commitment one step further. Exercise itself is chock full of benefits in its own right. However, it also has many secondary attributes that you might want to consider making your primary goal. Ever had a few too many? Or need a way to sleep better? Or pump up your bedroom mojo? The next section discusses how to solve those problems and more with the aid of specialised exercise. Keep reading to find out how your sweat can be a double-edged sword against life's problems.

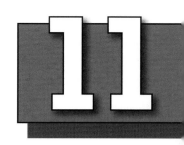

Double-Duty Workouts

Your workouts make you fitter and stronger and blast fat, but they should be giving you so much more. Here's how.

Multitasking is the knack of distracting yourself from two things—neither of which you enjoy enough to do by itself—by doing them simultaneously. It's about time your workouts follow your lead and hit more than one goal. The truth is that you already multi-task if you exercise. Getting sweaty gives you extra energy, more confidence and a stronger body and has made you a better man. But you deserve more. The exercise regimens in this chapter give you twice the payoff for the same effort. You'll find out how to boost your IQ and sex drive, beat stress, bust a hangover, get better sleep and live longer. Long after you've stopped exercising you can take comfort in the knowledge that you'll be multitasking away your problems without having to give them a second thought. Here are the best strategies for fixing some of life's more pressing problems.

Better-Sex Workout

Don't gamble on the muscles you think she likes. Better your odds with lady luck with this workout that will make you perform better in the bedroom.

When it comes to picking up girls, it's not all about abs. Yes, they may initially attract the fairer sex, but these modern times demand more versatility than the up-and-down sit-up. Building a physique for amazing sex has little to do with how much weight you can lift, press

or curl. It depends on how well your body can push and thrust. These actions are financed by your smaller muscles—the ones you can't see or feel. Luckily, they're easy to work and you can target most of them in a home gym setup. It doesn't take much to train these lesser-known muscles, but you'll have to work them with a mix of strength, flexibility and stamina exercises. The following plan will make you supple and strong enough to hold your body in positions for long periods of time—well, until she's finished, anyway.

How It Works

To train your bedroom mojo you can't just be excellent at curling heavy weights. You need to be good at everything. That's asking a lot, right? That's why this full-body workout mixes in strength-specific exercises as well as a few stretches. The key outcome: stamina. You'll do each exercise until failure, which is the point in the set at which you feel like your muscles have been injected with curry paste. When you're pushing out the reps and you reach this point, the thought of her (or the future her) should motivate you to keep going. Do all the moves as a nonstop circuit repeated one to three times and rest for one to two minutes after each one. You can even tack this circuit onto the end of your normal workout and do it as a finisher. Each circuit should take only 5 to 10 minutes, which is a small sacrifice for developing more stamina that could form the crux of a long-term relationship with the woman of your dreams.

Barbell Deadlift

This move will give you the strength to pick her up without any unnecessary grunting. You'll make her feel light and sexy.

Muscles

Quads, glutes, hamstrings, lower back, abs

Execution

1. Place a barbell (20 kilograms) on the ground in front of you. Stand with your feet shoulder-width apart.
2. Bend at your knees and hips and bring your upper body towards the bar. Grab the bar with an overhand grip (figure 11.1a).
3. Use your thighs to raise the bar until your legs are fully extended (figure 11.1b).

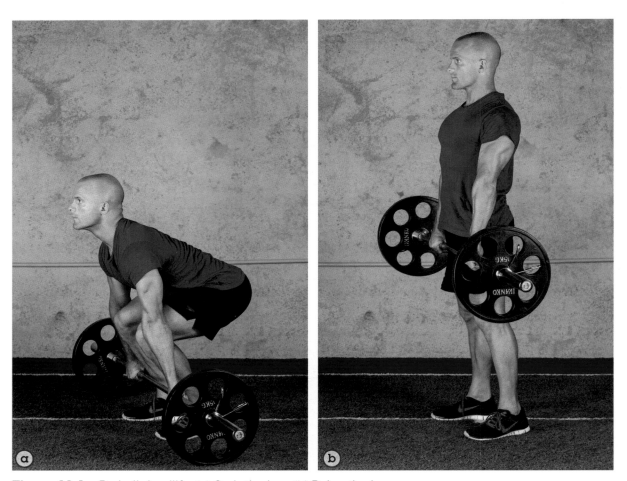

Figure 11.1 Barbell deadlift. *(a)* Grab the bar. *(b)* Raise the bar.

Swiss Ball Decline Push-Up

Learning to support your body weight with your hands will stop you from squashing her and will make it more likely you'll get a second serve.

Muscles

Shoulders, chest, triceps, abs

Execution

1. Kneel with a Swiss ball behind you. Place your hands flat on the floor shoulder-width apart.
2. Place your shins on the ball and get into the standard push-up position: arms straight, hands directly under your shoulders (figure 11.2a). Flatten your back and draw in your abs.
3. Tuck your chin. Leading with your chest, lower your body to the floor (figure 11.2b). Push yourself back up and repeat.

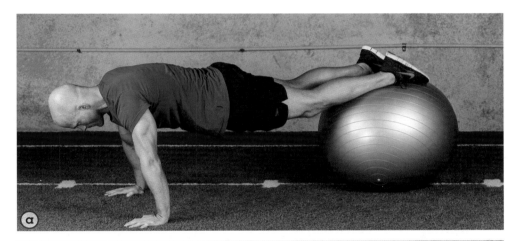

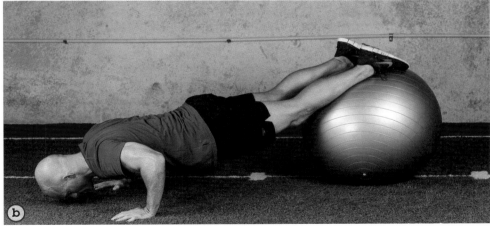

Figure 11.2 Swiss ball decline push-up. *(a)* Starting position. *(b)* Lower your body to the floor.

Lying Bridge

A strong core and pelvis are the cornerstones of the thrusting action. This exercise will improve your muscular stamina in all these areas.

Muscles

Glutes, core

Execution

1. Lie flat on your back with your knees bent and your feet flat on the floor. Place your arms at your sides.
2. Squeeze your glutes and slowly raise your glutes off the floor until your body forms a straight line from your knees to your shoulders (figure 11.3).
3. Hold this position for one to two seconds and then slowly lower yourself to the floor. Do three sets of as many reps as you can.

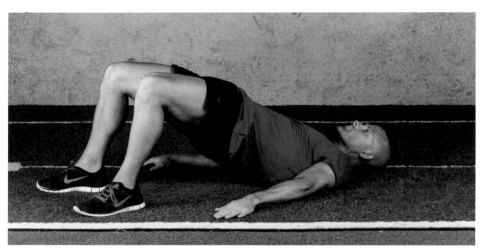

Figure 11.3 Lying bridge.

Weighted Overhand Pull-Up

This exercise creates a powerful, V-shaped back that offers the power to get creative in the bedroom without having to see the back cracker the next day.

Muscles

Back, biceps, abs, forearms

Execution

1. Use a belt to attach a small weight around your waist. Grab a pull-up bar with an overhand grip and place your hands shoulder-width apart. If you struggle to lift your body weight, use an assisted pull-up machine.
2. Hang so that your elbows are completely extended.
3. Bend your elbows and pull yourself up until your chin crosses the plane of the bar (figure 11.4). Pause, then slowly lower yourself to the starting position without allowing your body to sway. Do four sets of eight reps.

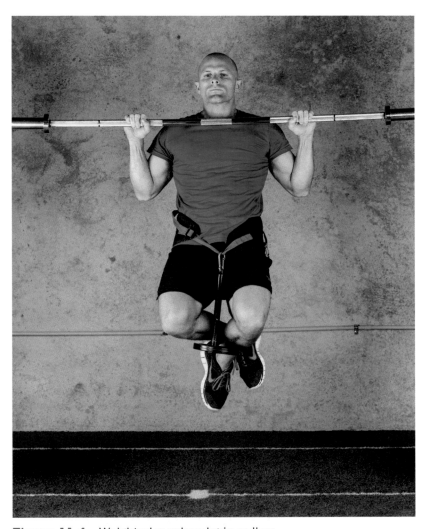

Figure 11.4 Weighted overhand-grip pull-up.

Standing Hip Thrust

You don't have to have a dirty mind to put your finger on the type of speciality strength this exercise is bound to create.

Muscles

Hip flexors

Execution

1. Stand with your feet together and place your hands on your hips. Step forward with one foot so that your feet are about half a metre apart. Point your toes forward and keep your knees slightly bent.

2. Gently push your pelvis forward until you feel a very mild stretch in your hips (figure 11.5). Although this move seems subtle, don't overdo it. The hip flexors are attached inside the legs in such a way that it takes very little effort to stretch them.

3. Hold the stretch for five seconds. Reverse leg positions and repeat.

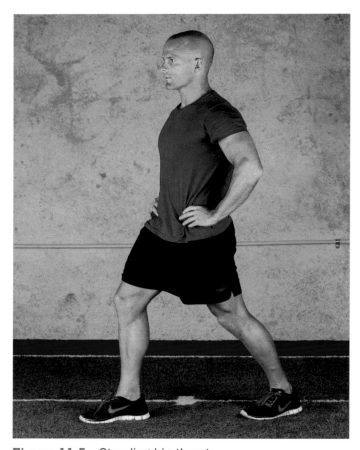

Figure 11.5   Standing hip thrust.

Plank With Raised Arm

Hands up if you want harder abs that both of you can enjoy.

Muscles

Abs

Execution

1. Lie facedown on the floor with your legs straight and together. Set your hands beneath your chest so that your body weight rests on your forearms. Raise up onto your elbows and toes so that your body forms a straight line from ankles to shoulders (figure 11.6a).

2. Raise your left arm in front of you and hold it there for 30 seconds (figure 11.6b). Repeat with your right arm.

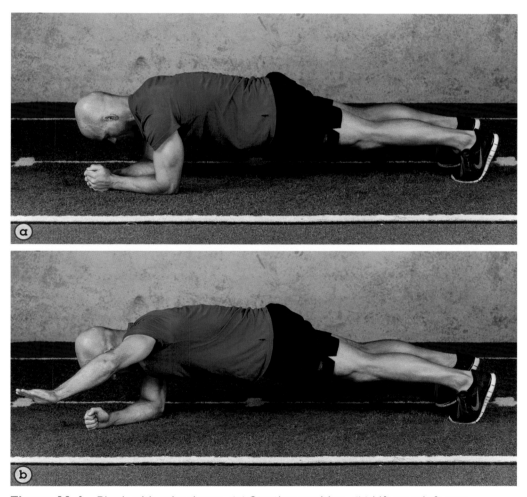

Figure 11.6 Plank with raised arm. *(a)* Starting position. *(b)* Lift your left arm.

Kneeling Leg Crossover

This exercise creates the kind of static strength in your legs that'll help you hold awkward positions for as long as she wants you to.

Muscles

Glutes

Execution

1. Get on all fours facing the floor and place your hands and knees shoulder-width apart (figure 11.7a). Straighten your right leg behind you and angle it to the right with your toes touching the floor.

2. Raise your right leg up and over your left leg (figure 11.7b), then lower it until your right foot touches the floor outside your left foot. Reverse the motion to get back to the starting position and repeat as many times as you can. Switch positions to work your left leg.

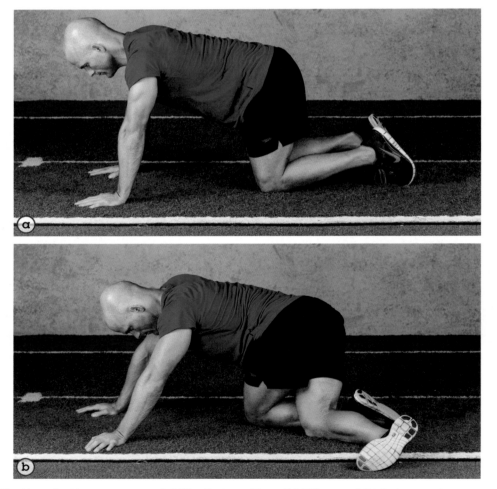

Figure 11.7 Kneeling leg crossover. *(a)* Starting position. *(b)* Lift your right leg up and over your left leg.

Side Plank With Raised Leg and Arm

Putting your hands in the air means you do care—about looking good, that is.

Muscles

Core

Execution

1. Lie facedown on the floor with your legs straight and together.
2. Get into the side plank position. Raise your top leg slightly off the ground and raise your top arm from your side into the air (figure 11.8). Hold that position and then switch sides. Resist the urge to wave to your reflection.

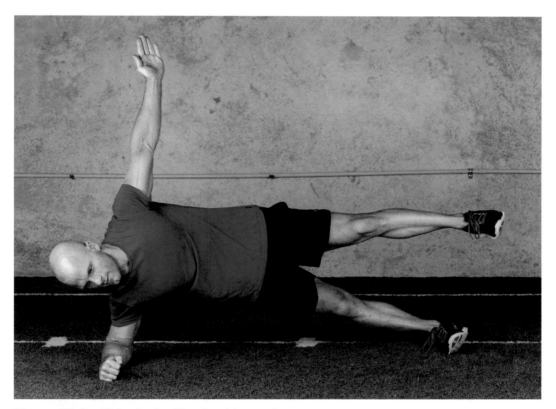

Figure 11.8   Side plank with raised leg and arm.

Lying Crossover Stretch

Cramps from overly tight muscles are never sexy. Here's how to put them to bed for good.

Muscles

Glutes

Execution

1. Lie on your back with your knees bent and your feet flat on the floor.
2. Slowly draw your right knee up to your chest. Grab the outside of your knee with your left hand and gently pull it towards your left shoulder as far as is comfortable (figure 11.9). Hold for 20 seconds and then lower your leg back to the starting position.
3. Repeat the move, this time raising your left knee and pulling it towards your right shoulder.

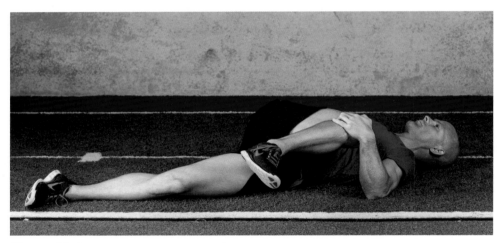

Figure 11.9 Lying crossover stretch.

Eat to Bolster Your Libido

You don't need pharmaceuticals to reclaim your manhood. All you need to do is step into the kitchen and eat the right foods. Here's what should be on your menu.

- Watermelon. It's a whole lot tastier than a pill and has the same effect. Researchers at the University of Texas (Jayaprakasha, Chidambara Murthy and Patil, 2011) found that the citrulline in watermelons makes more blood flow south. You don't even need a prescription.

- Dark chocolate. In a study from the University of California at San Francisco (Engler et al., 2004), blood vessel dilation increased by more than 10 per cent in participants who ate 50 grams of low-sugar dark chocolate per day.

- Berries. Forget about bringing coffee and toast to bed; bring the raspberries and strawberries. You lose 9 per cent of your daily zinc intake when you ejaculate. The berries will replenish the zinc you lose—five milligrams, or one third of your daily requirement—making them the perfect snack to eat between romps.

- Peanut butter. Sign on for the Skippy diet. Studies have found that men who ate diets rich in monounsaturated fat—the kind found in peanuts—had the highest levels of testosterone, which will help you grow big muscles and have firmer erections.

- Pomegranate juice. Turf the orange juice because a study at the University of California (Azadzoi et al., 2005) found that pomegranate juice boosts blood flow to your nether regions thanks to its high levels of antioxidants. It doesn't taste half bad, either.

Lifestyle Changes

Make these small changes to get some big results on the day.

- Go on holiday or down to the beach. The sun's rays increase your testosterone, found a study in *International Journal of Andrology* (Maggio et al., 2011). She may even find your darker skin more attractive. But don't overdo it—the boiled lobster look is out this year.

- Limber up to increase your endurance between the sheets. A study in *Journal of Sexual Medicine* (Dhikav et al., 2007) found that doing yoga for an hour a day tripled the length of time guys lasted in the sack.

- Think about doing some maintenance. A study in *Archives of Sexual Behaviour* (Prokop et al., 2012) found that women are most attracted to men who keep their fur coat in check. Women may be more attracted to hairless men because they are thought to be healthier, so get the Remington out.

Boost Your Circulation to Live Longer

Exercise has benefits beyond looking good at the beach. It can save your life. Here's how to boost your circulation for a better future as well as a better-looking physique.

Feeling healthy is not just about lack of sickness; it's about being in good nick inside and out. Unfortunately, some everyday quibbles can be a sign that something is awry under the hood. Your circulation could probably use a boost if you're prone to varicose veins or cold, numb or tingling hands and feet, if you regularly have leg cramps or if the colour doesn't jump back into your skin after it has been touched.

Don't ring the emergency number just yet because there is an easy solution: exercise. Flexing a muscle tells the nearby blood vessels that they need more blood to perform. The easiest way to force the flex? Lift heavy things. Regular strength training makes your blood vessels dilate and increases circulation throughout your entire body, which can even reduce cholesterol. The fastest remedy is performing exercises that work the muscles at either end of your body. In fitness circles this is called peripheral heart action, which is a fancy way of saying you do an exercise for legs then do one for chest or back. You rapidly circulate blood from top to toe. By the end of this workout you'll feel safe in the knowledge that you've trained your insides for the long game.

Circulation-Improving Workout

Alternate between workout 1 (table 11.1) and workout 2 (table 11.2) and leave at least a day of rest after every day of training. Perform 2 to 4 sessions a week. Do each exercise in a superset one after another without rest, then rest for 45 to 60 seconds and go again. To give your entire cardiovascular system a complete service, do 12 reps in each superset and repeat each superset 3 or 4 times. Consider the extra muscle you'll build and fat you'll burn a well-deserved bonus.

Table 11.1 Circulation-Improving Workout 1

Exercise	Sets	Reps
Superset 1		
1. Squat (barbell)	3-4	12
2. Dumbbell flat chest press	3-4	12
Superset 2		
3. Overhand-grip pull-up	3-4	12
4. Lunge	3-4	12
Superset 3		
5. Dumbbell deadlift	3-4	12
6. Dumbbell seated shoulder press	3-4	12
Superset 4		
7. Power clean	3-4	12
8. Lateral raise	3-4	12

Table 11.2 Circulation-Improving Workout 2

Exercise	Sets	Reps
Superset 1		
1. Inverted row	3-4	12
2. Step-up	3-4	12
Superset 2		
3. Lunge	3-4	12
4. Parallel bar dip	3-4	12
Superset 3		
5. Hammer curl	3-4	12
6. Split squat	3-4	12
Superset 4		
7. Seated calf raise	3-4	12
8. Dumbbell front raise	3-4	12

Improve Your Circulation Figures

Include these foods in your weekly diet to improve your circulation.

- Peppers, sweet potatoes, kiwifruit and strawberries. These foods have the high levels of vitamin C needed to make collagen, which keeps arteries supple.
- Walnuts, flaxseed and salmon. The omega-3 fatty acids act as natural anti-inflammatory agents for your muscles and arteries.
- Beans, brown rice, meat and poultry. You'll get the vitamins B_6 and B_{12} and folic acid needed to lower homocysteine, a risk factor for poor circulation.
- Green leafy vegetables, berries, watermelon and dairy. These are an excellent source of magnesium and vitamins A, C and E. They also provide selenium, which is necessary for keeping arteries supple and preventing them from cramping.

Do Nothing, Build Muscle

Going on holiday and want to come back bigger and tanned? Here's how you can do just that.

Once you've booked a holiday you know that your training quickly becomes focused on the day you clock off from work and hit the relax button. The focus of any preholiday training is usually looking your best for the entire vacation and earning yourself some food credits so you can tackle the odd buffet. Trouble is, you often come back looking a little smoother rather than more muscled after taking a few weeks off.

Fortunately, this doesn't have to be the case. You can come back from your holiday looking more chiselled and tanned and use the buffet line to your advantage. To accomplish this, the following programme will have you walking a tightrope between overtraining and overreaching. You've probably been warned about the former many times because it involves increasing your training but not increasing your rest and recovery. Your muscles struggle to keep up with all the added stress and release more cortisol, and testosterone—your muscle-building hormone—can also take a hit. So instead of growing and improving your performance you end up doing the exact opposite. It's common among overzealous athletes and has lots of pitfalls (see 'Signs of Overtraining'). But there is a way to use this training evil to your advantage.

Walk the Line

Overreaching is the step before you start to overtrain. When you overreach, you increase your training, put enormous stress on your muscles and bring them to a point just before overtraining. Here's the trick. Just before you feel the overtraining symptoms, pull out and completely stop training and start some well-deserved relaxation, whether at home or on an exotic beach. All you have to do is get stuck into enough high-protein food and do your sternest Homer Simpson impression at the buffet table. Then, while you're soaking up the sun, your muscles soak up the rest and nutrients. The damage from the heavy training load is repaired, which for you means growth. The end result? You'll bring back a holiday tan as well as more muscle.

Overreaching Workout

For the next 4 to 6 weeks you'll overreach by drastically increasing your training volume. You'll work each body part a few times a week and rest at least 24 hours between training sessions for each body part. This gives each part just enough time to recover before you work it again. Perform 3 sets of 10 repetitions of each exercise and take 30 to 60 seconds of rest between each set (tables 11.3 through 11.8). After the third exercise for every body part, perform a 6-rep drop set to completely finish off your muscles. On Sundays rest; you earned it.

Table 11.3 Overreaching Workout: Monday

Exercise	Sets	Reps	Rest
Chest			
1. Dumbbell flat chest press	3	10	30-60 sec.
2. Dumbbell incline chest press	3	10	30-60 sec.
3. Parallel bar dip	3	10	30-60 sec.
Shoulders			
4. Dumbbell seated shoulder press	3	10	30-60 sec.
5. Lateral raise	3	10	30-60 sec.
6. Dumbbell upright row	3	10	30-60 sec.
Triceps			
7. Close-grip bench press	3	10	30-60 sec.
8. Rope push-down	3	10	30-60 sec.
Abs			
9. Bicycle crunch	3	10	30-60 sec.

Signs of Overtraining

If you feel any of these symptoms, stop training completely or decrease your training load by one half.

MENTAL

Decreased desire to train

Depression

Apathy

Low self-esteem

Low concentration

Sensitivity to stress

PHYSICAL

Chronic fatigue

Sleeplessness

Lack of hunger

Headache

Upset stomach

Joint aches and pains

Table 11.4   Overreaching Workout: Tuesday

Exercise	Sets	Reps	Rest
Legs			
1. Squat (barbell)	3	10	30-60 sec.
2. Stiff-legged deadlift	3	10	30-60 sec.
3. Leg press	3	10	30-60 sec.
4. Good morning	3	10	30-60 sec.
Biceps			
5. Underhand-grip pull-up	3	10	30-60 sec.
6. Hammer curl	3	10	30-60 sec.
7. Cable rope curl	3	10	30-60 sec.

Table 11.5   Overreaching Workout: Wednesday

Exercise	Sets	Reps	Rest
Back			
1. Overhand-grip pull-up	3	10	30-60 sec.
2. Dumbbell bent-over row	3	10	30-60 sec.
3. Inverted row	3	10	30-60 sec.
Chest			
4. Dumbbell chest fly	3	10	30-60 sec.
5. Cable crossover	3	10	30-60 sec.
6. Dumbbell flat pullover	3	10	30-60 sec.
Abs			
7. Hanging leg raise	3	10	30-60 sec.

Table 11.6   Overreaching Workout: Thursday

Exercise	Sets	Reps	Rest
Legs			
1. Step-up	3	10	30-60 sec.
2. Lunge	3	10	30-60 sec.
3. Hamstring curl	3	10	30-60 sec.
4. Standing calf raise	3	10	30-60 sec.
Biceps			
5. Underhand-grip pull-up	3	10	30-60 sec.
6. Barbell biceps curl	3	10	30-60 sec.
7. Cable rope curl	3	10	30-60 sec.

Table 11.7   Overreaching Workout: Friday

Exercise	Sets	Reps	Rest
Back			
1. Power clean	3	10	30-60 sec.
2. Single-arm dumbbell row	3	10	30-60 sec.
3. Cable face pull	3	10	30-60 sec.
Shoulders			
4. Arnold press	3	10	30-60 sec.
5. Lateral raise	3	10	30-60 sec.
6. Incline reverse fly	3	10	30-60 sec.
Abs			
7. Plank			60 sec.
8. Side plank			60 sec.

Table 11.8   Overreaching Workout: Saturday

Exercise	Sets	Reps	Rest
Chest			
1. Dumbbell flat chest press	3	10	30-60 sec.
2. Dumbbell incline chest press	3	10	30-60 sec.
3. Parallel bar dip	3	10	30-60 sec.
Triceps			
4. Close-grip bench press	3	10	30-60 sec.
5. EZ-bar skull crusher	3	10	30-60 sec.
6. Triceps extension	3	10	30-60 sec.

Sleep Strong

Use this sleep-inducing exercise and nutrition plan to ensure that you wake up full of energy and live the dream.

Trouble getting on the nod? Ready your gown, nightcap and gym gloves. Research in *Journal of Sports Science and Medicine* (Ferris et al., 2005) found that doing three bouts of weight training a week improved people's ability to drop off and their sleep quality by 38 per cent. The participants were older, but that doesn't mean their routine won't work for spring chickens. Participants trained in the morning to give their bodies enough time to relax before they hit the sheets. Rest for 60 to 120 seconds between sets and do 2 sets of 10 to 12 reps of all the exercises to mimic their snooze-inducing workout. The idea is to exercise at a low intensity—only 50 per cent of the most weight you can push once on each of these exercises. Training at very high intensities does burn more calories but it can make you feel awake, especially if you do it at night. Low intensity and slow lifting speed are necessary to lull your body into becoming fitter, stronger and more accustomed to sleep. The workout (table 11.9) should take you only 30 minutes, which is a small price to pay for not having to sit through another rerun. Warning: The strength of the study participants increased by 52 per cent, so go easy on your alarm clock.

Table 11.9   Sheep-Counting Workout

Exercise	Sets	Reps	Rest
1. Dumbbell flat chest press	2	10-12	1-2 min.
2. Leg press	2	10-12	1-2 min.
3. Leg extension	2	10-12	1-2 min.
4. Dumbbell bent-over row	2	10-12	1-2 min.
5. Dumbbell seated shoulder press	2	10-12	1-2 min.
6. Hammer curl	2	10-12	1-2 min.

Run, row or cycle at a steady state for 10 to 15 minutes afterwards.

Sleep What You Sow

This pillow-time guide tells you how much shuteye does for your body.

Less than 4 hours a night: You'll reduce your stamina and endurance by 15 to 40 per cent, researchers found (Gundersen et al., 2006). Turn off the infomercials and you'll run farther tomorrow.

6 hours a night: When you work out after insufficient sleep, you exercise at an intensity that is lower than you realise and that feels higher than it is. Your muscles are less likely to receive enough of the stress they need to improve.

8 hours a night: You'll be raring to go and boost your recovery hormones. Research in

Journal of Clinical Investigation found that you release growth hormone while you kip, which repairs your muscles (Takahashi, Kipnis and Daughaday, 1968).

10 hours a night: You'll improve your sprint time by up to 8 per cent, found researchers at Stanford University (Mah et al., 2011). They also found that this amount of sleep increases power and improves reflexes—your new excuse to hit the snooze button faster.

12 hours a night: Now that's just plain lazy. Get a diary and fill it. A study in *Internal Medicine* (Gottlieb et al., 2005) found that snoozing this much will make you more likely to have diabetes, increasing your risk of obesity. Surprised? Now get the hell out of bed.

Eat Right to Sleep Tight

Sleeping isn't all pillows and dumbbells. How and what you eat is key to becoming a sleeping beauty.

- Eat green veggies, nuts, seeds and whole-grain cereals. These are rich in magnesium. A study in *Sleep* found that a healthy diet rich in magnesium improves the quality of your sleep (Hornyak et al., 1998).

- Avoid large meals. These will make you feel uncomfortable and bloated and will impede your sleep. However...

- Don't skip meals. If you do, you'll be focusing on the hunger in your stomach rather than on falling asleep.

- Avoid too much alcohol. Alcohol makes you wake up feeling groggy. However, some people do report sleeping better after a single nightcap.

Less Stress, More Chillaxing

Stress is responsible for 40 million lost working days in the United Kingdom each year, and 12 million people visit their general practitioners with stress-related problems annually. Here's the prescription for conquering life's worries with sweat.

Work, money, kids, exercise . . . . Ironically, everything that makes life worth living can also

What's So Bad About Stress?

Getting your knickers in a knot when somebody overtakes you produces excessive amounts of cortisol and adrenaline. These are necessary in small quantities, but having extended doses of them is like keeping your car at 10,000 rpm. This will make your engine burn out. Too much adrenaline accelerates heart rate, which increases blood pressure. Too much cortisol increases blood sugar levels, which inflates your belly, dampens your immune system and can eat away at your muscle. Do the following workout to destress, and try to remind yourself of the irony that anyone who drives faster than you is a maniac and anyone who drives slower than you is an idiot.

tear it down. If you experience stress you're not alone. The rate of workplace absenteeism due to stress is massively high across the globe. But don't fret. Instead, add two stress-busting tactics to your workouts: get outside to do cardio and take your sweet time when you do resistance exercise.

Researchers at the University of Wisconsin (Farrell et al., 1987) found that low-intensity weightlifting elevates mood better than medium- to high-intensity lifting does. Trying to exercise your demons simply won't work. To be relaxed you actually have to take a slightly relaxed attitude towards exercise, which you're probably not going to complain about. But that's not the only line of attack against your boss's annoying requests. The outdoors should play a part in your chill-out armoury. A mere five-minute canter in the open air near some greenery will improve your mood and self-esteem. Imagine what going for 15 minutes will do for your headspace. The following workout is built on these principles and will produce a body that feels relaxed but looks flexed. That's definitely one less thing to worry about.

Stress-Less Workout

Find a leafy park, beach or reserve and warm up with an easy 5-minute jog. Jog for 45 to 60 seconds before doing each bodyweight exercise (table 11.10). This strategy will relax you and hopefully eliminate any postworkout soreness. It'll also cut the time you exercise in half, so you get maximum rewards with a smidgen of effort.

Table 11.10 Stress-Less Workout

Exercise	Reps
Jog or cycle slowly for 12 minutes	
1. Squat (body weight)	6-8
2. Push-up	6-8
3. Plank	30 sec.
4. Lunge (body weight)	6 each leg
Jog or cycle slowly for 5 minutes	
5. Squat (body weight)	6-8
6. Push-up	6-8
7. Plank	30 sec.
8. Lunge (body weight)	6 each leg
Jog or cycle slowly for 10 minutes and then stretch	

Now call it a day. You'll be as calm as a Hindu cow and won't be sweating the small stuff.

Stress-Free Eating

Forget the chill pills. Here's how to feast away your worries.

- Spinach, peppers, cauliflower, mushrooms, asparagus, onions and tomatoes are rich in B vitamins that blunt the effects of the stress hormone cortisol.

- Eat oily fish or take fish oil tablets. A study in *Diabetes and Metabolism* found that cortisol levels were 20 per cent lower during stress tests in those who took a fish oil supplement (Delarue et al., 2003).

- Bananas contain high levels of the hormone melatonin, which promotes calm and sleep and helps you relax.

- Enjoy peanut M&Ms. The chocolate triggers the release of feel-good serotonin

Signs of Stress		
Fatigue	Poor concentration	Hair loss
Mood swings	More colds and flu	Slow wound healing
Inability to lose weight		

while the nuts provide protein that evens out your blood sugar and keeps you focused. Note: A bad day isn't an excuse to indulge in a whole bag for lunch.

Lifestyle Changes

Before you visit the doc for some happy pills, try these easy tips and tricks for max relaxing.

- Eat in a relaxed environment. Cortisol levels rise if you're stressed while eating. Avoid bad news by turning off the telly, putting down the paper and taking the time to enjoy your grub.
- Simplify your schedule. Cut out time-intensive activities that deliver little value and prioritise some relaxation into every day.
- Shift your perspective. How you perceive the world affects your stress levels. What stresses you might be brushed aside by another bloke. Don your rose-coloured glasses at all times.
- Surround yourself with positive, upbeat people. Social situations with demanding interactions bump up your stress hormones and increase your heart rate. Show that demanding girlfriend the outside of a slammed door.

Beat Your Hangover for Good

Big night on the town? Use this lunch-hour plan to feel like your old self without stumbling towards the golden arches of your nearest fast-food palace.

12:30: Get Some Energy

You're going to need fuel to beat your hangover. Your energy supply should be something that's easy on the palette and all natural; that'll make your meal less likely to drive the porce-lain bus. Your best bet is something soft such as a banana, which is rich in energy-yielding vitamin B_6. Even a bowl of fortified cereal is rich in this oomph-yielding vitamin, provided you can stomach the milk. Try to avoid sugar—your body has taken enough abuse already. Rather, sweeten up with honey, which is full of the sodium and fructose you need to get your hangover to buzz off (Stephens et al., 2008). It'll also give you the fast-acting pep you need to start your workout.

13:00 to 13:10: Get Out of the Office or House

Whether you're being paid to be hungover or doing it on your own time, after midday is a more-than-acceptable time to show your face to the world. If you're in the office it will also squash any rumours that you're too sick to be productive. The goal is to get to a leafy park away from busy roads and noises. This workout should take only about 10 minutes and you can do it by bike or on foot. Doing just a few minutes of outdoor exercise boosts fitness, gives you greater feelings of revitalisation, increases your energy and positive engagement and decreases in tension, confusion, anger and depression. Sounds like the recipe for curing a hangover. You're better off going green than choosing the glow of your gym's strip lighting.

13:10 to 13:30: Get an Energy Boost

Let's face it: Today is never going to be the day you break any personal records. Rather, work on pushing healing blood around your body so you can feel loose and energetic for the rest of the day. Do these exercises for about 10 to 20 minutes. Go longer if you can manage it and shorter if you can't. Rest for no more than 30 seconds between each move.

Leaning Lunge

This exercise will stretch your upper body and open up your lungs so you can breathe a little deeper.

Muscles

Glutes, hamstrings, quads, core

Execution

1. Stand with your feet together and your hands at your sides.
2. Raise your right arm above your head and then take a giant step forward with your right leg.
3. As you land, let your right arm touch your ear and try to get a stretch in your lats (figure 11.10). Step back to the starting position and repeat on your left side. Do six to eight reps on each side.

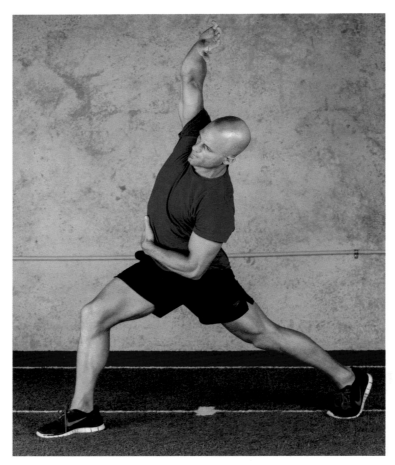

Figure 11.10 Leaning lunge.

Balance Deadlift

You may have lost your balance the night before, but this move is here to help you regain your composure.

Muscles

Hamstrings, lower back, core

Execution

1. Stand with your knees slightly bent.
2. Raise your right foot off the ground. Bend over and reach for your left foot with your hands (figure 11.11). Keep your back straight.
3. Alternate legs until you've done eight reps on each leg.

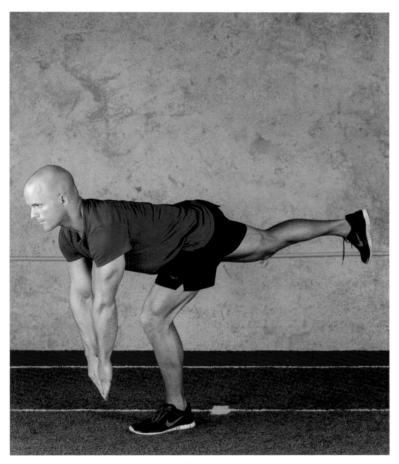

Figure 11.11   Balance deadlift.

Bird Dog

You may have had to assume this position only a few hours earlier. Get back into it and make sure it does some good this time.

Muscles

Abs, lower back

Execution

1. Get onto your hands and knees to give your best dog impression.
2. Lift your left arm and right leg off the floor and extend them away from your body (figure 11.12). Hold that position for five seconds, then switch sides and repeat. That's one rep. Do six to eight reps.

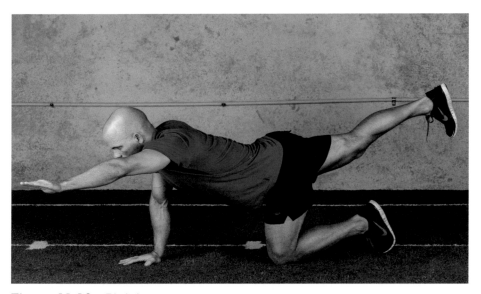

Figure 11.12 Bird dog.

Pushing Push-Up

This is the easy version of the regular push-up. Don't wimp out, even if you're feeling extremely weak, because it will help your strength return.

Muscles

Chest, shoulders, abs

Execution

1. Find a fence or a park bench that's about waist height.
2. Place your hands shoulder-width apart on the fence railing and extend your legs behind you so that your body is diagonal to the ground.
3. Bend your elbows and lower your chest to the railing (figure 11.13a). Then explode up and push yourself back to a standing position (figure 11.13b). Do 12 reps.

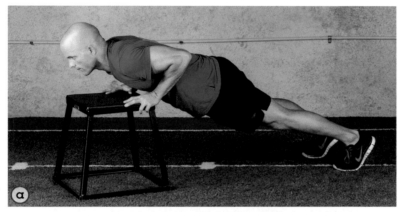

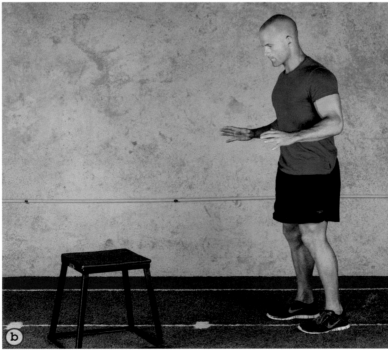

Figure 11.13
Pushing push-up.
(a) Lower your chest.
(b) Explode up to standing.

13:30 to 13:50:
You're Done; Now Get Some Food

Walk or ride briskly again for about 10 minutes until you've reached a café because by now your belly will be letting out some angry calls for grease. The best lunch? An egg, bacon and tomato muffin with a serving of orange juice will help you see the world sunny side up. The eggs are rich in cysteine, a substance that breaks down hangover-causing toxins in the liver. The tomato and juice team up to flush your body with vitamin C and fructose, which increase the clearance of alcohol from the blood. You'll feel like your old self by the last bite. The return of your memories is another story.

Use food to expel the marching band you in your head and heal the hurt from a night on the town. Here are some other hangover-busting foods that will help you recover.

- Pumpkin seeds. They may not be the first thing on your mind when you wake up, but the same could be said for the previous night's Tabasco sauce shooters. Pumpkin seeds are the richest source of magnesium, a mineral that alcohol leeches from your system. Magnesium is a natural headache reliever, so sprinkle these through your muesli to mute the bass drum in your noggin.

- Ginger. You might feel relaxed after a few toots, but your stomach will be doing more flicks-flacks than a box full of hamsters. Alcohol inflames your gut lining and increases the production of gastric acid. Fortunately, ginger beer—a nausea-relieving drink popular among pregnant lasses—acts as a ringmaster to your belly circus. If you're after a thirst quencher, ginger beer should be on the list.

- Isostar sport drink. You won't feel much like Usain Bolt, but any drink with taurine in it (such as a Powerade) will bring you back to the land of living. Researchers at the University of London's school of pharmacy found that taurine can reverse the liver damage caused by alcoholism (Kerai et al., 1999).

- Olive oil. Remember that craving for grease you get when you first wake up? Well, satisfy it with this oil. Your body craves fats to repair the damage from the previous night but it actually wants good fats, not the artery-clogging trans fats served by the greasy-spoon place. Olive oil is full of brain-boosting omega-3 fatty acids and liver-aiding unsaturated fats. Want eggs? Fry them in olive oil over low heat. You can even lob olive oil over a salad if you're brave enough to be healthy.

13:50 to 14:00:
Hit the Showers and Touch Up

During and after your shower be sure to drink as much water as you can stomach. Even if you don't feel like an athlete today, you're suffering from the same affliction they do: dehydration. Rehydrating will make your skin bounce back and give you an extra spurt of energy. That's it. You should be feeling like your old self—until the next Friday, that is.

Where Now?

Do these workouts as and when you need them rather than all the time—they're quick fixes for when these specific problems arise. At the end of these workouts you'll have learned how to do more than one thing at a time. Nowhere is that trait more on display than on a sport pitch. So if you fancy pitting your newfound skills against your fellow man, keep reading for the dish on sport training.

Sports Training

ap into your inner athlete. Embrace the sportsman in you to improve your fitness and skills and become your team's most valuable player, even if you're only a team of one.

If one thing is sure to push you past your old limits, it's competitiveness. Once you start trying to be better than the next bloke you'll realise that one of the greatest motivators for exercising and pushing past your former self is competition. The rivalry between you and the clock or another team can make you reach for that untapped energy in the depths of your muscles and force you to reach new heights, build bigger muscles, get fitter and become stronger.

Even if you think you're already fit because you burn a little fat here and lift a few weights there, you might not be truly fit—at least not in a total-body sense. You'll realise this only once you step onto a sport pitch. Sport fitness is more than just endurance, leanness and strength. It's about a combining them with power, acceleration and reaction time. This is what makes good athletes great and, more important, what makes sport fun. Variety provides balance, can prevent overuse injuries and breaks the monotony of stale, repetitive routines. The different degrees of effort in each session mean that you do both strength and aerobic work at the same time, which burns more fat than either form of exercise alone. Like the sound of those benefits? Step away from the Wii sports and find yourself a real opponent.

If you're a seasoned athlete or compete only in one particular sport, you might think it's best to specialise. Not always. Specialisation is for insects. Doing only one type of exercise repetitively strains the same muscles day after day, whereas cross-training helps you improve your fitness and overall conditioning. Involving yourself in a spectrum of activities conditions your body for everything rather than one specific thing. This better prepares you for the unexpected on the sport pitch and makes you stronger from a whole-body perspective.

Cross-training is a lot less complicated than you might think. If you're a persistent runner, try substituting one canter a week with a bike ride. Cross-training helps you recover because you won't be thrashing the same muscles, ligaments and tendons in your legs that running can abuse over time. What's more, research in *Sports Medicine* (Tanaka, 1994) found that cross-training is great for rehabilitating after an injury. The study also discovered that it boosts motivation, so if you're feeling lacklustre about your sport, try something new to get keen again.

With this in mind, is it possible to do a single routine that will condition you for all sports? Yes and no. The All-Sports Workout in this chapter gives you a baseline of fitness for every sport. If you want to specialise, sport-specific plans later in the chapter will help you condition yourself enough to get involved in a new sport or simply improve your performance in your current sport. If you want to outrun competitors, dogs or peeved girlfriends, use the workouts in this chapter to get a well-rounded sense of fitness. Stopped competing and started watching? Don't let the pursuit of money, women or a weed-free lawn stifle your natural competitiveness. There's a league for every age group, no matter how young or old. It's never too late to return to your competitive days. The steady purpose, banter and ability to fit into your pants are all worth fighting for. Unleash your inner sportsman. You can guarantee he's itching to go every time you tune your tube in to the match of the day.

All-Sports Workout

Build muscle, endurance and explosiveness that you can use to show off at your next match.

The basic needs of all sports are pretty much the same, unless you consider curling or chess athletic pursuits. For most sports you need a mix of speed, strength, muscle, explosiveness and endurance. You could attempt to build speed in one workout, strength in another, muscle in the next and so on, but this line of attack assumes that your body is able to segment its skills during a match. When you play sport you need the endurance to last the whole match coupled with the speed to reach the ball and the reaction time and explosiveness to do something productive with said ball. Combining all these skills in a few quick seconds without thinking about it is what separates the winners and losers. Rather than trying to fragment your body into its attributes you can train each one in every workout, making every sweat session more akin to an actual match. Adjust how much you eat to determine whether these workouts add bulk or reduce fat. They can and will do both, but teaming them up with the appropriate amount of calories will determine how your physique looks. How it performs is up to your natural, genetically given talent. Blame or thank Mom and Pop for that.

The all-sports workout is divided into three sections.

1. **Strength.** You'll do strength work at the start of the workout when you're fresher and stronger. The workout focuses on a single upper-body exercise and single lower-body exercise. In workouts 1 and 3 you'll start with a lower-body move and in workouts 2 and 4 you'll start with an upper-body move. This creates a balance of strength so that neither half of your body overpowers the other over time. The exercises in this section are structured as pyramids to allow you to push the maximum amount of weight. These let you safely increase the weight and reduce the repetitions. However, do try to rope help from a spotter to push the most weight you can manage. Rest for two to three minutes between each set, especially in the final sets of four reps; you'll need the rest to be stronger. Remember: The bigger the weight, the bigger the reward.

2. **Muscle-building endurance.** Do the exercises in this section as a single circuit using the same-size weight. If the first exercise calls for a barbell, use the most weight you can manage and don't put that weight down until you've done all the repetitions. The exercises work your smallest muscles, such as your biceps, first to maximise their strength. Towards the end of the set when you start to tire you can then use your bigger muscles, such as your legs, to help power through the reps. Rest for two minutes after each of these circuits. It's gut-wrenchingly tough and by the final set you'll be gagging for air, but remember that the more you hurt yourself in training the less you'll hurt during a match.

3. **Explosive speed.** Do the exercises in this section as a circuit and rest for 30 to 60 seconds afterwards. Fortunately, this section is nowhere near as tough as the previous superset because it calls for fewer reps. Concentrate on the speed of each rep and do each one as quickly as possible. This will leave your muscles poised to move quickly even when you're tired, which is what is demanded of you on a sports pitch.

Stick to this programme for four to eight weeks and then try one of the other workouts in the book, depending on whether your goal is fat burning or muscle building. This programme can be quite taxing on your nervous system. If you feel tired and stop making gains, take one to two weeks off from training and use a whole new set of exercises when you come back to this routine to keep challenging your body. Be sure to schedule enough rest between each workout.

Considering that most sports are played on weekends you'll do most of your training during the week. Do workout 1 (table 12.1) on Monday, workout 2 (table 12.2) on Tuesday, rest on Wednesday, workout 3 (table 12.3) on Thursday and workout 4 (table 12.4) on Friday.

Table 12.1 All-Sports Workout 1

Exercise	Sets	Reps
Strength		
1. Squat (barbell)	4	10, 6, 4, 4
2. Weighted overhand-grip pull-up	4	10, 6, 4, 4
Muscle-building endurance		
1. Barbell biceps curl	4	6
2. Squat press	4	6
3. Good morning	4	6
4. Dumbbell bent-over row	4	6
5. Deadlift	4	6
6. Close-grip bench press	4	6
Explosive speed		
1. Hanging leg raise	3	4
2. Medicine ball lying throw	3	4
3. Lying leg raise	3	4

Table 12.2 All-Sports Workout 2

Exercise	Sets	Reps
Strength		
1. Dumbbell incline chest press	4	10, 6, 4, 4
2. Lunge (barbell)	4	10, 6, 4, 4
Muscle-building endurance		
1. Hammer curl	4	6
2. Dumbbell upright row	4	6
3. Dumbbell flat pullover	4	6
4. Dumbbell seated shoulder press	4	6
5. Incline reverse fly	4	6
6. Dumbbell chest fly	4	6
Explosive speed		
1. Barbell rollout	3	4
2. Explosive push-up	3	4
3. Medicine ball slam	3	4
4. Barbell biceps throw	3	4

Table 12.3 All-Sports Workout 3

Exercise	Sets	Reps
Strength		
1. Dumbbell deadlift	4	10, 6, 4, 4
2. Parallel bar dip (weighted)	4	10, 6, 4, 4
Muscle-building endurance		
1. EZ-bar curl	4	6
2. Lateral raise	4	6
3. Power clean	4	6
4. Step-up	4	6
5. Cable crossover	4	6
6. Triceps push-down	4	6
Explosive speed		
1. Barbell rollout	3	4
2. Jumping split squat	3	4
3. Wrestles	3	4

Table 12.4 All-Sports Workout 4

Exercise	Sets	Reps
Strength		
1. Underhand-grip pull-up (weighted)	4	10, 6, 4, 4
2. Step-up (barbell)	4	10, 6, 4, 4
Muscle-building endurance		
1. Squat	4	12
2. Push-up	4	12
3. Lunge	4	12
4. Split squat	4	12
5. Pendulum	4	12
6. Superman	4	12
Explosive speed		
1. Explosive push-up	3	4
2. Bicycle crunch	3	4
3. Jumping split squat	3	4

You may want to taper the intensity of Friday's workout or leave it out altogether if you're playing a match on Saturday. This schedule is ideal if you're in the off-season of your sport. If you're midseason and playing matches on Saturday, you can work out four days in a row and rest on Friday. However, pay attention to how you feel because you might be too fatigued to train by Wednesday. The trick is to adjust your training schedule to how you feel on the day of training. Tired? That's a message from your body to take the day off. Don't ignore your body; it knows best and will perform at its best come game day.

Taking the Next Step: Speed

Speed might kill but it's also known to put winners on podiums. At the root of this match-winning trait is explosiveness, or the ability to move yourself or an object as fast as possible. Speed accelerates your pace and punches and gives you power you can use to fend off defenders and punch through gaps. The principle behind building speed involves harnessing the elastic energy of your muscles to increase strength, acceleration and explosive power. This process, which is beneficial to performance in all sports, fries an obscene amount of energy.

If you've been mixing your sport training with the sluggish pursuit of iron pumping, it's likely that you've actually been teaching your muscles to move slower. The workouts and tips that follow will make you faster and more elusive and will give you absolutely everything you need to know to improve your most prized asset: being a second ahead of your opponent. But that's not the only advantage of speed training. Explosive exercises, which use your fast-twitch muscle fibres, burn 11 per cent more calories during exercise and 5 per cent more calories after exercise compared with normal-speed reps performed with the same-size weight, found a study in *Medicine and Science in Sports and Exercise* (Mazzetti et al., 2007). This means that explosive exercises help you look leaner. So come on—what are you waiting for?

Do this full-body workout two or three times a week in conjunction with other training, such as a few runs, but don't team it with the all-sports workout. That's too much stress on your body. When you get started, leave a day's rest between each session. This programme will create explosiveness in the muscles you'll need for most sport movements such as punching, kicking, pushing and sprinting. The latter part of the workout uses a proven system called contrast training, where you do a strength move followed by an explosive exercise. A study at the University of Zagreb in Croatia (Markovic et al., 2004) found that contrast training makes athletes move up to 8 per cent faster. If this technique were a supplement, it would probably be illegal.

After you complete the all-sports workout and improve your speed you'll have a body that'll respond to competition and will probably feel pretty good about it all. Once you have the basics under your belt, you'll likely want to do something more specific to your sport. The coming sections give you all the ammunition you'll need for your chosen sport.

SPEED WORKOUT

Do this workout 1 or 2 times a week in conjunction with your normal weightlifting or cardio workout.

SECTION 1: STRAIGHT SETS

Finish all the sets of the first exercise—rest 60 seconds between bouts—and then move on to the next exercise (table 12.5).

Table 12.5 Speed Workout: Section 1

Exercise	Sets	Reps
1. Power clean	2	4
2. Squat press	3	4

SECTION 2: SUPERSETS

Do these moves (table 12.6) one after another. Rest for 1 to 2 minutes only after you've completed a set of each.

Table 12.6   Speed Workout: Section 2

Exercise	Sets	Reps
Superset 1		
1. Squat (barbell)	4	3
2. Jumping split squat	4	3
Superset 2		
3. Dumbbell flat chest press	4	4
4. Explosive push-up	4	4
Superset 3		
5. Split squat	3	4
6. Jumping split squat	3	4

SECTION 3: STRAIGHT SETS

Finish all the sets of the first exercise—rest 60 seconds between bouts—and then move on to the next exercise (table 12.7).

Table 12.7   Speed Workout: Section 3

Exercise	Sets	Reps
1. Medicine ball slam	3	4
2. Explosive push-up	3	4

Your Guide to Running

Gallop towards a fitter and slimmer self with the cheapest form of fitness.

The first thing we learn, before we even think about grumbling about our baby fat, is how to run. It is quite literally in our nature. A study published in *Nature* (Bramble and Lieberman, 2004) found that we are in fact born to run and that our physiology supports long-distance canters. The study's authors found that endurance running may have been so vital for our survival that it shaped our bodies. This proves that absolutely everyone—no matter what shape they're in—can lace up a set of trainers. And running is one of the most effective fat-burning activities you can do: The average 80-kilogram bloke nukes 594 calories during a 30-minute run. The only difficult bit is finding the right starting point. The following plans are for blokes who have better things to do than run but still need to shave a slice or two off the belly. One plan is for the bloke who can scarcely run a bath and the other is for the guy who can manage a 20-minute canter but wants to improve his performance. Find a stretch of pavement and start pounding it to get your excess to drop off.

Starter's Blocks

This plan will take you from loafing to running for 30 minutes continuously in just 3 running sessions a week for 8 weeks. After each session walk for 5 minutes to cool down and stretch gently for another 5 minutes. Don't worry about speed or distance—clocking time on your feet is your only concern.

START RUNNING PLAN

WEEK 1

Run for 1 minute and then walk for 90 seconds. Repeat 8 times. Do 3 times a week.

WEEK 2

Run for 2 minutes and then walk for 1 minute. Repeat 7 times. Do 3 times a week.

WEEK 3

Run for 3 minutes and then walk for 1 minute. Repeat 6 times. Do 3 times a week.

WEEK 4

Run for 5 minutes and then walk for 2 minutes. Repeat 4 times. Do 3 times a week.

WEEK 5

Run for 8 minutes and then walk for 2 minutes. Repeat 3 times. Do 3 times a week.

WEEK 6

Run for 12 minutes and then walk for 1 minute. Repeat 3 times. Do 3 times a week.

WEEK 7

Run for 15 minutes, walk for 1 minute and then run for 15 minutes. Do 3 times a week.

WEEK 8

Run for 30 minutes continuously.

Run a 5K Race

If you can manage 15 to 20 minutes of continuous running, this plan is your starter's gun for your first 5K race.

PREPARE FOR A 5K

WEEK 1

Monday: Rest.

Tuesday: Run for 20 minutes at an easy pace.

Wednesday: Rest.

Thursday: Run for 8 minutes at an easy pace. Run at a brisk pace for 45 seconds and then jog at a recovery pace for 2 minutes. Repeat this 4 times. Finish by running for 8 minutes at a slow pace.

Friday: Rest.

Saturday: Run for 20 minutes at an easy pace.

Sunday: Run for 25 minutes at an easy pace.

WEEK 2

Monday: Rest.

Tuesday: Run for 20 minutes at an easy pace.

Wednesday: Rest.

Thursday: Run for 8 minutes at an easy pace. Run at a brisk pace for 60 seconds and then jog at a recovery pace for 2 minutes. Repeat this 5 times. Finish by running for 8 minutes at a slow pace.

Friday: Rest.

Saturday: Run for 20 minutes at an easy pace.

Sunday: Run for 30 minutes at an easy pace.

WEEK 3

Monday: Rest.

Tuesday: Run for 25 to 30 minutes at an easy pace.

Wednesday: Rest.

Thursday: Run for 8 minutes at an easy pace. Increase the pace for a full 15 minutes and then jog at an easy pace for 10 minutes.

Friday: Rest.

Saturday: Run for 25 minutes at an easy pace.

Sunday: Run for 35 minutes at an easy pace.

WEEK 4

Monday: Rest.

Tuesday: Run for 8 minutes at an easy pace. Run 1 kilometre as fast as you can. Stretch and rest and then repeat. Run slowly for 7 minutes to recover and cool down.

Wednesday: Rest.

Thursday: Run for 10 minutes at an easy pace, 20 minutes at a moderate pace and then 10 minutes at an easy pace.

Friday: Rest.

Saturday: Run for 30 minutes at an easy pace.

Sunday: Run for 40 minutes at an easy pace.

WEEK 5

Monday: Rest.

Tuesday: Run for 25 to 30 minutes at an easy pace.

Wednesday: Rest.

Thursday: Run for 8 minutes at an easy pace. Run at a brisk pace for 2 minutes and then jog at a recovery pace for 2 minutes. Repeat this 3 times. Finish by running for 8 minutes at a slow pace.

Friday: Rest.

Saturday: Run for 35 minutes at an easy pace.

Sunday: Run for 40 minutes at an easy pace.

WEEK 6

Monday: Rest.

Tuesday: Run for 30 minutes at an easy pace.

Wednesday: Rest.

Thursday: Run for 20 to 25 minutes at an easy pace.

Friday: Rest.

Saturday: Rest.

Sunday: 5K race.

Running Q&A

Every runner has a few questions. Here are the answers.

Q: **How do I get started?**

A: Start walking for a time that feels comfortable—from 10 to 30 minutes. Walk to work, home or the store; it all counts. When you're able to walk for 30 minutes, sprinkle 1- to 2-minute running intervals into your walking. With time, make the intervals longer until you're running for 30 minutes straight.

Q: **Is it normal to feel pain when running?**

A: A little discomfort is normal, in a listening-to-Justin-Bieber kind of way, but running shouldn't be painful like a Slayer concert. If it hurts enough that you limp or alter your stride, you're probably injured. Stop running immediately and take a few days off.

Q: **What's the difference between running on a treadmill and running outside?**

A: A treadmill pulls the ground underneath your feet. You cover distance if you simply lift your feet and you don't meet any wind resistance. Running on a treadmill is easier, but you will burn fewer calories. However, most treadmills are padded, which is handy if you're a little heavy or injury prone and need to decrease the impact of your frame landing on the ground.

Q: **I always feel out of breath when I run. Is something wrong?**

A: Huffing and puffing a little harder is normal and will decrease as you get fitter. Concentrate on breathing from deep down in your belly. If you have to, slow down or take walking breaks. If it persists, ask your doc about the possibility that you have asthma.

Q: **I often suffer from a stitch when I run. Will this ever go away?**

A: Side stitches are common among beginners because the abdomen is not used to the jostling that running causes. These stitches will go away as you get fitter, but don't eat any solid foods during the hour before you set off. When you get a stitch, breathe deeply and concentrating on pushing all of the air out of your abdomen. This will stretch out your diaphragm muscle (just below your lungs), which is usually where a cramp hurts.

Put the Fun in Run

Many start running but only a few finish. Use these motivational tricks to keep you going.

- Have a regular slot in your day for running. If you try to squeeze running into an overloaded diary it just becomes another stress.

- Find a nice place to run. Two runs a week might have to be around the block, but a weekend run somewhere leafy will lure you back.

- Join a running club. Go to a running-shoe store or look online. Don't worry about being slow—someone else will always be slower.

- Set short-term goals. Aim first just to complete a distance, such as 5 or 10 kilometres, regardless of the speed. Improve your time once you reach the distance.

- Add variety to your training to avoid becoming a one-pace runner. Varying the surface on which you run or your speed and distance can help you work out countless training sessions.

- Compete against others or the clock. Competition is what makes the sport interesting. Get involved with a local club and look around for interesting races.

Avoiding Injury

Running can place a bounty of stress on your joints and muscles. Here's how to make sure it does more good than harm.

Warm Up, Cool Down

Your muscles are 10 per cent shorter when you're inactive than they are when you're warmed up. According to the laws of physics, muscles work better when they are longer. They can exert more force with less effort, meaning that longer muscles are much less prone to injury. Warm up by walking or slowly jogging for five minutes. Cooling down after your run helps gently push healing blood into your muscles and speeds up the recovery process. The extra time you spend warming up and cooling down leads to improved efficiency and decreased likelihood of getting injured.

Stretch Out

Without flexibility, you're an injury waiting to happen because tight muscles cannot go through a full range of motion. Inflexibility is the biggest cause of Achilles tendinitis and shin splints. Stretch for five minutes after a run when your muscles are warm and elongated.

Back Off

Training every day will wear your body down rather than build it up. You need to recover after a tough training session to help your muscles mend. Never do long runs two days in a row, and give yourself a day of easy running or rest between hard efforts.

Chill Out

The surest way to get injured is to train hard on a day when you're fatigued or feeling sore. Stress or lack of sleep can also take a toll. If you feel sluggish or have twinges, take a week off. Let your training schedule be your guide, not your jailer.

Branch Out

The wise runner explores cross-training options in order to be a stronger runner. Activities other than running rest your feet and legs and strengthen the muscles that running doesn't exercise. Cross-training will protect you from injury and improve your overall state of fitness. Swimming, cycling and rowing all complement a good canter.

Write It Down

A training log may seem obsessive–compulsive and boring, but charting your distance, pace, course and how you feel can give you an important perspective that makes it easy to spot and correct training errors.

Be Fit for Soccer

These soccer drills will help you beat defenders to bang in more goals.

The precision it takes footballers to consistently pilot a speeding object to within the exact centimetre of where they want it is a fine art that is unmatched in any sport. Control of pace demands balance and nimbleness. These footy drills will deliver you more grace and poise on any sport pitch. The first section focuses more on balance so that you can control the position of the ball with either foot, plus be sturdier on a surfboard and hit straighter drives with your golf swing. The second section includes a series of running drills that will improve the speed and agility of your footwork so that you can hot-step out of and around football, hockey and rugby tackles. Superior balance and nimbleness are qualities that transfer to every great sportsman. Read on to find how to improve yours.

Become More Balanced and Nimble

Do the workout a few times a week between your usual practise sessions to improve your game.

One-Footers

This exercise is good for off-balance and one-legged kicks.

Muscles

Calves; tendons and ligaments in ankle joints

Execution

1. Stand with your feet shoulder-width apart and arms horizontally out to your sides. Your hands should be in line with your shoulders.
2. Lift your left foot, bringing your left heel up towards the back of your left knee (figure 12.1). Close your eyes and hold the position for 30 seconds, then switch legs and repeat. Keep alternating legs for a period of 5 minutes.

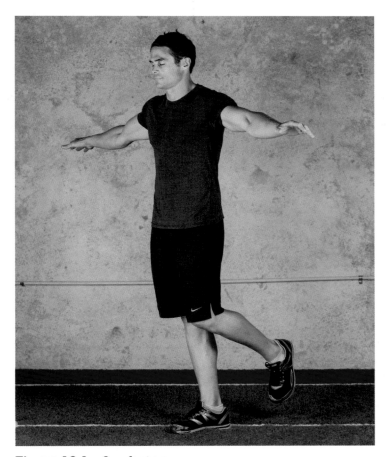

Figure 12.1 One-footers.

In and Out

This drill will improve your side step and your ability to weave through tackles.

Muscles

Quads, glutes, hamstrings, calves, core

Execution

1. Place 15 markers 30 centimetres apart in a straight line.
2. Stand to the left of the first marker. Step forward with your right foot so that it lands between the first two markers (figure 12.2a) and then spring out to the left with your left foot. Repeat the process until you reach the end of the markers. Slowly jog back to the starting position.
3. Repeat step 2 but step between the markers with your left foot and spring out with your right foot (figure 12.2b). Jog back to the starting position.
4. Stand in front of the markers. Step forward with your left foot and then step forward with your right foot so that your feet land between each marker (figure 12.2c). Jog back to the starting position. This completes one set. Perform five sets.

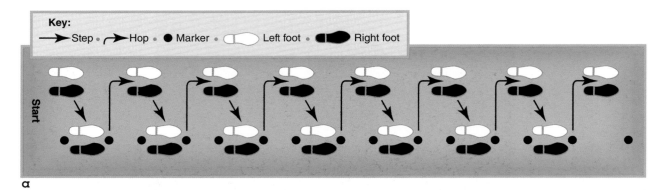

a

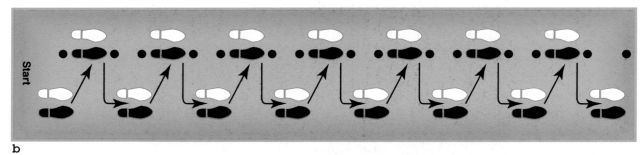

b

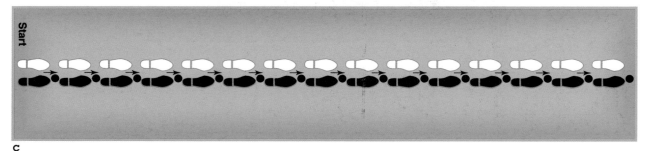

c

Figure 12.2 In and out. (a) Step your right foot between the markers and spring to the left. (b) Step your left foot between the markers and spring to the right. (c) Step both feet between the markers.

Single-Leg Raise

This move will improve your stationary jump for both kicking and heading balls.

Muscles

Calves, core

Execution

1. Stand on your right leg and lift your left leg towards your left knee. Rest your arms at your sides.
2. Rise onto your toes and rest your body weight on the ball of your right foot (figure 12.3). Hold that position for three seconds and then take two seconds to lower your heel back to the starting position. To increase the difficulty of the exercise, hold a dumbbell in your right hand. Perform four sets of five repetitions on each leg. Do not rest between sets.

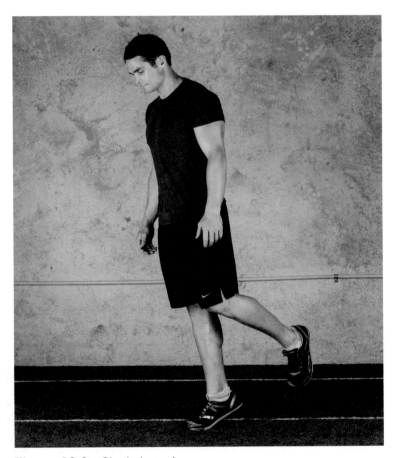

Figure 12.3 Single-leg raise.

Hurdle

This drill increases overall speed and will help you jump over and tackle.

Muscles

Quads, glutes, hamstrings, calves, core

Execution

1. Place five 30-centimetre hurdles or other obstacles 20 centimetres apart in a straight line. Place a marker in a straight line 14 metres away from the fifth marker (figure 12.4).

2. Spring over the five hurdles and then sprint at full pace to the marker. Slowly jog back to recover. This is one set. Perform five sets.

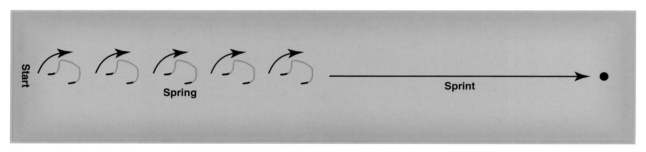

Figure 12.4   Hurdle.

Wall Kick

This drill will improve the accuracy and strength of your kicking in both legs.

Muscles

Glutes, hamstrings, quadriceps

Execution

1. Stand three metres away from a wall and face the wall.
2. Kick a football against the wall with your right foot (figure 12.5a) so that the ball rebounds towards your left foot (figure 12.5b). You shouldn't have to move to the left or right to retrieve the ball. Then kick the ball with your left foot so that it rebounds towards your right foot. This is one repetition.
3. Take a step back and repeat step 2. Keep taking a step back after each repetition until you miss the foot you are aiming for. When that happens, go back to the starting point. Repeat for five minutes or until you get so good you run out of space.

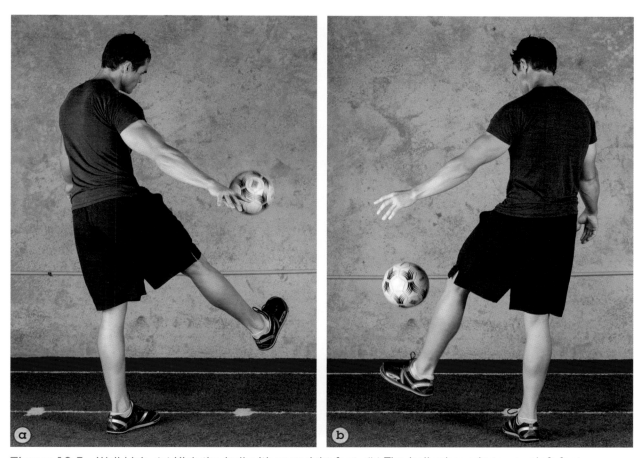

Figure 12.5 Wall kick. (a) Kick the ball with your right foot. (b) The ball rebounds to your left foot.

Diamonds

This drill will improve your ability to pounce on a counterattack opportunity or defend against one.

Muscles

Quads, glutes, hamstrings, calves, core

Execution

1. Place seven markers five metres apart in the formation of two diamonds (figure 12.6). The top of the first diamond should form the base of the second diamond.
2. Run forward from cone (c) 1 to C2 and then backward from C2 to C3. Turn around at C3 and run forward to C1. From C1 run backward to C4 and then forward to C2.
3. Repeat the same pattern in the second diamond by running forward to C7. This is one set. Perform three sets.

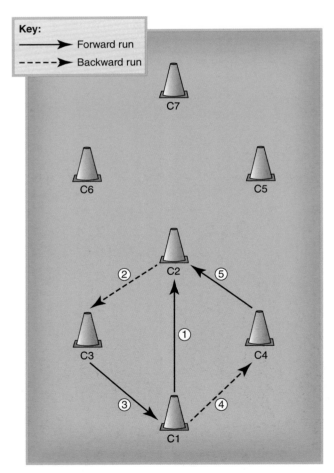

Figure 12.6 Diamonds.

Get Fighting Fit

Pack more power in your punches and arm up for any conflict.

If you look like you can take care of yourself chances are the day will come when you'll need to. Girls, football, a dirty glance—all the subtleties of a night out or a journey home can make the hairs on the back of your neck stand up. Whether it's your fault or his, blokes don't bawl over spilt beer—they brawl over it.

Big muscles are great for a pulling a biceps when you point to the gym, but bulky muscles have never won a fight. Speed is the winner in a tussle. A great fighter has a unique combination of strength, endurance, speed and flexibility. This workout develops the muscles you need for punching, kicking and throwing your rival to the ground. Sound like the kind of strength that you might find useful? Do this arse-kicking routine two or three times a week and mix it between your sparring, grappling, bag and speed work. Leave at least one day of rest between sessions to give yourself enough time to recover. It'll give you more muscle and explosive power and make you better than the United Nations in conflict resolution.

Duck Walk

This wrestling exercise builds power in the lower body. It conditions you to stand up if someone is on your back and to throw your opponent to the ground.

Muscles

Glutes, calves, thighs

Execution

1. Stand with your feet shoulder-width apart. Hold a single dumbbell or kettlebell under your chin.
2. Take a step forward and let the other knee drop to the ground (figure 12.7a). Stay in the crouched position and slide your other leg forward (figure 12.7b). Drop your knee and repeat. Once you get in motion stay in motion. Execute the move quickly and forcefully. Perform 3 sets of 10 steps on each leg and rest for 90 seconds between each set.

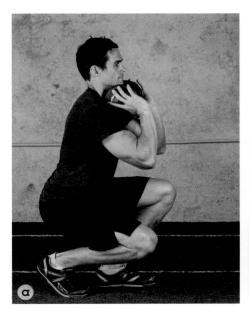 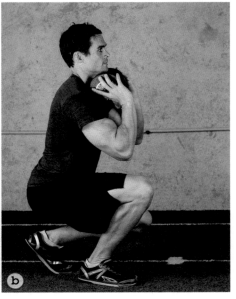

Figure 12.7 Duck walk. *(a)* Put your right knee down. *(b)* Slide your left leg forward.

Wrestles

This exercise strengthens the muscles you'll use when you grab your opponent by the scruff of the neck and throw him to the ground.

Muscles

Glutes, hamstrings, core, shoulders

Execution

1. Place a single weight plate on the end of an Olympic bar and wedge the weightless end of the bar into the ground or a corner of the gym. Stand with your feet shoulder-width apart on either side of the bar. Grip the end of the weighted portion of the bar with both hands. Hold it at arm's length in front of your chest.

2. Hold the bar in both hands. Lower it in an arc towards your left leg (figure 12.8a) while pivoting your feet and knees to your left. The weight plate should end up behind your left leg.

3. When the weight is 2.5 centimetres from the floor, pull the bar with your chest and arm in the form of a dumbbell fly and return to the starting position. Straighten your knees and pivot your toes back to the start. Repeat to your right side (figure 12.8b). The entire movement should make a semicircle. Perform three sets of five to seven repetitions on each side.

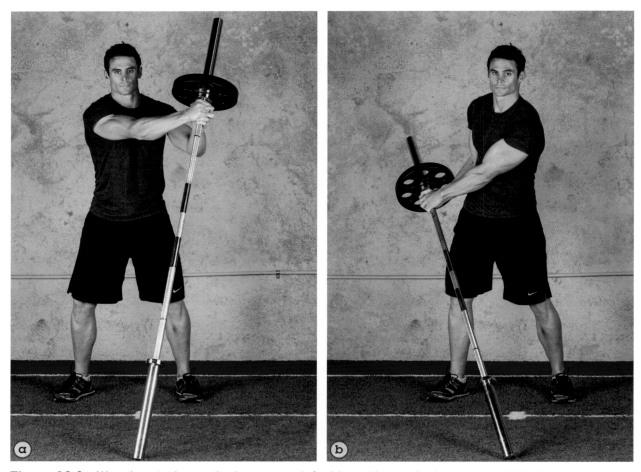

Figure 12.8 Wrestles. *(a)* Lower the bar to your left side. *(b)* Lower the bar to your right side.

Bounding

This exercise teaches you to generate power by pushing forward with your legs while you throw the punch, making your punches more deadly.

Muscles

Legs, upper body

Execution

1. Run for 5 minutes to warm up your muscles. Mark a distance of about 100 metres.
2. Run normally but drive up the knee that's being lifted until that thigh is parallel to the ground (figure 12.9). Jump in the air with each step. It should look like a bouncy run with longer-than-normal strides.
3. Run for 90 seconds after each 100 metres of bounding. Repeat 12 times.

Treadmill option: If you're on a treadmill, set it for intervals of 30 seconds of bounding and 2 minutes of normal running at a lower speed. Repeat 5 times and rest for 45 seconds between sets.

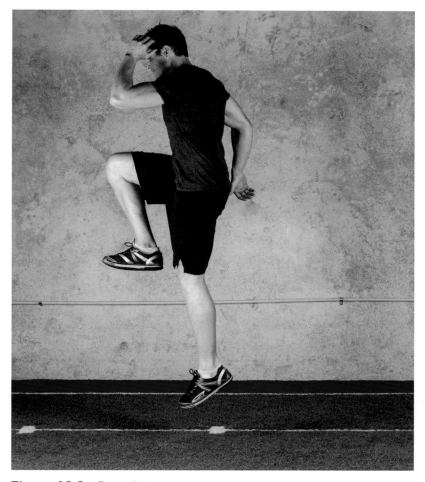

Figure 12.9 Bounding.

Medicine Ball Push-Up Shuffle

This exercise develops upper-body punching power and coordination simultaneously.

Muscles

Chest, triceps, abs

Execution

1. Lie facedown on the ground with a medicine ball beneath you. Support your body on the balls of your feet. Place your right hand on the medicine ball and your left hand on the ground. Keep your arms extended but not locked.

2. Keeping your back straight, bend your elbows and lower your body until your chest touches the ball (figure 12.10a). Explosively push up and off laterally with both hands so that your body passes over the ball and your left hand lands on the ball (figure 12.10b). Keep your feet hip-width apart and your core tight throughout the movement. Perform 3 sets of 5 repetitions on each arm. Rest for 60 seconds between sets.

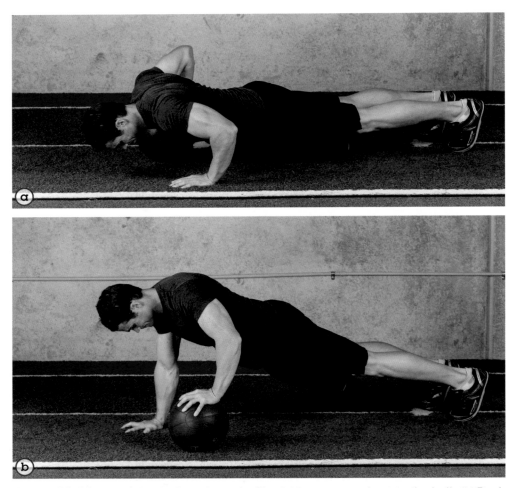

Figure 12.10 Medicine ball push-up shuffle. (a) Lower your chest to the ball. (b) Push up explosively and switch hands.

Pop-Up

You'll suffer the most damage if you get smacked while you're on the floor. This damage-control exercise will help you pop back to your feet.

Muscles

Legs, core, arms, chest

Execution

1. Lie face down on the floor with your hands on either side of your chest and your forearms perpendicular to the floor. Keep your toes on the ground and your feet perpendicular to the floor.

2. Bend your arms slightly (figure 12.11a) and push up with your hands and the balls of your feet. This will get you airborne. Bring your knees forward and hoist your upper body forward and upward. You should land on your feet in a crouching position (figure 12.11b). Perform this move 4 times and then sprint 10 metres; that's 1 set. Rest for 45 seconds between sets and complete 3 sets.

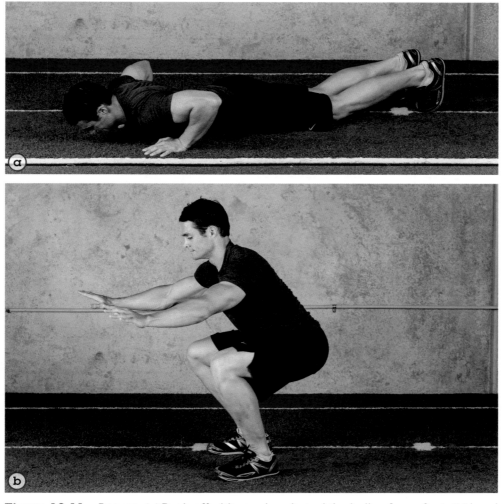

Figure 12.11 Pop-up. *(a)* Push off with your hands and the balls of your feet. *(b)* Land on your feet in a crouching position.

Medicine Ball Throw

This move both improves your reflexes and teaches you how to generate power from your upper body and release that power into an object.

Muscles

Chest, shoulders, triceps, abs

Execution

1. Stand about two metres away from a wall and face the wall. Stagger your feet and place them shoulder-width apart, bending your knees slightly. Hold a medicine ball to your chest with both hands and bend your elbows (figure 12.12a).

2. Straighten your elbows and throw the ball against the wall (figure 12.12b). Catch the ball as it rebounds; make sure to tense your abs a second before you catch the ball. Perform 3 sets of 12 repetitions and rest 30 seconds between sets. Do this move with one arm to make it more challenging.

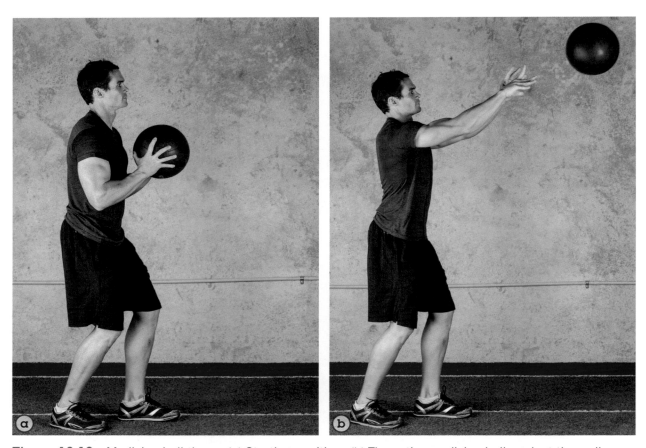

Figure 12.12 Medicine ball throw. *(a)* Starting position. *(b)* Throw the medicine ball against the wall.

Lateral Skaters

This drill develops quick foot action, which will help you dodge a punch and step into a position to land a punch.

Muscles

Inner thighs, ankles

Execution

1. Stand with both feet together. Push off laterally with one leg (figure 12.13a).
2. Upon landing, immediately push off in the opposite direction (figure 12.13b). Continue the drill for a specified amount of time. To develop quickness, perform as many reps as you can in 20 seconds. Jog slowly for 1 minute, then repeat and attempt to better the previous number of reps. Repeat 5 times.

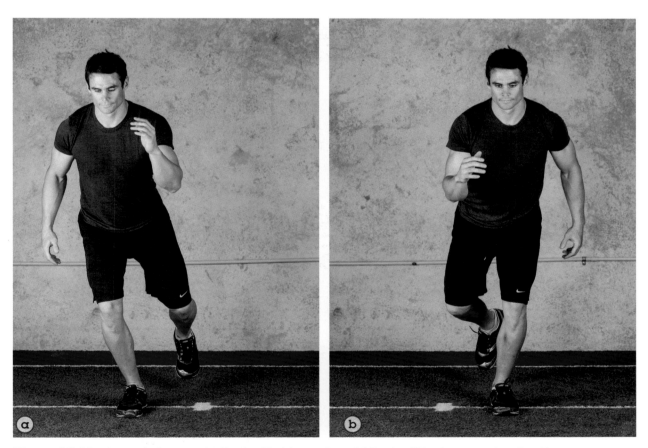

Figure 12.13 Lateral skaters. *(a)* Push off with one leg. *(b)* Push off in the opposite direction.

Super-Fly Push-Up

This exercise develops explosive power in the chest and arms that transfers into a quicker punch.

Muscles

Chest, triceps, abs

Execution

1. Get into the push-up position and place your hands slightly wider than your shoulders. Slightly bend your knees.
2. Keeping your back flat, lower your body until your upper arms are lower than your elbows (figure 12.14a). Quickly straighten your arms and knees and lift both your upper and lower body off the ground (figure 12.14b). If possible clap your hands together midair. Land on your hands and then let your feet touch the ground.
3. Perform 2 sets of 6 repetitions. Rest for 60 seconds between each set.

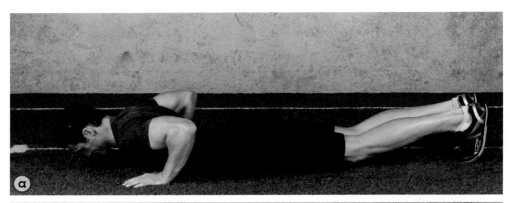

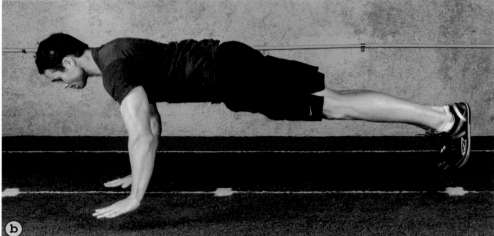

Figure 12.14 Super-fly push-up. *(a)* Lower your body towards the ground. *(b)* Push your hands and feet off the floor.

Get Ready for the Slopes

Soften the snow-season slip-ups and get flexible and balanced to be ski fit this winter.

Are aches and bruises your usual snow-season souvenirs? Skiing and snowboarding require core strength, balance, endurance and coordination so you don't end up arse down on the ice. This workout will ensure you get your money's worth of the cold stuff.

The most important thing for the average week-a-year boarder to do is stretch and get as flexible as possible. Regardless of your fitness, if you haven't trained specifically for skiing and snowboarding you'll work muscles you didn't know you had and be in agony for it after your first full day on the slopes. Most guys lose days of riding because they're stiff and in pain from their first day. The programme will help you hurdle the hurt and be both strong and supple in order to take advantage of every second you have on the slopes.

Get Balance and Strength

Do these weight-training exercises (see chapter 3 for descriptions) two or three times a week to improve your balance and put more spray into your turns.

- Squat (dumbbell): This exercise builds the strength and stamina you'll need in your upper legs to stay in a crouching position on the slopes. Do 3 sets of 20 repetitions and rest for 60 seconds between sets.

- Overhand-grip pull-up: This exercise builds strength in your upper body that will help you absorb the impact when you fall and offers some protection from common injuries such as broken wrists and collarbones. Do 3 sets of 8 repetitions and rest for 90 seconds between sets.

- Parallel bar dip: This exercise helps build strength in your upper body that transfers into improved balance on the slopes. Do 3 sets of 18 repetitions and rest for 60 seconds between sets.

- Push-up: This exercise promotes upper-body muscle balance, which will improve your balance on skis. Perform 3 sets of 15 repetitions and rest for 45 seconds between sets.

- Standing calf raise: This exercise is excellent for creating ankle strength and preventing an ankle injury. Do 4 sets of 15 repetitions and rest for 30 seconds between sets.

- Side plank: This exercise gives you a strong and flexible back that will help you in turns and twists. Do 3 sets of 30 seconds on each side and rest for 40 seconds between sets.

- Lying leg raise: This exercise improves your balance and builds the strength you'll need to consistently pull yourself up off the ice. Do 3 sets of 20 reps and rest for 60 seconds between sets.

Stretches

Do these stretches every second day starting a month before your flight and then every day during the two-week period before you go. Hold each stretch for 15 seconds if you are already flexible or 30 seconds if you are inflexible.

Quads

Sit on the floor and place your right foot in front, leg straight. Place your left foot behind with your knee pointing to the side. Grasp your left ankle with your left hand. Hold your left foot and pull it towards your glutes while pushing your hips forward (figure 12.15). Repeat with your other leg.

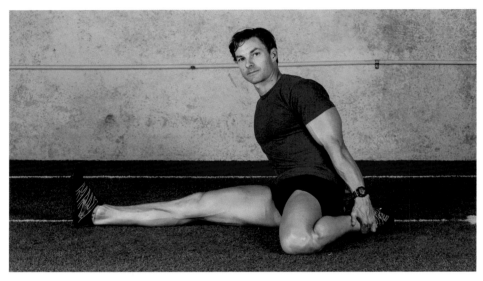

Figure 12.15 Quad stretch.

Hamstrings

Lie on your back and place your left foot on the floor. Straighten your right leg, keeping your knee slightly bent and your toes pulled towards your shin. Keeping your back and glutes on the floor, raise your right leg (figure 12.16) and hold it with both hands or a towel. Pull your leg towards your head. Repeat with the other leg.

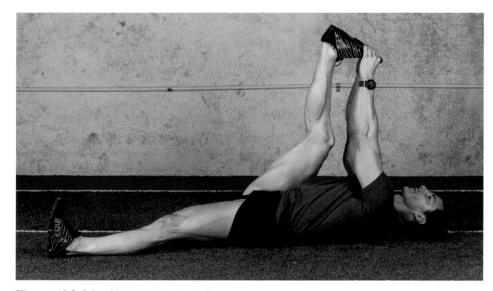

Figure 12.16 Hamstring stretch.

Groin

Sit on the floor with your knees bent. Place the bottoms of your feet together and bring them as close to your body as possible. Hold an ankle with each hand and rest your elbows on your thighs. Bend at the hips, move your upper body forward and push down on your thighs with your elbows (figure 12.17).

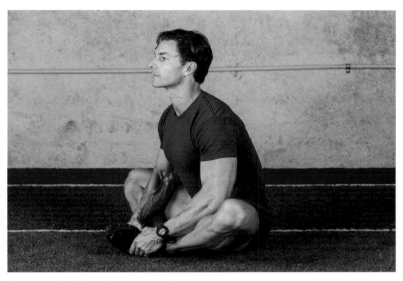

Figure 12.17 Groin stretch.

Glutes and Spine

Sit on the floor. Place your right leg straight out in front of you and cross your left leg over your right leg. Place your left foot flat on the floor on the outside of your right knee and rest your right arm on the outside of your left knee. Turn to the left and place your left hand behind you on the mat (figure 12.18).

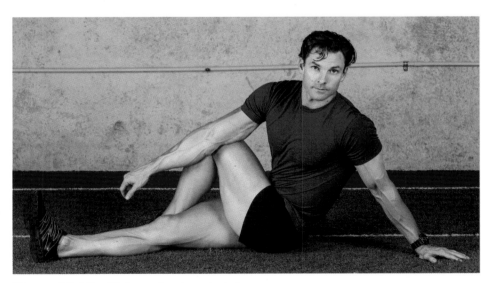

Figure 12.18 Glute and spine stretch.

Back

Stand with your legs together and knees slightly bent. Hold onto a pole or other stationary object at waist level with both hands. Bend forward at your hips until your upper body is parallel to the floor (figure 12.19). Pull your body slightly back and lean slightly to the left for 15 seconds, then repeat to the right.

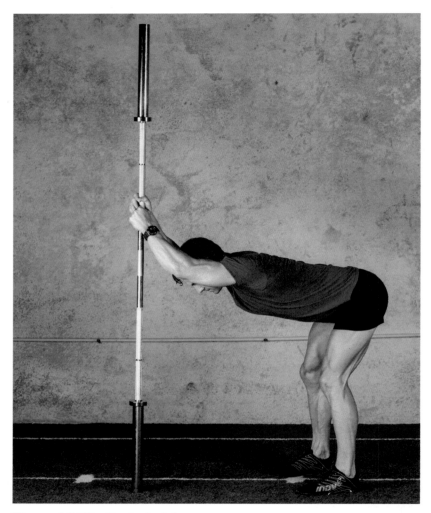

Figure 12.19   Back stretch.

Neck

Slowly roll your neck through 360 degrees at least 10 times. Place your right hand on the right side of your face and push against it for 10 seconds (figure 12.20) and then repeat on the left side.

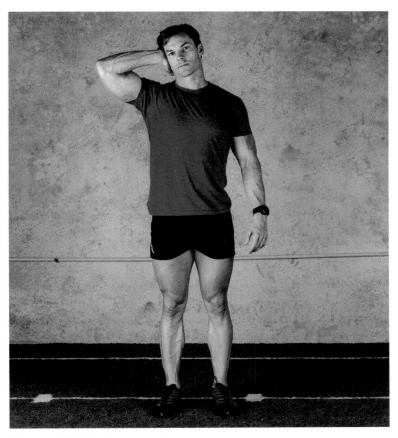

Figure 12.20   Neck stretch.

Get Fit for Rugby

Rugby is a blood, sweat and torn-ears sport that demands strength, power, speed and fitness. Here's how to get your body ready for it.

'Rugby is a good occasion for keeping 30 bullies far from the centre of the city,' Oscar Wilde once said. Perhaps that's because the goal of the game is to feign an interest in getting an oval ball across a white line while divvying your time between bashing, tackling and hurting a selection of 15 opponents. It's widely regarded as one of the most dangerous sports in the world, especially if you look at the injury rates

calculated by the labcoats. One study (Requa, DeAvilla and Garrick, 1993) rates rugby union as more dangerous than rugby league, Australian rules, soccer and ice hockey and found that, on average, in every English Premiership game at least two players from each side were lost for 18 days due to an injury. Those are some pretty tough odds to overcome, especially when even amateur scrumcap wearers play up to 35 games in a season. On top of that, rugby players are arguably the most highly conditioned athletes on the planet. They have to have foresight, incredible strength, feline agility and frighteningly fast reactions.

Do these drills one to three times a week in addition to your practise sessions to build a body that will excel in any pitch. In football, hockey, cricket and just about every sport you can think of, more speed is guaranteed to leave the opposition choking on your dust.

Outdoor Rugby Training

Do these whenever you can get outside. For the medicine ball power drills, all you need is a medicine ball and a few markers.

Medicine Ball Power Drill: Lateral Throw-Down

Stand with your feet about shoulder-width apart. Bend your knees slightly and hold one arm out to your side at shoulder height. Turn your palm up and hold a medicine ball in your hand. In one explosive movement, slide your hand over the top of the ball (figure 12.21) and slam the ball and your arm towards the ground. Aim to make the ball connect with the ground as hard as possible. The ball should land laterally in line with your feet. Perform three sets of five reps and rest for two to three minutes between sets.

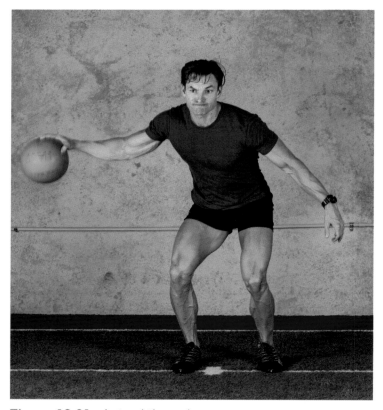

Figure 12.21 Lateral throw-down.

Medicine Ball Power Drill: Overhead Slam-Down

Stand with your feet shoulder-width apart and flat on the floor. Hold a medicine ball behind your head and cock your elbows 90 degrees backward (figure 12.22). Get onto the tips of your toes, flexing your calves in the process, and raise your body as high as possible. Bring the ball above the crown of your head and focus your eyes on where you want the ball to land. Using your shoulder strength, slam the ball into the ground as hard as you can. It should land at arm's length in front of you. Finish with your arms at your sides. Perform three sets of five reps and rest for two to three minutes between sets.

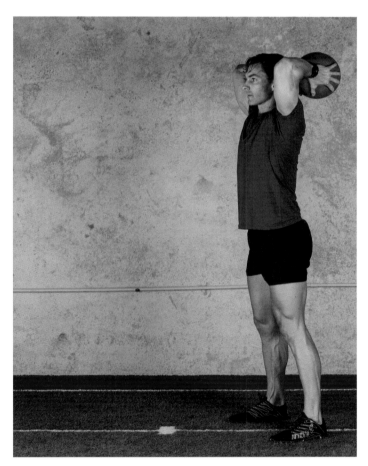

Figure 12.22   Overhead slam-down.

Medicine Ball Power Drill: Overhead Dumbbell Raise

Kneel on the ground and hold a single dumbbell between your legs with both hands. Keep your back straight and rest your feet flat on the ground. Keeping an arc in your elbows, bring the weight directly above your head in a swinging motion (figure 12.23). Pause for a second and then slowly lower the weight to the starting position. The lowering process provides resistance, so more muscles are recruited the longer you take. Perform three sets of five reps and rest for two to three minutes between sets.

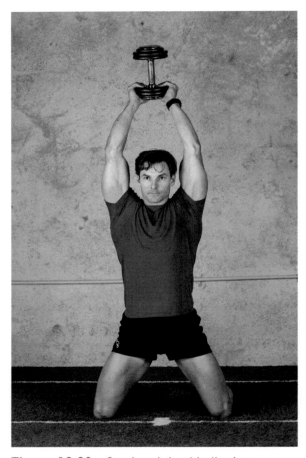

Figure 12.23 Overhead dumbbell raise.

Speed and Agility: Squares

Mark out a 10-metre square (figure 12.24). Start at the top left corner (cone 1). Sprint diagonally to the bottom right corner (cone 2) and perform a burpee. (For the burpee, begin in a squat position and place your hands on the ground in front of you. Kick your feet behind you so that you're in a push-up position. Quickly return your feet to the squat position, then leap up as high as possible from the squat position.) After performing the burpee, run backward to the top right corner of the square (cone 3) and pass a medicine ball or heavy sandbag to a partner. Then sprint forward to the bottom left corner (cone 4), complete another burpee and sprint directly to the top left corner (cone 1). To recover, jog for 30 seconds to a cone set up 15 metres away. Repeat for 6 sets.

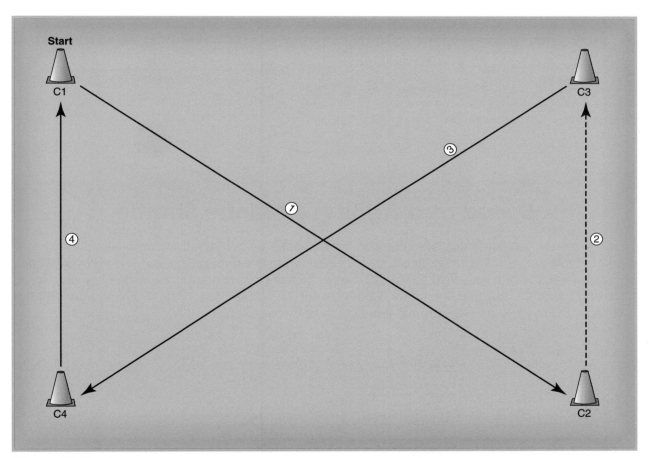

Figure 12.24   Squares.

Speed and Agility: 20-Metre Shuttle

This drill is best done on an open field. Place three sticks, cones, strips of tape or any other markers five metres apart in a row (figure 12.25). Stand with one foot on each side of the middle line. Squat and touch the line with your right hand. (This is the starting position.) Sprint to your right and touch that line with your right hand. Then sprint across to the far line and touch it with your left hand. Finally, sprint across the starting line. When you start over again in the middle, reverse the motion and sprint first to your left. Do the shuttle three times in each direction.

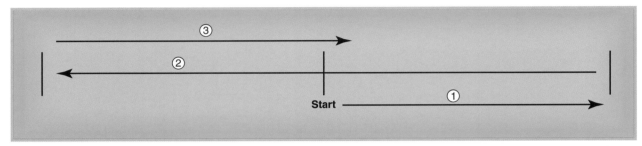

Figure 12.25 20-metre shuttle.

Speed and Agility: 60-Metre Shuttle

This drill builds your sprinting stamina and is best done on a football or rugby pitch. Place four markers 5 metres apart in a row (figure 12.26). Sprint 5 metres, touch the first line and sprint back and touch the starting line. Next, sprint 10 metres to the second marker, touch the line and sprint back and touch the starting line again. Finally, sprint 15 metres, touch the line, and sprint all the way back. Do the shuttle three to five times once or twice a week.

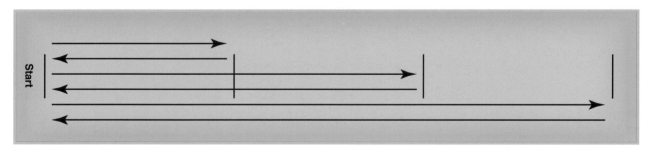

Figure 12.26 60-metre shuttle.

Gym Drills

Do these gym drills at least once a week to pack explosive power into your pace.

Box Blasts

Stand with your right foot on a plyometric box, step or bench and your left foot on the floor behind it. Place your arms at your sides. Push your right foot off the box with enough force so that both feet are in the air. As you jump, swing your arms overhead (figure 12.27). Land with your feet in the same position. Do a set of 10 repetitions and then repeat the move with your left foot on the box and your right foot on the floor. Do 2 sets of 10 reps with each leg.

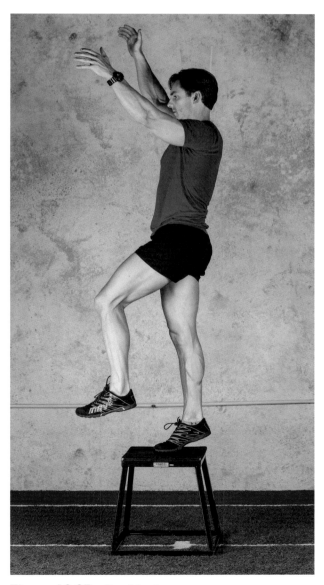

Figure 12.27 Box blasts.

Vertical Jump and Standing Long Jump

Chalk or wet your hands and reach up to touch the wall, making a mark. Jump as high as you can next to the wall (figure 12.28). If you want to measure the difference to get your vertical jump, touch the wall at the top of your jump. For a standing long jump, mark where your jump starts and lands and measure the difference. Write these measurements down and keep track of your progress.

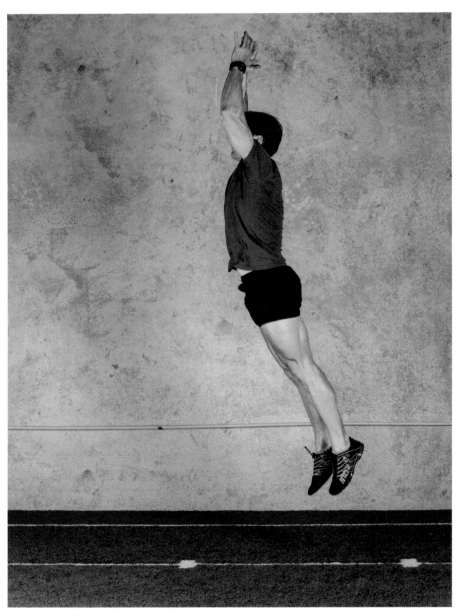

Figure 12.28 Vertical jump.

Box Jump

Stand in front of a box, exercise step or bench. Squat and lower your body about 8 centimetres. Jump up and land on the box (figure 12.29) in a squatting position with your knees bent and arms straight out in front of you for balance. Step back down to the starting position. Do 2 sets of 10 repetitions.

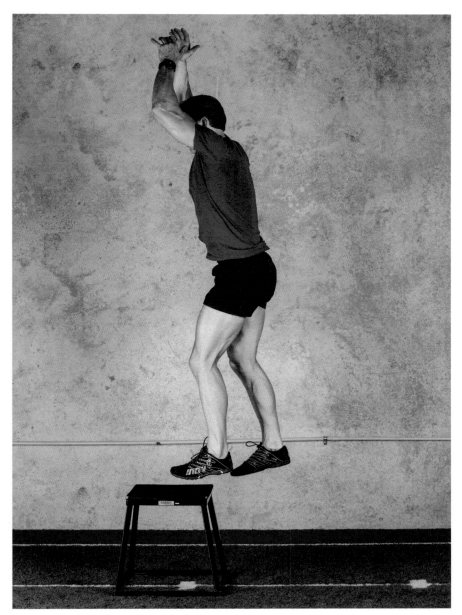

Figure 12.29 Box jump.

Long Jump

After doing box jumps do three to five rebound long jumps. Jump forward, land (figure 12.30a) and immediately spring up and out into your next long jump (figure 12.30b). Progress to doing both the box jumps and rebound jumps on one foot or with the added resistance of a weighted vest. Do two or three long jumps a few times a week.

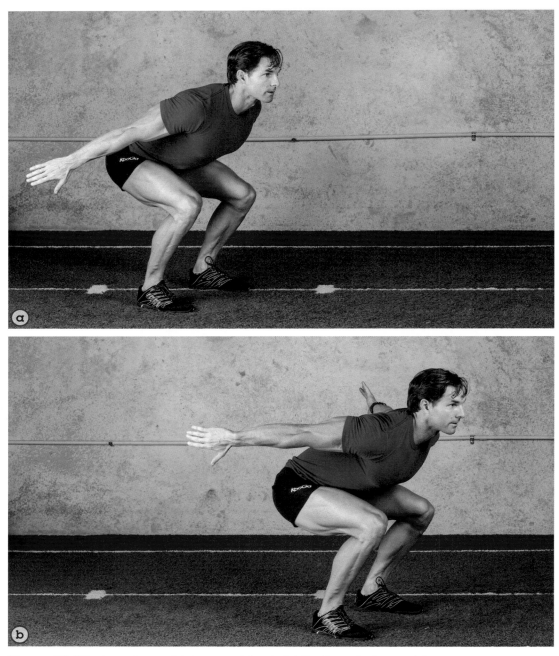

Figure 12.30 Long jump. *(a)* Jump and land. *(b)* Continue to the next jump.

Tum Tuck

Lie on your back with your knees bent and feet on the floor. Place your hands just below your navel. Inhale and let your stomach rise, then exhale as you take 4 seconds to pull your abs towards your spine (figure 12.31). Hold that position for 2 seconds. Repeat the move for a total of 10 to 12 repetitions. As your core strength improves, inch your feet farther out until you can perform this move with your legs straight and your back pressed against the floor.

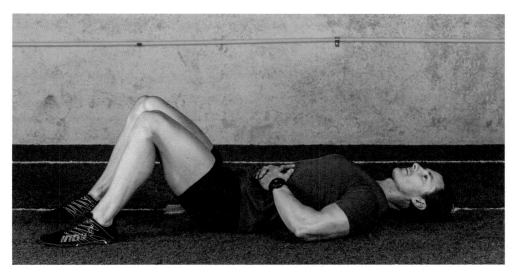

Figure 12.31   Tum tuck.

Standing Hammer Curl

Stand with your feet slightly less than shoulder-width apart. Hold a pair of dumbbells at your sides in a neutral grip with your palms facing each other. Keeping your abs drawn in, back straight, and elbows at your sides, begin to raise your forearms. Don't allow your shoulders or elbows to move forward, and watch that your elbows don't move out to your sides. When the dumbbells are just in front of your shoulders (figure 12.32), take 2 to 3 seconds to lower the weights until your arms are straight. Come to a full stop at the bottom of the movement and then go into your next curl. Do 3 sets of 10 repetitions and rest for 90 to 120 seconds between sets.

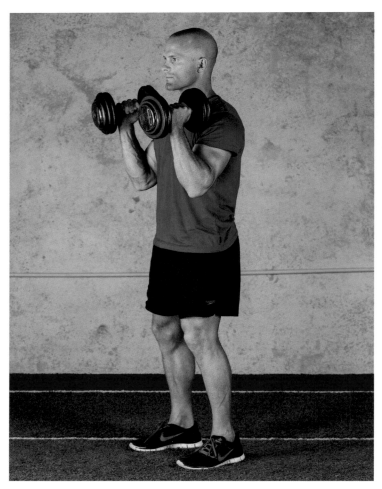

Figure 12.32   Standing hammer curl.

Get Rock-Solid Muscles for Climbing

Before you decide to become a rock star you should build a base level of strength that'll put you in good stead when you're dangling in the air. Here's the how-to.

A metre away is a 2-centimetre foot hole that you have to stretch your foot into. Win or lose pales in comparison; this is life or death. Agility, precision and careful coordination of your body weight is crucial to surviving the challenges climbing hands out. Improving this eye–hand coordination will benefit your climbing skills as well as sweeten the direction of your swing on the tee-off, add accuracy to your punches and blocks in martial arts and help you fling off opponents in contact sports or hang tight to any wind sail or sailing boat. The aim of this workout is to turn you into a master of your own body weight. That way you'll get your money's worth when you shell out to practise on the climbing wall. Do this workout twice a week in addition to your normal routine and your muscles will thank you for hitting the mark with your leap of faith.

Your Mini-Workout

Warm up by skipping for three to five minutes. Stand opposite a full-length mirror on a springy gym floor. Rest a jump rope at the back of your knees; look forward rather than down at your feet. Bounce lightly with no rope for a minute. Once you fall into a rhythm, bring the rope over your head and under your feet with each revolution.

Stretch next. Hold each stretch for 15 seconds.

- Fingers: Gently bend each finger back towards the top of your wrist and hold.
- Forearms: Bend your whole hand back towards the top of your wrist.
- Shoulders: Straighten one arm and move it across your upper chest. Hold the elbow of that arm with your opposite hand and pull your arm further across your body.
- Neck: Move your head gently from side to side and back and forth.
- Lats: Put one arm over your head. Bend your elbow and keep your forearm close to your upper arm. Pull your elbow towards your head and back. Repeat with your opposite arm.

Master Your Own Body Weight

If you own it you should be able to lift and shift it. Here's how.

Uneven Pull-Up

Loop a towel over a pull-up bar and hold both ends with your left hand. Grasp the bar with your right hand using an underhand grip. The vertical separation between your hands places greater stress on the arm of the upper hand. Pull up with both hands (figure 12.33).

Beginner: 3 or 4 sets of 5 repetitions holding both ends of the towel in one hand. Use the assistance pad if necessary.

Intermediate: 4 sets of 12 to 15 repetitions holding an end of the towel in each hand.

Advanced: 2 sets of 4 repetitions, 3 sets of 6 repetitions and then 2 sets of 8 repetitions. Use a weight belt to increase the resistance and decrease the weight accordingly for the sets with higher reps.

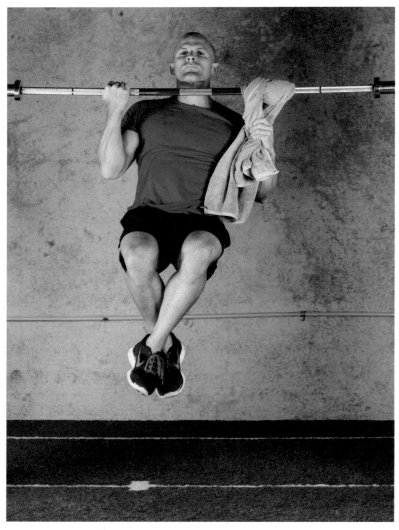

Figure 12.33 Uneven pull-up.

Hanging Knee Raise

Grab a pull-up bar and place your hands shoulder-width apart. Cross your ankles and, using just your abs, bring your knees up to your chest (figure 12.34). Don't start swinging; you want your abs to do the work, not momentum. Rock your pelvis slightly forward. Pause at the top of the movement and then slowly relax your abs and lower your knees. Don't lower your legs all the way. Repeat the movement.

Beginner: 3 or 4 sets of 10 to 15 repetitions.

Intermediate: 5 sets of 20 repetitions.

Advanced: Hang from the bar and raise your lower body horizontally to the front. Hold for 10 to 12 seconds and then lower. Repeat 5 times.

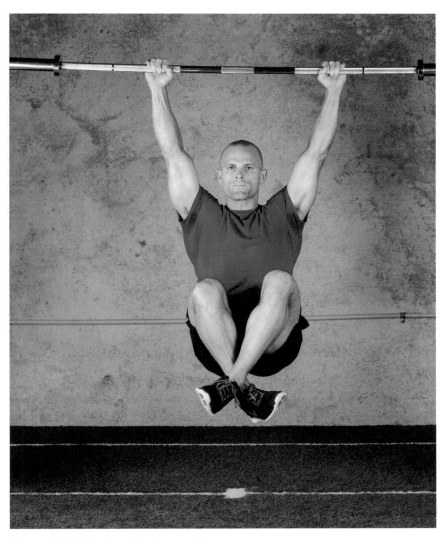

Figure 12.34 Hanging knee raise.

Dumbbell Curl

Hold two dumbbells at your sides with your arms straight and your palms facing in. Keeping your elbows at your sides, raise the dumbbells and rotate your forearms until the dumbbells are vertical and your palms face your shoulder (figure 12.35). Lower the weight to the starting position and repeat.

Beginner: 3 or 4 sets of 10 repetitions.

Intermediate: 4 sets of 12 to 15 repetitions.

Advanced: 2 sets of 2 to 4 repetitions, 3 sets of 6 repetitions and then 2 sets of 8 repetitions.

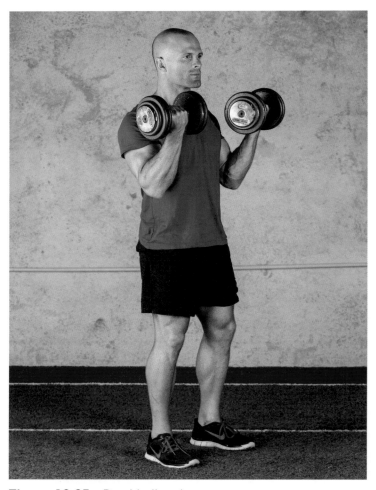

Figure 12.35 Dumbbell curl.

Deadhang

You'll need a purpose-built fingerboard, handy door frame (make sure it's secure!), or a chin-up bar. The edge should reach the end of your first finger joint. Keeping your arms straight, hang with both hands from a fingertip edge (figure 12.36) until you are forced to let go. Put chalk on your hands for improved grip.

Beginner: 3 sets of 3 to 4 seconds.

Intermediate: 4 or 5 sets of 5 to 7 seconds.

Advanced: 6 or 7 sets of 8 to 10 seconds.

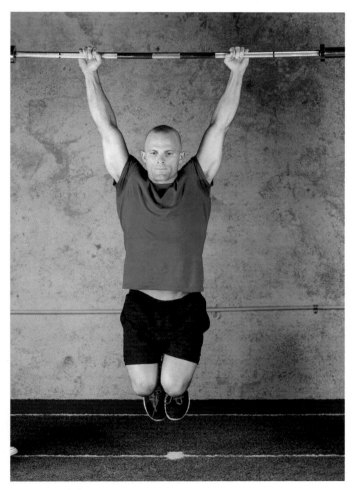

Figure 12.36 Deadhang.

Surf School

Get fit for the ocean with this workout that will give surfers of all abilities more balance and coordination.

Imagine an athlete who tackles opponents he knows he cannot beat. His rival is infinitely stronger, faster and angrier than he is. This is what Joe Average Surfer does every time he paddles out. Controlling a flimsy piece of fibreglass that's being propelled by the most unpredictable force on earth, we're sure you'll agree, takes talent and skill. And let's face it: That's why people consider surfing to be one of the coolest sports you can do. But don't just laze on the beach this summer. It's easy enough to get the hang of surfing's secrets if you're in the right kind of shape.

If you're tired of catching a tan, cull the beached-male impression and let this plan morph you from spectator to spectacular. Whether you're a rookie or are already up and riding this workout will improve your balance and coordination using Swiss balls and your body weight. Save yourself embarrassment by doing it in private before you go near a beach. When the sand hits your toes you'll look like you were born to ride. Add the routine to your normal training regimen twice a week three to four weeks before you go on a surf trip and you'll have the all moves—and a streamlined physique to match.

Warm-Up Circuit

Warm up by performing these three exercises without stopping. When you're done, rest for 90 seconds and then repeat.

Knee-Up

This exercise improves balance by teaching you to keep your upper body stable while your lower body moves independently. Lie faceup with your arms at your sides and your knees and heels together. Keeping your stomach tight, rock your legs up towards your chest (figure 12.37) while keeping your upper back and shoulders still. Do 2 sets of 12 reps.

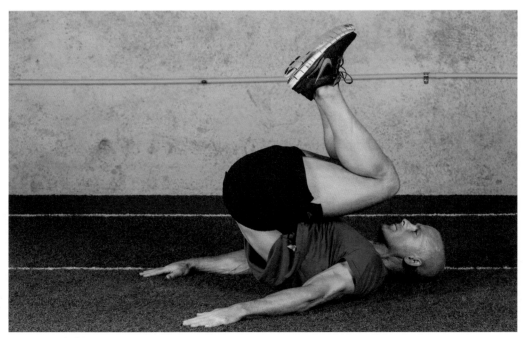

Figure 12.37 Knee-up.

Swiss Ball Back Stretch

This exercise stretches your lats, giving you a bigger range of motion that will help you paddle quicker for waves. Kneel in front of a Swiss ball and place the palms of your hands on the ball. Hold your chest up and your shoulders back and down and keep your stomach tight. Arch your back and roll the Swiss ball forward while keeping your hips back and your glutes on your heels (figure 12.38). Make sure you roll the Swiss ball forward rather than rolling your body forward over the ball. Do 2 sets of 20 reps.

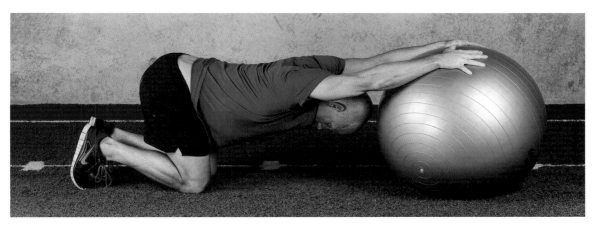

Figure 12.38   Swiss ball back stretch.

Hand Walk

This exercise teaches you to use your core to bring your upper and lower body closer together the way you would when doing tricks on a wave. Kneel and bend forward at the waist and place your hands on the floor. Keeping your stomach tight, walk your hands away from your legs (figure 12.39). Stop when your face is about eight centimetres above the ground and then walk your feet up towards your hands. Do two sets of six reps. To make it more difficult, stand with feet shoulder-width apart instead of kneeling.

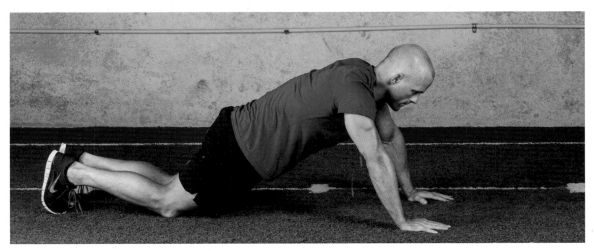

Figure 12.39   Hand walk.

Superset 1

Perform these three exercises without stopping. When you're done, rest for 90 seconds and repeat twice more.

Medicine Ball Step-Up to Overhead Press

This exercise gives you the strength in your legs, shoulders and core to stay upright and stable on an unstable object—your surfboard.

Execution

1. Stand with your feet shoulder-width apart in front of a box or step that's about 30 centimetres high. Hold a medicine ball at chest level.
2. Step onto the box with your right foot and push down from your heel (figure 12.40a). Balance on your right leg with your left leg elevated and press the medicine ball overhead (figure 12.40b).
3. Keeping your chest up and back straight, lower the ball and step back down to the starting position. Complete all reps for the right leg and then switch to the left leg. Do 2 sets of 12 repetitions.

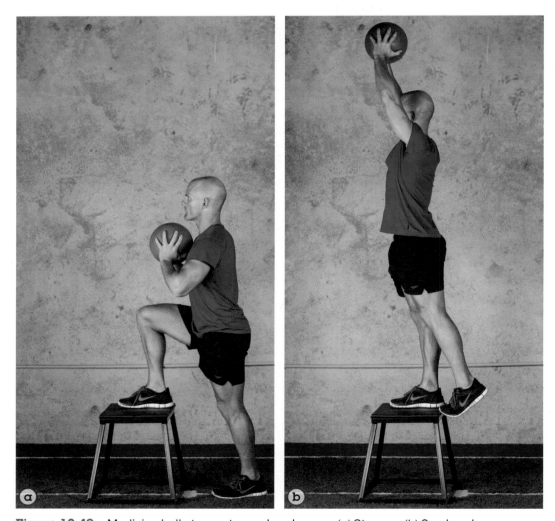

Figure 12.40 Medicine ball step-up to overhead press. *(a)* Step up. *(b)* Overhead press.

Twisting Lunge

This move develops coordination by forcing you to keep your balance when your lower half stays static while your upper body moves. This is crucial if you want to do tricks with more power and balance.

Execution

1. Stand with your feet about shoulder-width apart, arms crossed over your chest. Place your right foot about a metre in front of your left foot and get into a lunge position. Twist to the left, leading with your left shoulder (figure 12.41).
2. Return to the starting position and then place your left leg forward. Twist to the right, leading with your right shoulder. Do 2 sets of 10 reps on each leg.

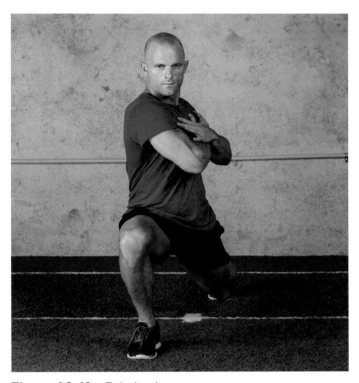

Figure 12.41　Twisting lunge.

Single-Leg Bridge

This exercise will improve your shoulder, hip and core stability, the three most important tools in surfing. These areas work together like a three-man basketball team to give you more balance.

Execution

1. Lie facedown in a push-up position. Place your forearms on the floor and under your shoulders.
2. Keeping your body in a straight line, press up on your elbows and tuck your chin so that your head is in line with your body. Lift one leg off the ground (figure 12.42) and then bring it back down. Alternate legs as you perform the repetitions. For more resistance, you can place a medicine ball on your lower back. Do 2 sets of 12 repetitions.

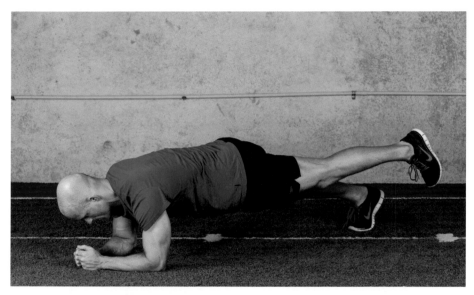

Figure 12.42 Single-leg bridge.

Superset 2

Perform these exercises one after another. When you're done, rest for 90 seconds and then repeat twice.

Russian Twist

This exercise gives you the rotational strength you need to hold your balance and manoeuvre up and down a wave.

Execution

1. Lie with your back on a Swiss ball and place your feet shoulder-width apart. Hold a medicine ball with both hands at arm's length.

2. Keeping your legs still, rotate your arms and trunk from your left side (figure 12.43) to your right side. Your head and spine should stay in the same position while your core rotates around them. If you don't have a Swiss ball, sit with your back 45 degrees to the floor. Raise your knees off the floor and bend them 90 degrees. Holding that position, rotate from left to right. Do 2 sets of 12 reps

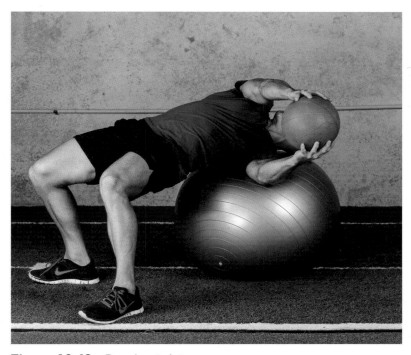

Figure 12.43   Russian twist.

Push-Up to Surf Stance

This exercise teaches you to get into a standing position on a surfboard as quickly and explosively as possible.

Execution

1. Lie facedown in a push-up position. Your body should form a straight line from your shoulders to your ankles.

2. Keeping your back flat, lower your body until your upper arms are lower than your elbows (figure 12.44a). Quickly straighten your elbows and explode up into a surfing stance with your feet hip-width apart and staggered. In this stance, your upper body faces forward (figure 12.44b). Return to the starting position and repeat. Do 2 sets of 12 to 15 reps.

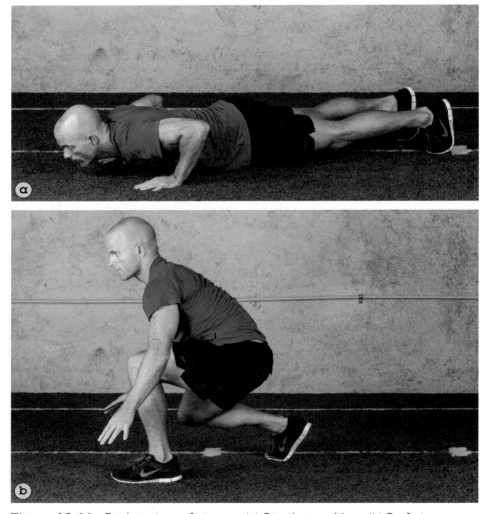

Figure 12.44 Push-up to surf stance. *(a)* Starting position. *(b)* Surf stance.

Swiss Ball Pike Push-Up

This exercise develops strength in your upper body while increasing your flexibility and coordination.

Execution

1. Place your hands on the ground in a push-up position. Place your shins on a Swiss ball.
2. Pull your glutes into the air and roll the Swiss ball towards your hands (figure 12.45), lifting up on your toes. Pause and then release back to the starting position. Do 2 sets of 12 to 15 reps.

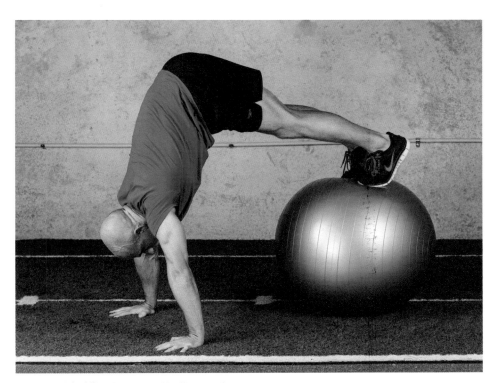

Figure 12.45   Swiss ball pike push-up.

The Best Cardio

The toughest part of surfing is the paddling, which demands incredible endurance. If you ask any surfer whether his sport is hard he'd probably just laugh. The reward of riding waves makes the slog of paddling pale in comparison, so surfers often forget how fit they actually are. But imagine trying to bulldoze yourself and a heavy board through waves that are intent on pushing you back. It's like running on a treadmill to reach the television at the end of it. Even once you're fit and can duck the board under the waves, there's always a chance you'll get stuck in a current that can suck you out to sea.

With that in mind only one type of cardio is worth doing: swimming. The best stroke? Front crawl. Backstroke works too because it's the reverse of the crawl, so mixing the two is your best option. Try to do as many laps as you can to improve your endurance and paddling power. It will condition the muscles you need to paddle and teach you to cope with being out of breath in water, which is one of the scariest things about being in the ocean. If you can keep your composure while under pressure from waves and a lack of oxygen, you'll get more waves and enjoy yourself a whole lot more. No pool? Rowing is your next best bet because it works your upper back and shoulders, which come into play when you paddle. Remember: The harder you work out of the water, the easier it'll be when you're at the beach.

Sports Talk

Here are some answers to the most common questions about sport training.

Q: **Will massage help me recover from a tough training session?**

A: Hippies everywhere will throw their rapeseed-oiled paws up in the air at the notion that massage does diddly for recovery. At least they're not a violent bunch. A study at Queen's University in the United States (Wiltshire et al., 2010) found that massage after exercise does not improve circulation to the muscle, nor does it assist in the removal of lactic acid and other waste products. The researchers discovered that massage actually impaired both the blood flow to the muscle after exercise and the removal of lactic acid from muscle after exercise. Unfortunately, not every massage has a happy ending.

Q: **I'm tired after Saturday's match. How can I still train when my joints and muscles are sore?**

A: Your local pool is your best place to do a Sunday or Monday training session after a Saturday match. Explosive, muscle-building exercises called plyometrics are the bread and butter moves for sportsmen looking to boost their performance, but they're famous for leaving you aching like you've been rolled in a car crash. When done in the water, however, plyometric exercise significantly decreases the level of muscle soreness you feel two to three days after a workout. To start strutting instead of hobbling, hit the pool and do three or four sets of six reps of jump squats after a tough leg workout.

Q: **Are postmatch ice baths really worth it for a knee problem?**

A: Yes, but you can localise the treatment rather than dunking yourself up to your neck. Research in *European Journal of Sport Science* (Brade, Dawson and Wallman, 2012) found that putting muscles in hot and then cold conditions enhanced recovery and hastened the return of muscle strength and power after a workout. Grab an ice pack, press it against the knee for a minute and then submerge that knee in hot water for a minute. Alternate for 12 minutes to be able to run two races in a row, even if they are just 5Ks.

Q: **I'm into surfing and snowboarding. What's the single best exercise I can do to improve my balance?**

A: For balance you need to work on your lower half, and the best exercise for this is squats. To give yourself impeccable balance, do the squats on one leg using your body weight. When you can do 3 sets of 10 single-leg, wobble-free squats while standing on a hard floor, bring in a very unlikely workout aid: your pillow. Standing on a cushy surface forces your hip and leg muscles to work much harder. Do the squats first thing in the morning and you'll get stronger legs and improved balance that will help you stand strong on every board you pick up.

Q: **I play rugby competitively but struggle to balance the demands of weight training, cardio and rugby practise. Can I train when I'm still a bit sore?**

A: Avoiding the gym when you're aching is a pretty sensible thing to do. Stiffness usually means that you've trained hard and that your body is still recovering. You can still train if you're not so stiff that you can't move. A little stiffness is good, and once your muscles are warmed up you probably won't feel the aches. Be wise about it and try to alter your diet so that it supports your heavy training load. Skip training the day before a match so that your muscles are fully recovered when it's time for them to perform.

Q: **After watching the World's Strongest Man competition I want to start training like the contestants do to get more powerful for sport. What's a good starting point?**

A: Take it one step at a time because you don't want a garden full of tractor tires that haven't been flipped in months. One of the best exercises you can do involves your car. Take it to an empty car park and have a friend sit in the driver's seat. Get behind the car and take turns pushing your ride. You'll build incredible strength in your legs and improve your cardiovascular fitness, which you'll find useful on every sport pitch. Leave the treadmill to the blokes on the losing team.

Q: **I want to add some distance to my golf swing. How can I do it?**

A: Do workouts that focus on rotational power and flexibility. Also, follow a strict stretching routine for all your muscles so that you can let your swing flow as naturally as possible and not start tensing up over time. When you're in the gym work on two muscle groups. The first is your core. Work your core one to three times a week using some of the abs routines in this book. The second is your chest. A powerful chest improves a golf swing, found scientists at East Stroudsbury University in the United States (Gordon et al., 2009). Surprisingly, chest strength had a greater effect on club head speed—an important indicator of driving distance—than body rotation did because the pecs are highly active during the acceleration phase of the downswing. Feel free to ask your opponent how much he benches before you put a wager on the next game.

Q: **How important are team talks? Should we spend more time warming up or talking?**

A: Take the time to warm up your mouth. A study at Florida State University (Tenenbaum, Sar-El and Bar-Eli, 2000) found that winning teams talked strategy twice as much as losing teams did and that teammates on winning teams vocally encouraged each other nearly three times as frequently as those on losing teams. Whatever team sport you're playing, try to discuss strategy and express encouragement between every play. When in doubt, cite the *Cool Runnings* mantra: 'I see pride. I see power. I see a bad-ass mother who don't take no crap off nobody!'

Q: **I'm a triathlete. Is there anything I can do after a race to boost my recovery when my entire body aches?**

A: The research is conflicting. Ice baths can help reduce swelling and inflammation. If your local pub won't lend you their machine, alternate between 30 seconds of hot and 30 seconds of cold in the shower. Once you're relaxing on the couch, put your feet up at least as high as your heart. Gravity will move fluids from your legs to the rest of your body and will help boost your recovery rather than let the blood pool in your legs.

Q: **Should I bother with really expensive running shoes?**

A: No; just get a pair that you feel comfortable in. Expensive shoes are a waste of money. The debate about whether expensive running shoes are necessary can be settled by asking whether running shoes themselves are necessary. Running shoes didn't actually appear until the 1970s. What did guys do before that? They still ran. They still broke world records. They were still a lot fitter than most people today. Running shoes are somewhat of a farce. No shoe company has ever funded or produced research that outlines the benefits of running shoes, purely because no benefits exist. However, research in *PM&R* (Kerrigan et al., 2009) discovered that running shoes may actually cause damage to the knees, hips and ankles. The researchers found that running shoes exerted more stress on these joints than running barefoot does. Nike isn't going to boast about that; instead, it will tell you how much you need the extra cushioning because it feels softer. Unfortunately, softer means instability that can roll your ankle.

That's it. You now have all the tricks, training plans and rock-solid information you need to excel on the sport pitch and in day-to-day life. By finding enjoyment in exercise you've given your body and soul a lifelong gift. To get an idea of how much you've progressed, dig out the training diary you began when you first started reading this book. No doubt some big changes have occurred, mentally as well as physically. Your hard work and relentless consistency have probably taught you a bit more about yourself and the incredible feats you perhaps didn't think you were capable of before you decided to make a change. You've learned several lessons along the way. Some were likely tough and some may have come easy. The most important lesson is that of self-respect because when a body is strong the mind becomes equally strong. So stick to it, find your passion and live the dream while sporting the physique you deserve. The dead man floats with the current but the strong man swims against it. Never wait for your ship to come in—swim to it.

References

Ainsworth, B.E., W.L. Haskell, M.C. Whitt, M.L. Irwin, A.M. Swartz, S.J. Strath, W.L. O'Brien, D.R. Bassett Jr., K.H. Schmitz, P.O. Emplaincourt, D.R. Jacobs Jr., and A.S. Leon. 2000. Compendium of physical activities: An update of activity codes and MET intensities. *Med. Sci. Sports Exerc.* 32(9 Suppl.):S498-S504.

Amigo, I., and C. Fernandez. 2007. Effects of diet and their role in weight control. *Psychol. Health Med.* 12(3):321-327.

Azadzoi, K.M., R.N. Schulman, M. Aviram, and M.B. Siroky, M.B. 2005. Oxidative stress in arteriogenic erectile dysfunction: Prophylactic role of antioxidants. *J. Urol.* 174(1):386-393.

Bandy, W.D., J.M. Irion, and M. Briggler. 1997. The effect of time and frequency of static stretching on flexibility of the hamstring muscles. *Phys. Ther.* 77(10):1090-1096.

Bell, G.J., D. Syrotuik, T.P. Martin, R. Burnham, and H.A. Quinney. 2000. Effect of concurrent strength and endurance training on skeletal muscle properties and hormone concentrations in humans. *Eur. J. Appl. Physiol.* 81(5):418-427.

Bell, N.H., R.N. Godsen, D.P. Henry, J. Shary, and S. Epstein. 1988. The effects of muscle-building exercise on vitamin D and mineral metabolism. *J. Bone Miner. Res.* 3(4):369-374.

Børsheim, E., and R. Bahr. 2003. Effect of exercise intensity, duration and mode on post-exercise oxygen consumption. *Sports Med.* 33(14):1037-1060.

Brade, C., B. Dawson, and K. Wallman. 2012. Effects of different precooling techniques on repeat sprint ability in team sport athletes. Available: www.tandfonline.com/doi/full/10.1080/17461391.2011.651491.

Bramble, D.M., and D.E. Lieberman. 2004. Endurance running and the evolution of *Homo*. *Nature*. 432(7015):345-352.

Bryner, R.W., I.H. Ullrich, J. Sauers, D. Donley, G. Hornsby, M. Kolar, and R. Yeater. 1999. Effects of resistance vs. aerobic training combined with an 800 calorie liquid diet on lean body mass and resting metabolic rate. *J. Am. Coll. Nutr.* 18(2):115-121.

Childs, J.D., D.S. Teyhen, P.R. Casey, K.A. McCoy-Singh, A.W. Feldmann, A.C. Wright, J.L. Dugan, S.S. Wu, and S.Z. George. 2010. Effects of traditional sit-up training versus core stabilization exercises on short-term musculoskeletal injuries in US Army soldiers: A cluster randomized trial. *Phys. Ther.* 90(10):1404-1412.

Cooper, K.H. 1968. A means of assessing maximal oxygen uptake. *J. Am. Med. Assoc.* 203:201-204.

Davis, W.J., D.T. Wood, R. Andrews, L.M. Elkind, and W.B. Davis. 2008. Elimination of delayed-onset muscle soreness by pre-resistance cardioacceleration before each set. *J. Strength Cond. Res.* 22(1):212-225.

Delarue, J., O. Matzinger, C. Binnert, P. Schneiter, R. Chiolero, and L. Tappy. 2003. Fish oil prevents the adrenal activation elicited by mental stress in healthy men. *Diabetes Metab.* 29(3):289-295.

Dhikav, V., G. Karmarkar, M. Gupta, and K.S. Anand. 2007. Yoga in premature ejaculation: A comparative trial with fluoxetine. *J. Sex. Med.* 4(6):1726-1732.

Engler, M.B., M.M. Engler, C.Y. Chen, M.J. Malloy, A. Browne, E.Y. Chiu, H.-K. Kwak, P. Milbury, S.M. Paul, J. Blumberg, and M.L. Mietus-Snyder. 2004. Flavonoid-rich dark chocolate improves endothelial function and increases plasma epicatechin concentrations in healthy adults. *J. Am. Coll. Nutr.* 23(3):197-204.

Farrell, P.A., A.B. Gustafson, W.P. Morgan, and C.B. Pert. 1987. Enkephalins, catecholamines, and psychological mood alterations: Effects of prolonged exercise. *Med. Sci. Sports Exerc.* 19(4):347-353.

Ferris, L.T., J.S. Williams, C.-L. Shen, K.A. O'Keefe, and K.B. Hale. 2005. Resistance training improves sleep quality in older adults—A pilot study. *J. Sports Sci. Med.* 4:354-360.

Gallagher, D., S.B. Heymsfield, M. Heo, S.A. Jebb, P.R. Murgatroyd, and Y. Sakamoto. 2000. Healthy percentage body fat ranges: An approach for developing guidelines based on body mass index. *Am. J. Clin. Nutr.* 72(3):694-701.

Golding, L.A., C.R. Myers, and W.E. Sinning. (Eds.) 1989. *Y's way to physical fitness: The complete guide to fitness testing and instruction.* 3rd ed. Champaign, IL: Human Kinetics.

Gordon, B.S., G.L. Moir, S.E. Davis, C.A. Witmer, and D.M. Cummings. 2009. An investigation into the relationship of flexibility, power, and strength to club head speed in male golfers. *J. Strength Cond. Res.* 23(5):1606-1610.

Gottlieb, D.J., N.M. Punjabi, A.B. Newman, H.E. Resnick, S. Redline, C.M. Baldwin, and F.J. Nieto. 2005. Association of sleep time with diabetes mellitus and impaired glucose tolerance. *Arch. Intern. Med.* 165(8):863-867.

Gundersen, Y., P.K. Opstad, T. Reistad, I. Thrane, and P. Vaagenes. 2006. Seven days' around the clock exhaustive physical exertion combined with energy depletion and sleep deprivation primes circulating leukocytes. *Eur. J. Appl. Physiol.* 97(2):151-157.

Herbert, R.D., M. de Noronha, and S.J. Kamper. 2010. Stretching to prevent or reduce muscle soreness after exercise. Available: http://onlinelibrary.wiley.com/doi/10.1002/14651858.CD004577.pub3/abstract;jsessionid=96D334E88F323A4A4239BC01A24E07A6.d03t02.

Hornyak, M., U. Voderholzer, F. Hohagen, M. Berger, and D. Riemann. 1998. Magnesium therapy for periodic leg movements-related insomnia and restless legs syndrome: An open pilot study. *Sleep.* 21(5):501-505.

Hunter, D., and F. Eckstein. 2009. Exercise and osteoarthritis. *J. Anat.* 214(2):197-207.

Jayaprakasha, G.K., K.N. Chidambara Murthy, and B.S. Patil. 2011. Rapid HPLC-UV method for quantification of L-citrulline in watermelon and its potential role on smooth muscle relaxation markers. *Food Chem.* 127(1):240-248.

Johnstone, A.M., G.W. Horgan, S.D. Murison, D.M. Bremner, and G.E. Lobley. 2008. Effects of a high-protein ketogenic diet on hunger, appetite, and weight loss in obese men feeding ad libitum. *Am. J. Clin. Nutr.* 87(1):44-55.

Karila, T.A., P. Sarkkinen, M. Marttinen, T. Seppälä, A. Mero, and K. Tallroth. 2008. Rapid weight loss decreases serum testosterone. *Int. J. Sports Med.* 29(11):872-877.

Kelleher, A.R., K.J. Hackney, T.J. Fairchild, S. Keslacy, and L.L. Ploutz-Snyder. 2010. The metabolic costs of reciprocal supersets vs. traditional resistance exercise in young recreationally active adults. *J. Strength Cond. Res.* 24(4):1043-1051.

Kerai, M.D., C.J. Waterfield, S.H. Kenyon, D.S. Asker, and J.A. Timbrell. 1999. Reversal of ethanol-induced hepatic steatosis and lipid peroxidation by taurine: A study in rats. *Alcohol Alcohol.* 34(4):529-541.

Kerrigan, D.C., J.R. Franz, G.S. Keenan, J. Dicharry, U. Della Croce, and R.P. Wilder. 2009. The effect of running shoes on lower extremity joint torques. *PM&R.* 1(12):1058-1063.

Kindermann, W., A. Schnable, W. Schmitt, G. Biro, J. Cassens, and F. Weber. 1982. Catecholamines, growth hormone, cortisol, insulin and sex hormones in anaerobic and aerobic exercise. *Eur. J. Appl. Physiol. Occup. Physiol.* 49(3):389-399.

Kolata, G. 2001. "Maximum" heart rate theory is challenged. *The New York Times,* April 24.

Lally, P., C.H.M. van Jaarsveld, H.W.W. Potts, and J. Wardle. 2010. How are habits formed: Modelling habit formation in the real world. *Eur. J. Soc. Psychol.* 40(6):998-1009.

Leidy, H.J., M. Tang, C.L.H. Armstrong, C.B. Martin, and W.W. Campbell. 2010. The effects of consuming frequent, higher protein meals on appetite and satiety during weight loss in overweight/obese men. *Obesity.* 19(4):818.

Loprinzi, P.D., and B.J. Cardinal. 2011. Association between objectively-measured physical activity and sleep, NHANES 2005-2006. *Ment. Health Phys. Act.* 4(2):65.

Maggio, M., G.P. Ceda, F.G.P., Lauretani, F., C. Cattabiani, C.,E. Avantaggiato, E.,S. Morganti, S.,F. Ablondi, F.,S. Bandinelli, S.,L.J. Dominguez, L.J.,M. Barbagallo, M.,G. Paolisso, R.D. G., Semba, R.D., and L. Ferrucci, L. 2011. Magnesium and anabolic hormones in older men. *Int. J. Androl.* 34(6 Pt. 2):E594-E600.

Mah, C.D., K.E. Mah, E.J. Kezirian, and W.C. Dement. 2011. The effects of sleep extension on the athletic performance of collegiate basketball players. *Sleep.* 34(7):943-950.

Maresh, C.M., M.J. Whittlesey, L.E. Armstrong, L.M. Yamamoto, D.A. Judelson, K.E. Fish, D.J. Casa, S.A. Kavouras, and V. Castracane. 2006. Effect of hydration state on testosterone and cortisol responses to training-intensity exercise in collegiate runners. *Int. J. Sports Med.* 27(10):765-770.

Markovic, G., D. Dizdar, I. Jukic, and M. Cardinale. 2004. Reliablity and factorial validity of squat and countermovement jump tests. *J. Strength Cond. Res.* 18(3):551-555.

Mazzetti. S., M. Douglass, A. Yocum, and M. Harber. 2007. Effect of explosive versus slow contractions and exercise intensity on energy expenditure. *Med. Sci. Sports Exerc.* 39(8):1291-1301.

McLester, J.R., P. Bishop, and M. Guilliams. 1999. Comparison of 1 and 3 day per week of equal volume resistance training in experienced subjects. *Med. Sci. Sports Exerc.* 31(5 Suppl.):S117.

Mjølsnes, R., A. Arnason, T. Østhagen, T. Raastad, and R. Bahr. 2004. A 10-week randomized trial comparing eccentric vs. concentric hamstring strength training in well-trained soccer players. *Scand. J. Med. Sci. Sports.* 14(5):311-317.

Okada, T., K. Huxel, and T. Nesser. 2011. Relationship between core stability, functional movement and performance. *J. Strength Cond. Res.* 25(1):252-261.

Paffenbarger, R.S. Jr., R.T. Hyde, A.L. Wing, and C.C. Hsiegh. 1986. Physical activity, all-cause mortality, and longevity of college alumni. *N. Engl. J. Med.* 314(10):605-613.

Pereles, D., and E. McDevitt. 2011. Proceedings of the American Academy of Orthopaedic Surgeons Meeting, February 15-19.

Prokop, P., M.J. Rantala, M. Usak, and I. Senay. 2012. Is a woman's preference for chest hair in men influenced by parasite threat? *Arch. Sex. Behav.* Sept. 13 (epub ahead of print).

Purslow, L.R., M.S. Sandhu, N. Forouhi, E.H. Young, R.N. Luben, A.A. Welch, K.T. Khaw, S.A. Bingham, and N.J.

Wareham. 2008. Energy intake at breakfast and weight change: Prospective study of 6,764 middle-aged men and women. *Am. J. Epidemiol.* 167(2):188-192.

Requa, R.K., L.N. DeAvilla, and J.G. Garrick. 1993. Injuries in recreational adult fitness activities. *Am. J. Sports Med.* 21(3):461-467.

Robergs, R.A., and R. Landwehr. 2002. The surprising history of the "HRmax = 220 – age" equation. *J. Exerc. Physiol. Online.* 5(2):1-10.

Rogers, R.A., R.U. Newton, K.P. McEvoy, E.M. Popper, B.K. Doan, and J.K. Shim. 2000. The effect of supplemental isolated weight-training exercises on upper-arm size and upper-body strength. Muncie, IN: Human Performance Laboratory, Ball State University.

Sherman, K.J., D.C. Cherkin, J. Erro, D.L. Miglioretti, and R.A. Deyo. 2005. Comparing yoga, exercise, and a self-care book for chronic low back pain: A randomized, controlled trial. *Ann. Intern. Med.* 143(12):849-856.

Shrier, I. 2004. Does stretching improve performance? A systematic and critical review of the literature. *Clin. J. Sports Med.* 14(5):267-273.

Shrier, I., and K. Gossal. 2000. Myths and truths of stretching: Individualized recommendations for healthy muscles. *Phys. Sports Med.* 28(8):57-63.

Siri-Tarino, P.W., Q. Sun, F.B. Hu, and R.M. Krauss, R.M. 2010. Meta-analysis of prospective cohort studies evaluating the association of saturated fat with cardiovascular disease. *Am. J. Clin. Nutr.* 91(3):535-546.

Slotterback, C.S., H. Leeman, and M.E. Oakes. 2006. No pain, no gain: Perceptions of calorie expenditures of exercise and daily activities. *Curr. Psychol.* 25(1):28-41.

Smith-Spangler, C., M.L. Brandeau, G.E. Hunter, J.C. Bavinger, M. Pearson, P.J. Eschbach, V. Sundaram, H. Liu, P. Schirmer, C. Stave, I. Olkin, and D.M. Bravata. 2012. Are organic goods safer or healthier than conventional alternatives? A systematic review. *Ann. Intern. Med.* 157(5):348-366.

Stallknecht, B., F. Dela, and J.W. Helge. 2007. Are blood flow and lipolysis in subcutaneous adipose tissue influenced by contractions in adjacent muscles in humans? *Am. J. Physiol. Endocrinol. Metab.* 292(2):E394-E399.

Stephens, R., J. Ling, T.M. Heffernan, N. Heather, and K. Jones. 2008. A review of the literature on the cognitive effects of alcohol hangover. *Alcohol Alcohol.* 43(2):163-170.

Sullivan, E.L., and J.L. Cameron. 2010. A rapidly occurring compensatory decrease in physical activity counteracts diet-induced weight loss in female monkeys. *Am. J. Physiol. Regul. Integr. Comp. Physiol.* 298(4):R1068-R1074.

Sunkaria, R.K., V. Kumar, and S.C. Saxena. 2010. A comparative study on spectral parameters of HRV in yogic and non-yogic practitioners. *Int. J. Med. Eng. Inform.* 2(1):1-14.

Takahashi, Y., D.M. Kipnis, and W.H. Daughaday. 1968. Growth hormone secretion during sleep. *J. Clin. Invest.* 47(9):2079-2090.

Tanaka, H. 1994. Effects of cross-training. Transfer of training effects on $\dot{V}O_2$max between cycling, running and swimming. *Sports Med.* 18(5):330-339.

Tenenbaum, G., T. Sar-El, and M. Bar-Eli. 2000. Anticipation of ball location in low and high-skill performers: A developmental perspective. *Psychol. Sport Exerc.* 1(2):117-128.

Thompson Coon, J., K. Boddy, K. Stein, R. Whear, J. Barton, and M.H. Depledge. 2011. Does participating in physical activity in outdoor natural environments have a greater effect on physical and mental wellbeing than physical activity indoors? A systematic review. *Environ. Sci. Technol.* 45(5):1761-1762.

Tremblay, A., J.-A. Simoneau, and C. Bouchard. 1994. Impacts of exercise intensity on body fatness and skeletal muscle metabolism. *Metabolism.* 43(7):814-818.

Uribie, B.P., J.W. Coburn, L.E. Brown, D.A. Judelson, A.V. Khamoui, and D. Nguyen. 2010. Muscle activation when performing the chest press and shoulder press on a stable bench vs. a Swiss ball. *J. Strength Cond. Res.* 24(4):1028-1033.

Warden, R., and K. Fuchs. 2007. Exercise when young may reduce risk of fractures later in life. *J. Bone Miner. Res.* 22(2):251-259.

Weston, A.R., K.H. Myburgh, F.H. Lindsay, S.C. Dennis, T.D. Noakes, and J.A. Hawley. 1997. Skeletal muscle buffering capacity and endurance performance after high-intensity interval training by well-trained cyclists. *Eur. J. Appl. Physiol.* 75:7-13.

Wiltshire, E.V., V. Poitras, M. Pak, T. Hong, K. Rayner, and M.E. Tshcakovsky. 2010. Massage impairs post exercise muscle blood flow and lactic acid removal. *Med. Sci. Sports Exerc.* 42(6):1062-1071.

Yamaguchi, T., and K. Ishii. 2005. Effects of static stretching for 30 seconds and dynamic stretching on leg extension power. *J. Strength Cond. Res.* 19(3):677-683.

About the Author

Ray Klerck is a well-known personal trainer and former fitness editor for *Men's Health* magazine in the UK. He has also appeared as a fitness model on the cover of that publication. Today he continues as a *Men's Health* fitness and nutrition advisor on a freelance basis. He writes and edits an 18-page section of the magazine titled Personal Trainer and contributes regular in-depth features on health and fitness for other popular publications such as *FHM*, *GQ*, *Fighters Only*, and *Men's Fitness*.

After qualifying as a Register of Exercise Professionals (REPs) level 4 master personal trainer and nutrition specialist with Premier Global (equivalent to NASM CPT), Klerck joined *Men's Health* UK in 2001. Over the next seven years he became the most successful fitness editor in the magazine's history, combining his expert knowledge with the latest scientific research to create award-winning exercise and nutrition programmes.

Klerck has trained clients from all backgrounds—celebrities, athletes, *Men's Health* staff and readers—helping ordinary people build muscle and burn fat for remarkable before-and-after results featured in the magazine. Klerck's influence helped *Men's Health* become the UK's best-selling men's magazine, and his workouts continue to reach large audiences in Australia and the UK. *Men's Health* UK has been voted best edition of that global publication (48 editions total) for four years in a row. It has also won accolades as UK Magazine of the Year.

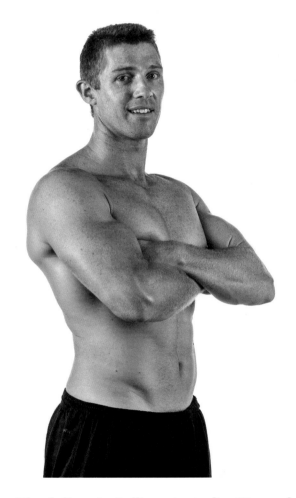

Klerck lives in Ballina, Australia. His work continues to appear in multiple international *Men's Health* editions and is followed by millions of readers each month. Klerck recently coauthored *A Fist Full of Food* with Matt Lovell, the UK's leading sport nutritionist.

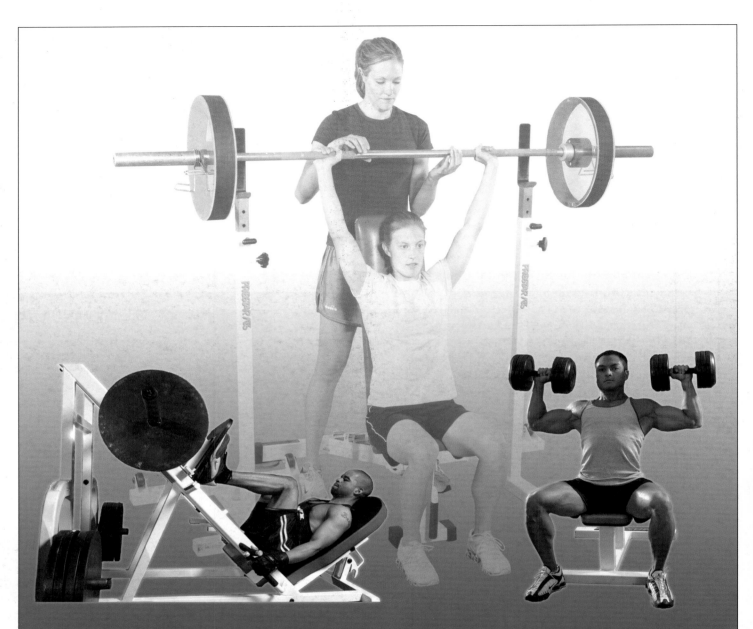

You'll find other outstanding strength training resources at

www.HumanKinetics.com/strengthtraining

In the U.S. call 1-800-747-4457

Australia 08 8372 0999 • Canada 1-800-465-7301
Europe +44 (0) 113 255 5665 • New Zealand 0800 222 062

HUMAN KINETICS
The Premier Publisher for Sports & Fitness
P.O. Box 5076 • Champaign, IL 61825-5076 USA